160
Seas/9a

Cajal and de Castro's Neurohistological Methods

Cajal and de Castro's Neurohistological Methods

MIGUEL A. MERCHÁN, MD, PHD

PROFESSOR OF HISTOLOGY
FACULTAD DE MEDICINA
INSTITUTO DE NEUROCIENCIAS DE CASTILLA Y LEÓN
UNIVERSIDAD DE SALAMANCA
SALAMANCA, SPAIN

JAVIER DeFELIPE, PHD

RESEARCH PROFESSOR
CONSEJO SUPERIOR DE INVESTIGACIONES CIENTÍFICAS
INSTITUTO CAJAL
AND
CENTRO DE TECNOLOGÍA BIOMÉDICA
UNIVERDIDAD POLITÉCNICA DE MADRID
MADRID, SPAIN

FERNANDO de CASTRO, MD, PHD

TENURED SCIENTIST
GRUPO DE NEUROBIOLOGIA DEL DESARROLLO-GNDE
CONSEJO SUPERIOR DE INVESTIGACIONES CIENTÍFICAS
INSTITUTO CAJAL
MADRID, SPAIN

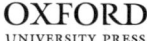

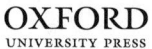

Oxford University Press is a department of the University of Oxford. It furthers
the University's objective of excellence in research, scholarship, and education
by publishing worldwide.Oxford is a registered trade mark of Oxford University
Press in the UK and certain other countries.

Published in the United States of America by Oxford University Press
198 Madison Avenue, New York, NY 10016, United States of America.

© Oxford University Press 2016

First Edition published in 2016

All rights reserved. No part of this publication may be reproduced, stored in
a retrieval system, or transmitted, in any form or by any means, without the
prior permission in writing of Oxford University Press, or as expressly permitted
by law, by license, or under terms agreed with the appropriate reproduction
rights organization. Inquiries concerning reproduction outside the scope of the
above should be sent to the Rights Department, Oxford University Press, at the
address above.

You must not circulate this work in any other form
and you must impose this same condition on any acquirer.

Library of Congress Cataloging-in-Publication Data
Merchán, Miguel A., author.
Cajal and de Castro's neurohistological methods / by Miguel A. Merchán, Javier DeFelipe,
and Fernando de Castro.
   p. ; cm.
Includes translation of "Elementos de Técnica Micrográfica del Sistema Nervioso" (Principles of
Micrographical Technique for the Nervous System), originally published in Spanish in 1933.
Includes bibliographical references.
ISBN 978-0-19-022159-1 (alk. paper)
I. DeFelipe, Javier, author.   II. de Castro, Fernando,— , author.   III. Merchán, Miguel. Elementos
de Técnica Micrográfica del Sistema Nervioso. English.   IV. Title.
[DNLM: 1. Ramón y Cajal, Santiago, 1852-1934.   2. de Castro, Fernando, 1896-1967.
3. Histological Techniques—history.   4. Nervous System—anatomy & histology.   WL 101]
QP355
612.8—dc23
2015030544

9 8 7 6 5 4 3 2 1

Printed by Sheridan, USA

This material is not intended to be, and should not be considered, a substitute for medical or other
professional advice. Treatment for the conditions described in this material is highly dependent on
the individual circumstances. And, while this material is designed to offer accurate information
with respect to the subject matter covered and to be current as of the time it was written, research
and knowledge about medical and health issues is constantly evolving and dose schedules for
medications are being revised continually, with new side effects recognized and accounted for
regularly. Readers must therefore always check the product information and clinical procedures
with the most up-to-date published product information and data sheets provided by the
manufacturers and the most recent codes of conduct and safety regulation. The publisher and the
authors make no representations or warranties to readers, express or implied, as to the accuracy or
completeness of this material. Without limiting the foregoing, the publisher and the authors make
no representations or warranties as to the accuracy or efficacy of the drug dosages mentioned in the
material. The authors and the publisher do not accept, and expressly disclaim, any responsibility
for any liability, loss or risk that may be claimed or incurred as a consequence of the use and/or
application of any of the contents of this material.

*To the Illustrious Doctor D. Rafael Segarra
and other colleagues of the Republic of Argentina, who have so generously provided
the funds for the publication of this little book. This work is dedicated to them by
their devoted friends and fellows.*

The authors

CONTENTS

Preface xi
Foreword xiii
Preliminary Information xxi
List of Plates xxiii

SECTION ONE Historical Context

1. The Authors and Their Backgrounds 3
   Jaime A. Merchán and Jorge Prieto

SECTION TWO Basic Histological Techniques

2. The Microscope and the Fixatives 21
   Microscope 21
   Fixatives 22

3. Decalcifying Agents 35

4. General Dissociation Procedures 39
   Embedding Techniques and Agents (Celloidin, Paraffin and Gelatin) 39
   Dissociation 39
   Sectioning 40
   Frozen Section Procedure 40
   Celloidin and Collodion Embedding 41
   Paraffin Embedding 43
   Gelatin Embedding 45
   Superficial Paraffin Imbedding 45

5. Handling and Mounting Serial Sections 47
   Sections of Celloidin-embedded Material 47
   Sections of Paraffin-embedded Material 50

6. General Staining Methods 51
   Some Remarks on the Staining Process 51
   Sources and Composition of Dyes 53

7. Formulae for Carmine and Hematoxylin: Substantive and Adjective
   Coloration with Aniline Stains 55
   Bichromic and Trichromic Methods 55

Double and Triple Stains   57
Modifications of the Iron-Hematoxylin. Methods for the Staining of Mitochondria   58

8. Section Mounting and Preservation   65
Mounting Sections that Require Previous Dehydration and Clarification   65
Section Mounting without Dehydration and Clarification   67

SECTION THREE Special Techniques

9. Methods for the Demonstration of Neuronal Morphology: Golgi's Procedures and Their Variations   71

10. Continuation of the Methods for Demonstrating the Morphology of Neurons   85
Ehrlich's Methylene Blue and its Variations (*EN 19*)   85
Fixation, Sectioning, and Mounting Techniques for Methylene Blue Stained Material   89

11. Methods to Study the Structure of the Nerve Cell   97
Nissl Chromatic Bodies   97
Methods for Staining the Neurofibrils   99
Silver Impregnation Methods   101
Impregnation of the Golgi Apparatus   114
Demonstration of Plastosomes, Centrosomes, Oxidases, and Pigmentary Spherules   118
Nucleus and Cell Membrane   122

12. Staining of Neuronal Axons in the Centers   125

13. Myelin Staining   127

14. Coloration of the Macroglia, Microglia, and Oligodendroglia   133
Macroglia   133
Demonstration of the Gliosomes and Mitochondria   146
Impregnation of Oligodendroglia and Microglia   149

15. Methods to Demonstrate the Connective Tissue   157
Methods for Staining the Connective Tissue   157
Impregnation Methods for Connective Tissue   158
Supravital Staining with Acidic Dyes   161

16. Methods for the Demonstration of Substances Produced by Alterations of the Cell Metabolism   163
Demonstration of Some Cell Granules   164
Demonstration of Fats and Lipoid Substances   165
Demonstration of Ferric Pigments   167
Demonstration of non-Ferric Pigments   168

Glycogen Demonstration   169
Demonstration of Amyloid Substance and Corpora Amylacea   170
Demonstration of Hyaline Degeneration   171
Calcareous Substances   171

17. Methods for the Demonstration of the Peripheral Nerves under both Normal and Pathological Conditions   173
Demonstration of Ranvier Nodes   174
Methods to Stain the Schwann Cells   174
Methods for Myelin Staining   178
Lantermann Incisures; Spiral Apparatus; Spinous Double Bracelet; Neurokeratin Network (*EN 47*)   179
Demonstration of the Cylinder-Axis and Neurofibrils   181
Demonstration of the Connective Tissue of Nerve Trunks (Endoneurium, Perineurium, and Epineurium)   184

18. Methods for the Demonstration of Peripheral Nerve Endings   187
Gold Chloride Methods   187
Demonstration of Nerve Endings with the Golgi Method   189
Demonstration of Peripheral Nerve Endings with Ehrlich's Methylene Blue Procedure   189
Neurofibrillary Methods Capable of Demonstrating the Nerve Endings   190
Methods to Demonstrate the Nerve Trunks and Nerve Endings in Organs Protected by Bone Tissue   194
Procedures for Staining the Sympathetic and Dorsal Root Ganglia   197

19. Techniques for the Demonstration of the Nervous Tissue of Invertebrates   201
Methods Capable of Revealing the Morphology of Neurons   201
Methods for Staining Neurofibrils   202

20. Methods for Demonstrating Some Pathogenic Microorganisms   205
Demonstration of the Syphilis Treponema   205
Demonstration of the Trypanosomes in Sleeping Sickness   208
Coloration of Negri Bodies in Rabies   208
Demonstration of the Tuberculosis Bacillus   209

Editors' Notes   211
Vocabulary   223
Notes   231
Bibliography   237
Index   241

PREFACE

After the premature death of Professor Jaime Merchán in 2011, the text for the present edition was rescued from among his computer files by his brother and pupil Miguel, co-editor of the present publication. This book has been published thanks to the generous help and enthusiastic support of Drs. de Castro Soubriet (grandson of Fernando de Castro) and DeFelipe. The editors are especially thankful for the contribution of Dr. Constantino Sotelo, probably the last active member of the school of Neurohistology created by Santiago Ramón y Cajal. We wish to emphasize, however, that it was Jaime Merchán Cifuentes and his younger pupil Jorge Prieto Cueto who were truly responsible for this publication. Due to his long personal experience of working with Fernando de Castro, Merchán was able to produce far more than just a literal translation of Cajal's original book of micrographic techniques.

Jaime Merchán was born in Madrid in 1946 and was a pupil at the British Council School before studying medicine at the Universidad Complutense, in Madrid. He became Professor of Histology at the Universidad Complutense between 1978 and 1980, and was later appointed to the Histology Chair at the Universidad Miguel Hernández, in Alicante. Since his medical student days, he worked in de Castro's research laboratory, first at the medical school and later at the Instituto Cajal and was to remain by de Castro's side until the latter's death in 1967. During the years in which histological research of the nervous system was still based almost exclusively on silver nitrate staining methods, de Castro and Jaime Merchán used all, or nearly all, the methods described in this book. Their invaluable practical experience enabled them to provide the data and clarifications essential to understand the historical context of the methods employed by Cajal and his followers, thus establishing the basis for the study of brain function.

As Nobel Prize scientist Dr. Erik Kandel pointed out, the neuron theory, the dynamic polarization law, and the specificity of the connections theory were undoubtedly the result of hard work, persistence, and imagination on the part of Cajal and his disciples, who formed the Spanish School of Neurohistology. Neuroscientists of today can only fully understand the origin and importance of these pioneers by looking at them in their historical context and appreciating their outstanding command of chemistry, physics, and staining reactions. Thanks to his hands-on experience while working with de Castro, Jaime Merchán was able to make the subject and translation accessible to the modern reader of this book, for which Cajal had chosen Fernando de Castro to compile the advances in methodology achieved during the second half of the nineteenth century and the first decades of the twentieth century—advances which were used by Cajal and his disciples to dismantle the reticular theory.

The editors of the present volume wish to pay homage to Jaime Merchán in particular but also to an entire generation of scientists who fulfilled Cajal's dream, a dream that is illustrated by one of his most famous sayings:

"So often has it been said that the problem with Spain is a cultural one. Indeed, if we wish to be part of the civilized world, it is mandatory that we cultivate the barrenness of our land and of our minds, rescuing for posterity and for the motherland all the rivers that are lost in the sea and all the talent that is wasted in ignorance."

There is no doubt that today Spain is a competitive country in almost all fields of science and particularly in nervous system research. It is important to emphasize, however, that this is not due solely to the political and economic changes that occurred after the death of Franco. We believe it would not have happened without the impulse of the pioneering scientists in the late nineteenth and early twentieth century: Tello, Achúcarro, Del Río-Hortega, de Castro, Lorente de Nó, Pedro Ramón y Cajal—all direct disciples and collaborators of Santiago Ramón y Cajal. With this monograph we would like to show the importance of their legacy, their sacrifice, their enthusiasm, and their titanic effort in kindling the flame of scientific research amid political and social cataclysm. The editors want to acknowledge the efforts of Dr. Heather Fulwood and Dr. Francisco Nogales in the revision of the manuscript, in particular, for having succeeded in preserving the terminology used by the authors in the original edition.

M. A. Merchán
J. DeFelipe
F. de Castro Soubriet

FOREWORD

BY CONSTANTINO SOTELO ■

It seems obvious that to understand the way our brain functions, we are first required to know how it is organized. This prerequisite might explain why neuroanatomy has been at the forefront of advances in our knowledge of neuroscience. There is no doubt that the conceptual revolution introduced by Santiago Ramón y Cajal in his "Neuron Doctrine," providing morphological evidence that the nervous system was made up of billions of independent, richly and precisely interconnected nerve cells, gives Cajal the well-deserved title of the founder of modern neuroscience.

In neuroscience, as in many other experimental sciences, the most important advances often have been generated by the use of new analytical methods, because technical improvements make it possible to choose between opposing theories supposedly explaining the same facts. The introduction of a revolutionary technique by Camillo Golgi (1873) made an enormous contribution to most of Cajal's studies on the architectural organization of the brain and spinal cord. It was with Golgi impregnation that Cajal gathered his most important evidence for the contiguity of nerve cells (contacts between neurons), in opposition to the then generally accepted concept of nerve cell continuity through protoplasmic bridges (reticularism).

The period covered by the highly creative work of Cajal (1887–1934) was a period of rich technical innovation. William Windle, in the presentation of a book devoted to neuroanatomical techniques, published in 1957 (*New Research Techniques in Neuroanatomy*, C. Thomas, Springfield, Illinois), proposed naming this period the "Cajal epoch," which embraces the technical contributions of many renowned neuroanatomists, in addition to Cajal and Golgi. Among these investigators who have greatly helped to unravel the complexity of the central nervous system (CNS) with their original techniques, I will mention: Paul Erhlich, Louis Ranvier, Vittorio Marchi, Alois Alzheimer, Max Bielschowsky, Frank Nissl, Carl Weigert, Jean Nageotte, and many others. The "Cajal epoch" extended beyond Cajal's death, up until the 1950s, when new technical advances introduced by Walle Nauta—his selective impregnation of degenerating axons—and Sandy Palay—the intracardiac perfusion technique for the electron microscopic study of the brain—inaugurated another epoch. This new period could be named the "Neurocytology and Tract Tracing epoch," and it lasted until the 1980s.

Cajal not only contributed to this technical breakthrough with his modifications of the Golgi method, but he created valuable techniques to study intraneuronal organelles (reduced silver impregnation, 1903), and astroglial cells (gold chloride-sublimate impregnation, 1913). In their excellent review, Javier DeFelipe and Ted Jones (Santiago Ramón y Cajal and methods in neurohistology, 1992, *TINS* 15: 237–245) emphasized that Cajal in his early years of work on the CNS from 1887 to 1892 (during which time he published thirty of his best papers) was not very prolific in describing the modifications of the Golgi method he used. In 1889, however, he published a technical note on the modifications required to obtain successful Golgi impregnation in the embryonic CNS. More importantly, in his monograph *La Rétine des Vértébrés* (La Cellule 9: 121–255; 1892), Cajal provided a detailed description of his "double impregnation" procedure, which was named the rapid Golgi method.

One of the most important human accomplishments of Cajal was to awaken the scientific curiosity of young scientists who, motivated by Cajal's discoveries, were attracted to the investigation of the nervous system. Thus, in a country like the Spain of the end of the nineteenth and beginning of the twentieth century, devoid of scientific traditions, young researchers began to work directly under Cajal's supervision, whereas some others such as Nicolás Achúcarro and his pupil Pío Del Río Hortega were affiliated with his laboratory. Cajal brilliantly succeeded in changing Spanish mentality and founded what is known as the "Spanish School of Neurohistology," with exceptionally good people such as Francisco Tello, Domingo Sánchez, and his last two pupils Fernando de Castro and Rafael Lorente de Nó. The zenith of the "Spanish School of Neurohistology" occurred at the end of the golden period of Cajal's analytical studies with Golgi impregnated material. The Golgi method, although it has been and remains a powerful tool for studying the morphology of neuronal cell bodies, and axonal and dendritic arbors, is not appropriate for the study of subcellular components (nucleus, cytoplasmic organelles). New questions emerged, particularly after the studies by S. Apáthy in the leech, and A. Bethe in vertebrates, of some components of the neuronal cytoskeleton (called the neurofibrils).

These investigators, based upon poor preparations obtained with unreliable techniques for the staining of neurofibrils, considered these structures to be the elements that conducted nervous activity and reported that they formed continuous networks, passing from neuron to neuron—thereby transiently reviving the decaying reticular hypothesis. From 1901 to 1903, Cajal worked very hard to develop a reliable method of staining neurofibrils, particularly in axons. He finally succeeded, and in 1903 he published the reduced silver technique. From this point on, a large part of his research and most of that of his pupils was carried out using this new technique. Numerous variants were published, each one adapted to the material used, and the reduced silver method became a "must" in the study not only of neurocytology, but in the analysis of the degeneration and regeneration of the nervous system. Francisco Tello mastered this method in his studies of the action of hibernation on neuronal cytoskeleton and, particularly, of the development of the embryonic CNS. Fernando de Castro used the reduced silver method and modified it with the addition of new hypnotic compounds to the fixatives, resulting in a new variant with which to impregnate neurons and axons within their bony envelopes. These methods were used in most of his studies of the peripheral nervous system, particularly in his excellent investigations of the innervation of chemoreceptors and baroreceptors.

The staining of neuroglial cells was also one of the main activities of the "Spanish School of Neurohistology." Although Cajal himself was extremely motivated by the study of neuroglial cells, and participated in it extensively by developing his method of gold chloride-sublimate to stain astroglial cells, he was not as successful as some of his collaborators. Achúcarro, an eminent neuropathologist, was devoted to the study of the glial cells in normal and pathological conditions. He spent years trying to develop a "pan-glial" reduced silver method specifically for the study of all classes of neuroglial cells. In 1911, Achúcarro succeeded in developing the tanin-ammoniacal silver method to stain rod-like cells (stäbchenzellen), showing that these cells had phagocytic activity. But his premature death at the age of thirty-eight prevented him from finding such a "pan-glial" method. This prize fell to his pupil Río Hortega. His ammoniacal silver carbonate technique (1919) allowed him to make the most important discoveries in the field of glial cells. I agree with Marcus Jacobson (*Foundations of Neuroscience*, 1993, Plenum Press, New York) when he wrote: "In historical perspective [. . .] what Cajal is to the neuron, Río Hortega is to the neuroglia." Indeed, Río Hortega with the modifications of his silver carbonate method was able to dissociate within the "third element" of Cajal (a category of uncharacterized cells that, in addition to the fibrous and protoplasmic astrocytes, occurs in the CNS), two different classes of glial cells, oligodendroglial and microglial cells, each with a completely different function and embryonic origin.

Cajal, although faithful to the idea that technical innovation was essential for scientific progress, did not impose the use of new techniques just to be modern. For him, the important thing was to have technical tools adequate to answer the questions being investigated. When such tools were missing, Cajal spent a lot of time and energy in their development. Thus, under Cajal's leadership, a group of highly motivated young researchers (those of the "Spanish School of Neurohistology") greatly contributed to a repertoire of reliable techniques for analyzing the normal and pathological histology of the nervous system. It is, therefore, understandable that one of the last tasks of Cajal's life was to record for posterity his own compilation of universally developed techniques, used by him and his pupils. Of course, well-deserved priority would be given to the technical achievements of the "Spanish School of Neurohistology." For this important endeavor, Cajal decided to associate himself with Fernando de Castro, his youngest and beloved pupil. Thus, in 1933, a year before Cajal's death, there appeared an important book titled, *Elementos de Técnica Micrográfica del Sistema Nervioso*, namely, this book, which is now published for the first time in English.

This preface gives me the chance to remember the great man that was Fernando de Castro, my mentor and friend, to whom I will always be in debt. Fernando de Castro, one of the most brilliant pupils of Cajal, started his work on the nervous system in 1916. He was a twenty-year-old medical student at the University of Madrid when he joined the Cajal laboratory. He began his training working first on gustatory receptors. Following Cajal's instructions, to become acquainted with the general techniques of histology, and with those more specific for neuromorphology, de Castro was exposed to several kinds of material ranging from the olfactory bulb (neuroglial cells) to the cerebellum (aberrant climbing fibers). Soon, he discovered his real vocation, and devoted himself to the study of the peripheral sensory and sympathetic systems. His thesis, on the *Study of the Human Sensory Ganglia in Normal and Pathological Conditions. Typical and Atypical Cellular Forms,* became a classic when—translated into English—it was published by Wilder Penfield (1932) in his *Cytology and Cellular Pathology of the Nervous System*. After the sensory ganglia, de Castro undertook the study of sympathetic ganglia (1922 to 1926), also included by Penfield in his treatise.

The golden epoch of de Castro's work stretched from 1925 to 1928, when he was working on the innervation of the carotid sinus and, particularly, the glomus caroticum. His mastering of the methylene blue and reduced silver methods was essential for the analysis of nerve fibers and terminal axonal arbors in these two carotid structures. During these years, the sinus area was a relatively well-known structure. Because of the early work by the group of H. E. Hering and later on by Corneille J. F. Heymans, the carotid sinuses were shown to contain receptors that, by a reflex mechanism, regulate the activity of the cardiovascular and respiratory centers. In this reflex, afferent signals to the medullary cardiovascular region inhibit sympathetic tonic activity to blood vessels and the heart, while increasing the vagal effect to the heart. Much less studied was the area called carotid glomus, although its existence had been known since the eighteenth century. Its texture, composed of very fine intertwining capillaries, prompted some investigators to consider it as a sort of endocrine gland, similar to the medulla of the suprarenal gland. In his important paper of 1926, Fernando de Castro showed that the glomus could not be considered as a glandular structure. On the contrary, the richness of the innervation of the glomic cells and the existence of its special vascular organization suggested that the glomus was a sensory organ aimed at reacting to variations in the chemical composition of the blood. As clearly stated, however, by Antonio Gallego (in *Cajal y la Escuela Neurológica Española*, Universidad Complutense, Madrid, 1981) in his portrait of de Castro, he was more interested by function than by mere structure. Thus, de Castro, despite the deficiency in physiological tools and experience, worked hard (hosted by the Laboratories of Physiology and Pharmacology of the Medical School) to obtain some evidence in favor of his own ideas regarding the function of the carotid glomus.

In 1928, de Castro published his second important paper on this topic. In this publication, he completed his anatomical studies and reported that the sensory receptors in the glomus were terminal axonic fields of the glossopharyngeal nerve. Using an old kymograph, he was able to record changes in cardiac frequency and blood pressure just by electrical stimulation of the "intercarotidien" nerve or, as published some years later, by changing some parameters in the composition of the blood. De Castro was, therefore, able to show that the carotid glomus had a chemoreceptor function. From histology, he changed direction and became an accomplished physiologist, still driven by the same concept: the significance does not lie in the research method used but rather in the question that is to be answered.

The Spanish Civil War (1936–1939) marked a complete halt to the scientific development of Spain. De Castro, who was at the peak of his scientific production (at forty years of age), decided to remain in Spain, a decision that proved very significant for the future of his career. The victory of General Francisco Franco in the Spanish Civil War imposed a return to darkness, paralleled by an increase in the power of the Catholic Church. As de Castro himself often commented to me during those days, those in power believed that agnostic people must be systematically wrong because—of course—they did not deserve God's support. Thus, Cajal and most of the members of the "Spanish School of Neurohistology" were wrong in their ideas in defense of the "Neuron Doctrine." This illogical thinking explains why it was in Cajal's own country that obsolete reticularist ideas began to flourish again. Simultaneously with this radical change of ideas, Fernando de Castro was dismissed from his chair as Professor of Histology at the University of Madrid, and his laboratory space at the Cajal Institute was reduced. For almost fourteen years, de Castro was obliged to exert his abilities as pathologist and surgeon to sustain his family, without abandoning his own research, which in those years was concerned with the study of nervous and synaptic plasticity (heterologous peripheral nerve anastomosis) and pursuing his work on chemoreceptors.

I first met Fernando de Castro in October 1955, when I was one out of over 1,000 students, who (in a crowded manner) attempted to follow his teaching at the Medical School. At that time, Madrid had only one medical school, and the number of students was unbelievably high. (Over 800 students started every first-year course, although fewer than 300 completed the course.) De Castro was a great teacher but a very demanding one. Thus, a high percentage of students took two or more years to pass their examinations, which explains the accumulation of students and the overcrowding at his classes. Although I was more taken by the "modern" biochemistry than by the "old" histology, I very soon was attracted by de Castro's personality, and decided that I must try to be trained in his laboratory. My first encounter with him was a real disaster. I requested an appointment, and, taking advantage of a family acquaintance, I tried to make my dream a reality. Don Fernando, as he was affectionately known, was very angry with me, and explained that to be trained in his laboratory was an honor that had to be earned.

A year later, after being lucky with my examination marks in histology, I was finally admitted to the laboratory. What started as a complete failure became not only the beginning of a wonderful human relationship, but an excellent training period that engendered my love for neuroscience, particularly neuromorphology. Thus, from 1957 to 1961, when I finished my medical studies and decided to emigrate to start a free life in France, was one of the most important periods of my life. During these years, I devoted most of my spare time to Don Fernando's laboratory, despite the unusual schedule of work imposed by him (from 7 PM to 11 PM every day). His politeness and gentle dedication to teaching and care of his students made him the gentleman of Spanish neuroscience.

For four years, I was trained in the techniques developed by Cajal and his pupils (with the exception of the rapid Golgi method, because osmic acid was a luxury too expensive just for training). During those days, when—following the recommendations of Don Fernando—I was working on the granule cells of the olfactory bulb (strange neurons devoid of axons that could participate in bulbar microcircuits through their dendrites) the book *Elementos de Técnica Micrográfica del Sistema Nervioso* was my dear companion, my bible. When the book appeared in 1933, its main purpose was to provide Spanish-speaking students and scientists with a complete repertoire of methods used for the analysis of the morphology of neurons and glial cells, in the normal and pathological nervous system. Twenty-five years later, the book had kept its relevance, only the selective silver methods to impregnate degenerating axons and, of course, electron microscopy were missing. The attraction of the book lies in the fact that it describes techniques accurately, discussing the preferential fixatives to be used, the way to obtain the most convenient sections and, principally, offers detailed step-by-step technical protocols. How lucky we were to be guided by such a book, written by two masters of neuromorphology, who had invested a great deal of their time in developing and/or improving most of the techniques reported. This was particularly true in my case, because my preparations were systematically evaluated by the critical eye of Don Fernando, who constantly helped me with his advice to improve the results. Thus, when I left Spain, my only belongings were my knowledge of and skills with most of the silver methods, and a copy of the book given to me by Joaquín Rodríguez, the laboratory attendant, a copy that I still use.

What is the point of publishing an English version almost eighty years after the book was published in Spanish? The fact that this repertoire of techniques has never been published in English prevented it from becoming the standard reference in the field of neuromorphology during its early golden period. It is, therefore, essential from a historical viewpoint to provide free access to all the classical techniques that have marked the history of neuromorphology, especially now that we are living a new golden epoch of the field. Indeed, the technical progress made during the last twenty years with new advances emerging from physics, chemistry, and molecular biology has once again pushed neuromorphology to the forefront of modern neuroscience.

An almost constant dream of neuromorphologists has been to correlate the chemical constituents of the neuron with their structural counterparts, to better appraise neuronal function and organization. This desire gave rise to classical "histochemistry," a field that has now changed completely with the development of several technical approaches, such as (1) Autoradiography and the diversity of its applications, from the study of tracing connections based upon axoplasmic transport, to identification of neurotransmitters and receptors; (2) Immunocytochemistry, with its multiple applications for the study of neuronal and neuroglial constituents; (3) In situ hybridization for detection of messenger RNAs, to study gene expression and regulation; and (4) Gene transfer with the cDNA of genes coding for exogenous proteins (for instance, Lac Z and, particularly, "green fluorescence protein") that allows the complete morphological study of the transfected cells.

The progress in physical sciences and informatics has generated new tools for the study of the organization of the brain and the examination of the dynamic aspects of the neuron. For instance, the development of computer-assisted image-analysis has promoted new kinds of quantitative studies, such as three-dimensional (3-D) morphology of Golgi impregnated neurons with their dendritic and axonic fields, or 3-D reconstruction of neuronal compartments from electron micrographs. The development of confocal laser-scanning microscopy (CLSM) has provided an enhanced resolution, compared with classical fluorescence microscopy, and has allowed the 3-D reconstruction of thick sections. Advances in laser technology during the last ten years have permitted the development of a new type of CLSM, which, while keeping all the advantages of the confocal microscopy (ability to penetrate scattering tissues), has the added advantage of greatly reducing phototoxicity and photobleaching. This is two-photon laser-scanning microscopy (TPLSM), where fluorescence excitation above or below the plane of study is practically nonexistent. Thus, it can be used to study thick brain slices in organotypic culture or even neuronal compartments located several hundreds of micrometers deep in the living brain (e.g., functional imaging of calcium concentrations in small dendritic spines). In addition, the explosion of noninvasive brain imaging techniques, like positron emission tomography (PET-scan) and functional magnetic resonance imaging (fMRI), have allowed investigators to analyze functional aspects of activity of the same brain region repeatedly and over extended periods of time. These noninvasive imaging techniques underlie the modern revolution in cognitive neuroscience and have opened up a virgin territory in the exploration of human brain function. It is obvious that we have now entered a new golden period, that of the "Chemoanatomy and Functional Neuromorphology epoch."

The English version of Cajal and de Castro's neuroanatomical techniques offers the whole neuroscience community a simple way to compare modern and classic morphological methods applied to the study of the nervous system. Thus, as stated above, the main interest of this book lies in its historic value. It is worthwhile recalling, however, that some of the techniques described have maintained their relevance and can be extremely useful for training students seeking a vocation in neuroscience research. More importantly, even some of the classical techniques, particularly the Golgi method and its variants and the reduced silver impregnation, remain as valuable as—and often cheaper than—the most sophisticated immunocytochemical methods. Can an anti-neurofilament immunostained neuron appear brighter and better depicted than a reduced silver impregnated neuron? I still enjoy the memory of a meeting in France (Fontevraud Abbey) during the early 1980s, when Heinz Wässle opened the presentation of his work on the retina simply by saying: "In 1911, Max Bielschowsky with his new monoclonal antibody had beautifully stained displaced ganglion cells. . .." This introductory statement was accompanied by the projection of a superb micrograph showing displaced ganglion cells in whole-mount retinas impregnated with the Bielschowsky silver method. A wonderful demonstration of the imperishable value of the classical techniques reported in this book.

With this English translation, the *Técnica Micrográfica del Sistema Nervioso* by Santiago Ramón y Cajal and Fernando de Castro will now start a second life. I hope that this second life will become as fruitful as the first one. Let me finish these incomplete introductory remarks, with another personal memory. In 1995, four years before his death, my French advisor and teacher for almost forty years, the late René Couteaux, offered me his personal copy of the Spanish edition of this book (with an autograph of Don Fernando). René Couteaux, the founder of French neurocytology, wrote, "A mon ami Constantino Sotelo, je transmets ce livre très fatigué, mais chargé de souvenirs et de sentiments." Readers of this book, do not forget this dedication; you have in your hands a book that has existed for a long time and is charged with the memories and feelings of generations of neuromorphologists who have been initiated in the nervous system through this compilation of techniques. I hope it will also help you in your search for knowledge of the organization and function of the CNS.

Paris

PRELIMINARY INFORMATION

Spanish enthusiasts of the Normal and Pathological Histology of the nervous system voiced the need for a technical book that dealt specifically with the analysis of the texture and morphology of neurons; thus we have gathered a fairly complete repertoire of the methods and formulae most frequently used nowadays. This handbook is for physicians, and thus it would have been unforgivable to overlook those procedures that reveal the fine pathological anatomy of neurons and glial cells and consequently lesions of paramount importance for the exact diagnosis of diseases of the cerebrospinal axis. We only have excluded here some (but not all) of the general methods that are usually described in general Histology and Pathology textbooks and also formulae that, although useful in the past, now have been surpassed by more consistent and powerful techniques.

We would be ungrateful if we did not acknowledge the sponsorship that Doctor D. Rafael Segarra, an eminent Spanish physician in the Republic of Argentina, and a group of enthusiastic compatriots have generously provided for the publication of this treatise. To all of them, our hearty gratitude.

S. Ramón y Cajal, F. de Castro
Madrid, January 1933

LIST OF PLATES

Plate 1. Cajal's trichrome (triple staining with fuchsin or magenta, picric acid and carmine indigo) used by de Castro to stain the glomus caroticum. The ground substance stains light green, collagen bundles and nuclear chromatin dark blue, and the cytoplasm of glomus cells pink. Pericytes and basement membranes stain very dark blue (almost black), highlighting the relationship between cell nests and blood vessels (X20). Photograph obtained from an original slide from Professor Fernando de Castro (Archivo Fernando de Castro).

Plate 2. Mounting and conservation of tissue sections. Illustration of original histological slides from the early twentieth century. The sections were covered according to the staining technique. The first slide on the left in the top row has a thin coverslip using Canada balsam as the cover medium, the usual method at the time. The adjacent slide, however, had no coverslip, the tissue being painted over with several layers of Dammar resin dissolved in benzol or xylol. The next slide on the right has a circular coverslip sealed with gum or lacquer.

The lower part of the photograph shows a detail of Section 5 from the top row in order to illustrate the labeling system over sections. The stain is a fast Golgi method of the vertebral axis of an embryo (thick serial sections probably cut with at least a 200 µm setting on the microtome). The label at the slide reads: "Sympathetic axons leading to the rachideal and commissural pairs." In the lower part, next to the trident symbol, the text reads: "Sympathetic axon with collateral branching." Ink lines highlight the most interesting areas, such as the entrance of collaterals in a rachideal ganglion (Figure 2). Photographs obtained from original slides from Professor Fernando de Castro (Archivo Fernando de Castro).

Plate 3. Mosaic of microphotographies (at X10) from the histological slide shown in Figure 1 (bottom part) as a track of the method of study followed by the Cajal school. Arrowheads show the spinal ganglia and the red arrows the chain of sympathetic ganglia. Vertebrae and apophysis clearly define the conjunction holes where ganglia are hosted (white dotted line). The inset shows the sympathetic collateral branches (green arrows, on the left: stellate neurons) and their relationship with the spinal ganglion (rounded neurons: green arrows, on the right). All the images were taken at X10. Photographs obtained from original slides from Professor Fernando de Castro (Archivo Fernando de Castro).

Plate 4. Methods for the demonstration of neuronal morphology. Golgi method and variants—Fast Golgi. Staining of cerebellar grains and parallel fibers of the molecular layer (X10). Photograph obtained from an original slide from Professor Fernando de Castro (Archivo Fernando de Castro).

Plate 5. Methods for the demonstration of neuronal morphology. Golgi method and variants—Cox's method. Clear staining allowing the study of various types of neurons in the cerebellum. 1. Purkinje's cell. Arrowhead shows axonal root. 2. Deep stellate cell (basket cell). 3. Lugaro's fusiform cell (X10). Photographs obtained from original slides from Professor Fernando de Castro (Archivo Fernando de Castro).

Plate 6. Methods for the demonstration of neuronal morphology. Golgi method and variants—Cox's method applied to the study of cat cerebral cortex (top X5, bottom X10). Photograph obtained from an original slide from Professor Fernando de Castro (Archivo Fernando de Castro).

Plate 7. Methods for the demonstration of neuronal morphology. Ehrlich's method and variants using methyl blue. Intravital staining with methyl blue carried out by Professor Fernando de Castro in order to study the fibers of the carotid sinus. (Modification of Cajal's method. Fixed in ammonium molybdate. Adult cat carotid.) In the upper part there is an original pen and ink wash drawing by the author (published in de Castro. F.: "Sur la structure et l'innervation du sinus carotidien de l'homme et des mammifères. Nouveaux faits sur l'innervation et la fonction du glomus caroticum." Trav. Lab. Rech. Biol. 25: 331–380, 1928). Below is a terminal field of fibers in the aortic wall clearly showing characteristic barosensitive meniscus of these fibers. The background blue staining is due to the intravital diffusion of the stain (X20). Photograph obtained from an original slide from Professor Fernando de Castro (Archivo Fernando de Castro), to whom the original drawing also belongs.

Plate 8. Intravital staining with carmine to analyze blood vessel distribution in the gastric mucosa of the rabbit (X10). Photograph obtained from an original slide from Professor Fernando de Castro (Archivo Fernando de Castro).

Plate 9. Nervous cell structure. Demonstration of the tigroid substance (Nissl chromatic granules) using anilines (Cresyl violet—top) and silver impregnation (cold silver carbonate –bottom) (X100). Slides from Professor Jaime Merchán Cifuentes.

Plate 10. Nervous cell structure. Silver impregnation of neurofibrils. Lamb spinal medulla stained with Bielschowsky's standard procedure (Mosaic X40 –top; X100 –bottom). Slides from Professor Jaime Merchán Cifuentes.

Plate 11. Nervous cell structure. Silver impregnation of neurofibrils. Intramural ganglion (dog esophagus); Gros's method, optimal effect. Top: axonal pathways strongly stained in black; glial capsule, formed by spindle-shaped cells, stained violet (mosaic, X10). Bottom: neuron with somatic cytoplasm and dendrites packed with neurofibrils and surrounded by glial cells (X100). Photographs obtained from original slides from Professor Fernandode Castro (Archivo Fernando de Castro).

List of Plates

Plate 12. Upper cervical ganglion from a cat (autonomic nervous system) Cajal–Castro's reduced silver impregnation (mosaic X10). On the right, an original sketch by de Castro showing the special features of the dendrites of the cervical sympathetic neurons (published in de Castro. F.: "Sobre la fina anatomía de los ganglios simpáticos, vertebrales y prevertebrales de los simios." Bol. Soc. Esp. Biol. XI: 171–177, 1926). Photograph obtained from original slides from Professor Fernando de Castro (Archivo Fernando de Castro), to whom the original drawing also belongs.

Plate 13. Coronal section from mouse embryo. Cajal–Castro's reduced silver impregnation using somnifene as fixative. These slides were used in the study of morphology and connections of the glomus caroticus. Top: the fibrillary tracts can be clearly seen stained in black against a golden background (X5). Bottom: a high magnification of neurons showing neurofibrils (X40). Photographs obtained from original slides from Professor Fernando de Castro (Archivo Fernando de Castro).

Plate 14. Section of cerebellum impregnated with a hydroquinone-based technique (Ramón y Cajal. S.: "Une formule pour colorer dans les coupes les fibers amedullées et les terminaisons centrales et périphériques." Trab. Lab. Invest. Biol. Univ. Madrid, 23: 237, 1925). The horizontal pathway of the axons of deep stellate cells from the molecular level and the brush axons of Purkinje cells can be clearly seen (X10). Photographs obtained from original slides from Professor Fernando de Castro (Archivo Fernando de Castro).

Plate 15. Section of human brain impregnated with an ammonium alcohol (the label reads "brain from an old female"). Lipofuscin granules are seen in the cytoplasm of the neurons from the cortical pyramid (X10). Photographs obtained from original slides from Professor Fernando de Castro (Archivo Fernando de Castro).

Plate 16. Cajal–Castro's method for the study of peripheral nerve regeneration. Longitudinal section of the sciatic nerve. Arrows show the lesion produced by a suture below the proximal and above the distal end. Green boxes contain details from the right, organized from bottom to top, in a proximal to distal direction (Mosaic X5). Meniscus and dilations possibly represent cones of axonal growth (X20). Photographs obtained from original slides from Professor Fernando de Castro (Archivo Fernando de Castro).

Plate 17. Tangential section of the mucosa and the muscular wall of the stomach of a three-month-old puppy (Mosaic X5). Cajal–Castro's reduced silver impregnation. The intramural plexus make a continuous network of nonmyelinated nerve fibers (Center, X20). Packed cells can be seen in each node of the plexus. Some of these cells may correspond to those named in the current literature as the "interstitial cells of Cajal," which represent motility pacemakers of the intestinal tract (high magnification in the top right corner, X100). Photographs obtained from original slides from Professor Fernando de Castro (Archivo Fernando de Castro).

Plate 18. Impregnation of the cellular Golgi complex. Cajal's method using formalin-uranyl nitrate (Ramón y Cajal. S.: "Un sencillo método de coloración selectiva del retículo endoplásmico y sus efectos en los diversos órganos." Trab.

Lab. Invest. Biol. Univ. Madrid, 2: 129, 1903). The internal reticular apparatus (terminology in use at the time) is shown. Cajal used this method in exocrine gland cells and proposed, for the first time, its role in cellular secretion (X 100). Original slides from Professor Jaime Merchán Cifuentes.

Plate 19. Myelin staining. Del Rio Hortega's method for staining ganglionar glia. Sympathetic ganglion from a cat (X5, X20). Photographs obtained from original slides from Professor Fernando de Castro (Archivo Fernando de Castro).

Plate 20. Bolsi's method using Cajal's ammonium silver oxide (Ammonium bromide). Average staining quality. Astrocytes and their "sucking feet" (end feet) attached to a blood vessel wall can be seen (X40). Original slides from Professor Jaime Merchán Cifuentes.

Plate 21. Myelin staining procedures. Osmic acid. Top: low-power image of a peripheral nerve (X10). Bottom: magnification of nodes and paranodes, Schmidt-Lantermann's incisures and spiny bracelet of Nageotte (top left corner X100). Photographs obtained from original slides from Professor Fernando de Castro (Archivo Fernando de Castro).

Plate 22. Optimal staining of Kluver Barrera's trichrome method for myelin in a rat auditory nerve. Nitric acid formalin decalcification "used by Cajal for the study of the ear." Top left: cochlear nuclei of rat brain. Right: overview in a sagittal plane of the entire pathway of the cochlea, auditory nerve, and cochlear nuclei. This method highlights the difference in staining between Schwann cells (turquoise) and oligodendrocytes (light blue) (X 10). Bottom: transition zone between central and peripheral glia can be clearly seen (X20). Original slides from Professor Miguel Merchán Cifuentes.

Plate 23. Average quality staining using Fink and Heimer's method for the study of axonal degeneration. Rat's cochlear nuclei subsequent to a small lesion in the cochlea (after seven days). Arrowheads show the fragmented axonal pathway following Wallerian degeneration. Degeneration buds can be selectively seen with this method, which was widely used to analyze nervous system connections before the introduction of tract tracing methods (X 40). Original slides from Professor Miguel Merchán Cifuentes.

SECTION ONE

Historical Context

1

The Authors and Their Backgrounds

JAIME A. MERCHÁN AND JORGE PRIETO
Professors of Histology, University of Alicante, Spain

Every great work is the result of a great idea carried out with great passion.
—Cajal

Santiago Ramón y Cajal is such a well-known figure internationally that any attempt to present an exhaustive account of his life here would only repeat his autobiography[1] or numerous biographies. Therefore, we will merely highlight the chief landmarks of Cajal's and de Castro's lives in the context of their social and scientific backgrounds.

Cajal was born in 1852, in Petilla de Aragón, a small village in one of the poorest regions of Spain, a country which at that time lagged far behind the socioeconomic development of the major Western countries. Although Spain had been the center of a rich empire until only a few years before Cajal's birth, it had not invested its wealth in modernization. The industrial and transport revolutions taking place elsewhere did not occur in Spain and the economy remained dependent mainly on agriculture. While neighboring countries were experimenting with liberalism and enjoying economic growth, Spain's serious internal political struggles anchored the country firmly in the past.

Unsurprisingly, this economic and political backwardness affected scientific development. At a time when Faraday, Gay-Lussac, Ampere, Poisson, Ohm, Dalton, Oersted, Gauss, Wöhler, and others were working elsewhere in Europe, Spain produced no major scientific work. The main reason was the Spanish government's attitude toward education; there were only ten universities in Spain at this time, the majority of which were still looking back to their past glories rather than trying to shape the future with authentic scientific projects. Even the ancient and prestigious University of Salamanca only had five hundred students. The lack of resources was not the only thing responsible for this stagnation; the University system itself impaired many kinds of research because all scientific activity had to be carried out in Madrid, while the other nine universities were limited to teaching, because they lacked the necessary infrastructure and funding. Generally, professorships were awarded through local political influence; only in Madrid was there a structured procedure for considering the scientific merit of the candidates' work.

Primary and secondary schools fared no better. Although the Constitution of 1812 established that everyone had a right to education and a network of schools managed by the City Councils had been built, in reality, the lack of public funding meant that only the children of well-to-do families could attend secondary school (high school). Primary teachers were so poorly paid that often they depended on donations from the pupils' families; this, together with poor teaching conditions, led to low standards in the public schools. Thus, children from wealthy families were often educated at home with private tutors.

Cajal's tutor was his father, who was a doctor in a small village. He not only taught him arithmetic, geography, grammar, and physics but also endowed in him a deep love for nature. From an early age, Cajal was gifted at drawing and accumulated a huge collection of sketches of landscapes, animals, and plants. This hobby lasted throughout his life; later he was to illustrate his papers with freehand drawings in Indian ink on gouache,[1] which he transferred himself to the plates for the etchings. Only by doing this himself could he be assured of the high standards he required.[2] Furthermore, he expected his disciples to be adept at drawing. He also enjoyed painting still lifes, portraits, nudes, and other types of paintings and eventually also became interested in the newly discovered art of photography.

His artistic leanings proved useful when, still only a teenager, his father started to prepare him for a future medical career and began by teaching him anatomy. Day after day Cajal carefully sketched the bones that his father had obtained from the village cemetery. After Cajal had retired, he reminisced how "the future professor and modest, but stubborn and active, researcher that I became, was the result of those anatomy lessons taught in the barn."

After finishing high school, he studied at the Medical School in Zaragoza from 1869 to 1873. His first job as a physician in the Spanish colonial army took him to Cuba, where he contracted malaria and had to return to Spain after two years. He was very ill for more than two years; during his convalescence he worked as an assistant professor in the Anatomy Department at Zaragoza Medical School. Subsequently, he was put in charge of the anatomical museum, during which time he studied histology, then a new subject not included in the undergraduate medical curriculum. Histology only was taught in postgraduate programs and mostly as a theoretical subject because there were no laboratory facilities in Zaragoza. This was true of all Spanish universities except the Central University in Madrid. However, thanks to Professor Aureliano Maestre de San Juan, a disciple of Schwann and Ranvier,[3] for the first time in his life, Cajal examined histological preparations under the microscope. He was so fascinated that he spent his scarce savings on a Verick microscope and set up a rudimentary laboratory in the attic of his house. In these modest conditions, while living on a small salary, Cajal began his long and successful scientific career.

At first, his research was somewhat disappointing. He published only two papers in six years, one of which ("Microscopical observations on the nerve endings in the voluntary muscles of the frog," [1881]) suggested that nerve fibers were continuous with muscle cells. He published his doctoral thesis (*Origins of Inflammation*) two years later, at the time he was appointed to the Chair of Descriptive Anatomy at the Faculty of Medicine at the University of Valencia.

During the four years he spent in Valencia, Cajan's research was strongly influenced by an epidemic of cholera, which affected the whole country. Physicians of all specialties were expected to work toward controlling the spread of the disease. The first report of an anti-cholera vaccine was published by Dr. Jaime Ferrán, triggering a fierce controversy in the medical world. Under the pseudonym "Dr. Bacteria," Cajal published two papers on the cholera bacillus, as well as a number of newspaper articles. The Zaragoza County Council printed his results as a reference for the prevention of cholera and awarded him a cash prize, which he refused. In addition, however, the Council bought him a Zeiss microscope, the best then available, which he went on to use in the research that eventually established his neuron theory.

Two milestones in his career occurred at this time; he had a paper accepted for the first time by an international journal, the *International Monatschrift für Anatomie und Histologie* (founded by Krause)[4] and he met Dr. Luis Simarro, a psychiatrist who had worked with Ranvier. Simarro introduced Cajal to the Weigert-Pal (**157**) method and the recently discovered Golgi technique. Although Simarro was not convinced of the utility of the latter, Cajal recognized its great potential and immediately put it to use in an intensive exploration of the central nervous system, which he carried out in collaboration with his successor at Valencia, Dr. Bartual.

Cajal acknowledged that his initial results were disappointing, because it was mandatory "strictly to determine the conditions of the chromoargentic reaction and adapt it to each particular case. And, if the encephalon and other central organs of the adult human and other vertebrates prove too complex to allow their structure to be scrutinized by these means, why not use the method systematically on lower animals or early developmental stages of ontogenetic evolution, in which the nervous system must show a simple, and even schematic, organization? That was the research plan we set ourselves."

He embarked on his ambitious project while in Valencia, but he had to continue it in Barcelona when he was appointed to its newly created Chair of Histology in 1887. Undoubtedly, the subsequent four years were the most important of his career. He described the basic organization of many areas of the central nervous system and established the neuron doctrine, confirming the cell theory for the nervous system in a paper published in 1888, in which he demonstrated the anatomical and functional independence of nerve cells in the cerebellum of pigeons.

The scientific world did not readily accept, or often even seriously consider Cajal's hypotheses even though they had been published in international journals, such as the *International Monatschrift für Anatomie und Histologie,* and the *Anatomischer Anzeiger.* Frustrated by the lack of interest in his findings, Cajal decided to present his results in person in Berlin in 1889, at the prestigious meeting of the Deustche Gessellschaft für Anatomie. He received a cold response, however, due to both a distrust of his methods and misgivings about a Spanish scientist. (He was described as "exotic.") Van Gehutchen, Professor of Histology at the University of Louvain, wrote some years later: "The facts described by Cajal in his first publications were so shocking that the histologists treated them with skepticism. The distrust was such that in the Berlin meeting in 1889 Cajal, who later became the great histologist from Madrid, was cut off, evoking only incredulous smiles. I can still remember him taking Kölliker, the then undisputed master of Histology in Germany, to show him his admirable microscopic slides in order to convince him of the veracity of his findings" (Livre Jubilaire du A. Van Gehutchen. Le Neuraxe, 1911). Kölliker was so impressed with what he saw that he decided to sponsor this unknown scientist from Spain, saying to him: "Your results are so beautiful that I plan to take on a series of confirmatory studies immediately. I have discovered you, and I want to share my discovery with Germany."[5] Subsequent studies were published in Kölliker's own journal and in the *Anatomischer Anzeiger* in 1890 and 1891.[(2)]

We should clarify that confirmatory studies were often performed in order to check that results were bona fide. Such distrust stemmed from various factors in research methods, such as inconsistency, a lack of standardization in the purity of reagents and the use of the light microscope, which often was used at its limit of resolution.[6] Every result had to be confirmed by other researchers in different laboratories and the more famous the director of the laboratory, the better. Furthermore, photomicrography was not sufficiently developed to be used as a scientific tool and articles were not reviewed as thoroughly as they are today. In addition, interchange of ideas and results between scientists could only be done by handwritten letters sent by a sluggish postal system. And last, but not least, it was not easy to attend international meetings; travel was arduous and time-consuming, even within Europe. Thus it was difficult to demonstrate personally the validity of results. In summary, at the turn of the nineteenth century, research was only accepted by the scientific community if it was supported by an authority in the field. Thus, the importance of Kölliker's decision to back Cajal, an unknown Spanish scientist, cannot be underestimated.

After the Berlin meeting, Cajal's ideas became accepted by the most famous histologists of the time: His, Schwalbe, Déjérine, Kupffer, Krause, Weigert, Eddinger, Retzius, Van Gehutchen, Waldeyer (who coined the term, "neuron"), Von Lenhossék, Lugaro, Mathias Duval,[7] and others. Skeptics remained, however, the most notorious being Camillo Golgi, Professor at the University of Pavia. Ironically, the very person who had developed the method that Cajal used in proposing the neuron theory was a "reticularist"; he believed that axons formed a continuous network linking the cellular somata, although he did acknowledge that the dendrites terminated freely in the neuropil, near the blood vessels. He considered that the axonal endings described by Cajal were artifacts, caused by the incomplete impregnation staining of the meshwork. Regrettably, this argument persisted even in their lectures at the Nobel Prize award ceremony, causing tempers to rise, not only of both laureates but also of the jury.[8]

Cajal's scientific contributions in his years in Barcelona were published as *The New Concept of the Histology of the Nervous System* (El nuevo concepto de la histología del Sistema Nervioso), which was translated into German shortly afterward (Ramón y Cajal, R.: Neue Darstellungen von Histologischen bau des Zentralnervensystems. Archiv für Anatomie und Physiologie, 1893). Professor Léon Azoulay asked Cajal for a revised version, which he translated into French and published under the title *Les Nouvelles idées sur la structure du Système Nerveux chez l'Homme et chez les Vertebrés*, a reference work on the microscopical organization of the nervous system. It was such a success that three editions were published in the first three months, and most neuroscientists of the time used it to learn about the cellular architecture of the nervous system ("each cell is a completely independent physiological area"), the existence of the synapse ("The nervous action is transmitted by contiguity, by means of a series of induction phenomena through interneuronal joints"), and neuronal polarization ("The transmission of the nervous impulse always take place from the protoplasmic branches and neuronal soma toward the cylinder-axis"). Together with these basic principles, the book included a large amount of new data about the nervous system, from rather simple concepts, such as the innervation of the neuromuscular spindles, to extremely complex ones, such as the organization of the cerebral and cerebellar cortices, retina, olfactory bulb, and the spinal cord.

The wide acclaim for this book encouraged Cajal to undertake a more ambitious project, aimed at gathering "[...] all the infinite details about the morphology and structure of cells, although not just as a collection of microscopical details and minute facts with no regard for the physiological significance. On the contrary, the purpose is to build, as far as possible, theoretical science." The outcome was the publication, fourteen years later, of *The Texture of the Nervous System in Man and the Vertebrates* (Textura del Sistema Nervioso del Hombre y los Vertebrados), which Cajal later enlarged (1909) and which was translated into French by Léon Azoulay under the title, *Histologie du Système Nerveux de l'Homme et des Vertebrés*.[9]

In 1892, Cajal was appointed to the Chair of Histology at the Central University in Madrid. His arrival in Madrid was totally different from his arrival in Barcelona; he was now well-known, both nationally and internationally (although he had yet to receive his many prizes, such as Moscow, 1900; Helmholtz, 1905; and Nobel, 1906). He was respected in the academic world, especially by the Dean of the Medical School, Professor Julián Calleja, who provided him with greatly improved working conditions.[10] Not only did he now have well-equipped laboratories, assistants, and technicians, he was eligible for public funding for his research, which he had previously paid for out of his salary, a difficult task for a father of six children.

Cajal rapidly proved his worth; almost immediately he wrote the well-known paper on the retina published in *La Cellule,* the studies on the thalamus, Ammon's horn, and fascia dentata, whose illustrations are still reproduced in modern treatises, and the report on the nuclei of the cranial nerves. He also published extensive theoretical articles, such as the paper, "Laws of the morphology and dynamics of the nerve cells" and others discussing the optic pathways. He also started using the methylene blue method, modified from a technique originally developed by Bethe. This method rendered a wealth of new findings, such as the Cajal-Retzius cells of the cerebral cortex, the distribution of the central expansions of dorsal root ganglion cells, and, most importantly, the confirmation of the images obtained by means of the Golgi method.

The reason for using the methylene blue staining as a control for the Golgi images is that, although both techniques render similar results, they are based on completely different chemical processes. In the Golgi method the tissue is fixed with osmium and potassium dichromate, before being impregnated with silver nitrate, so that a crystallization of silver chromate takes place inside the neurons. Methylene blue is a well-recognized proton acceptor (**87**). If a tissue capable of redox processes is exposed to methylene blue, the dye will be reduced to a colorless base, mainly by the mitochondria. If the base is then exposed to a strong oxidant, for example, atmospheric oxygen, the color reappears. Therefore, the methylene blue can be used as a vital (**93**) or supravital (**89, 91, 92**) stain, thus avoiding fixation artifacts. Once stained, the tissue can be studied without the need for aggressive treatment; indeed, dehydration is unnecessary as the sections can be mounted in glycerol and, if the specimens are thin enough, even sectioning can be avoided. Even handmade, medium-thick sections of tissue are sufficiently transparent to allow microscopic examination.

Cajal's work soon gained national and international acceptance: He was made a member of the Spanish Royal Academy of Exact and Natural Sciences and Physics,[11] and the Spanish Royal Academy of Medicine. The Royal Society of London asked him to give the Croonian Annual Lecture in 1894, after which he received an honorary degree from the University of Cambridge. His stay in Britain was very important to him; not only was it his first trip abroad since the Berlin meeting in 1889, it was the first time he had been welcomed as a foremost scientist and invited to speak as a peer before leading researchers in a meeting presided by Lord Kelvin. He also met the leading British physiologists of the day (e.g., Langley, Schaffer, and Ferrier) and had the opportunity to witness their experiments, such as cortical ablations and the subsequent examination of their degenerating axons using Marchi's method. During his stay in England he was a house guest of Charles Scott Sherrington, with whom he became lifelong friends; indeed, their friendship extended to their disciples.

Some years later, in 1897, he was invited to the tenth anniversary of Clarke University in Worcester, Massachusetts. Only two years after the Spanish-American war, which had ended with the defeat of the Spanish navy in the Philippines and Cuba and the consequent loss of these Spanish colonies, Cajal left for America from a country infused with anti-American feeling. It is not surprising, therefore, that he was taken aback when he discovered that the United States was totally different from the jaundiced picture painted by the Spanish press. His visits to the Universities of Clarke, Columbia, and Harvard, the exquisite education and culture of his hosts, and the dynamism of that young society convinced him that although the United States had not yet reached the cultural and economic standards of Germany and England, the country was in the process of becoming the world's industrial and intellectual leader. His anti-American feelings were transformed into sincere admiration and he began to blame Spanish politicians for the recent humiliating military defeats. Subsequent to his trip to the United States, Cajal, a liberal and an agnostic, became deeply involved in the movement for social regeneration in Spain, which sowed the seeds of the Second Republic.

Upon his return to Spain, he learned that the International Medical Conference had awarded him the Moscow Prize for the most outstanding medical research over the previous three years. With this prestigious prize, Cajal acquired a social status to match his professional one and used his new influence to promote scientific research in what was still a backward nation. Both in his autobiography and in his book, *Advice for a Young Investigator*, Cajal stated that the chief aim of his work was to bring Spain up to the level of the most advanced countries, regardless of the sacrifices he would have to make in order to achieve this. He advised young researchers that "[...] the gratitude of your country is above that of your family. One's offspring perishes and forgets, whereas the Motherland lasts and remembers. You have to use your life so that your children call you a fool but your fellow citizens consider you great." Such humility and noble ideals in a man who invested both his talent and rather meager means into his internationally acclaimed research, converted Cajal into a national hero. Even now, there is not a city in Spain without a street named after him. He promoted several institutions for the advancement of science, one of which, the Board of Further Education (*Junta de Ampliación de Estudios*), became the present Council of Scientific Research (*Consejo Superior de Investigaciones Científicas*).

The Moscow prize also had great repercussions on his own research; the Institute for Biological Research was founded at the University of Madrid, but was independent from the University and had a separate budget. (Upon Cajal's death it became known as the Cajal Institute.) After twenty years of intense, solitary work he could at last create his own research team. Previously, except for Bartual, Claudio Sala, and a few more, he had not even had any graduate students due to lack of funding at Valencia and Barcelona. It was not until he was at the new Institute that he could work with and train other scientists. His brother, Pedro Cajal, and Domingo Sánchez were the first to join him, followed by Tello, who enrolled at the Institute in 1902 as an undergraduate medical student and later became Cajal's foremost pupil. Achúcarro (who had worked with Pierre Marie, Alzheimer, Babinski, and Kraepelin) became part of his team in 1910, Del Río Hortega in 1912, Lafora (who had been head of the pathology laboratory at Washington's Mental Asylum) in 1914, de Castro (still a medical student) in 1916, and Lorente de Nó some years later. Cajal considered these coworkers to be true disciples who would continue his work in the future. He also trained Calleja, Lavilla, Olóriz, Márquez, and Aguilera, as well as Ramón Terrazas and Blanes Viale, who died when they were 21 and 22 years old, respectively, and his own son, Jorge Ramón Fañanás, who later worked in bacteriology, although he had had a promising start in histology.[12] Other, less well-known students, included Villaverde, Sanz Ibáñez, Estable, Martínez Pérez, and Rodríguez Pérez.

During the first years by the beginning of the twentieth century, Cajal had turned his attention to neuroglial cells, which, although not a new line of research, as he had described the glia in almost all of the areas where he had used the Golgi method, with stains astrocytes fairly well, it was a collateral line of research. His brother, Pedro, was specifically interested in invertebrate glia and formed the hypothesis that glial cells prevented the free diffusion of the "neural current."

When Achúcarro came to work at the Institute in 1910, he introduced a new research aspect. He was a clinical psychiatrist who believed in a pathological basis for psychiatric disorders, as opposed to the current philosophical explanations inherited from the previous century.[13] While working in Alzheimer's laboratory, Achúcarro had noticed that many psychiatric diseases concurred with changes in the glial cells. The changes had not been properly studied, however, because the methods then available, such as those of Weigert (**165**), Held (**171**), or Alzheimer (**172**) were not sensitive enough. The Golgi method stained glial cells much better but only demonstrated a few cells, which was a severe obstacle for rigorous pathological analysis. Achúcarro developed a staining method, using ammoniacal silver oxide (**177**), which stained the *rod cells* in the syphilitic brain. He was determined to convince Cajal of the importance of the glial cells, which he saw as a diffuse endocrine gland that could play a part in diseases such as schizophrenia.

Cajal then was working on the existence of a network described by Holmgren, which would connect the Golgi complex with the extracellular space, and he had invented a method using uranyl nitrate (**136**). This technique consistently stained the Golgi apparatus, but also stained astrocytes, although rather sporadically. It showed cytoplasmic granules in the glial cells, suggesting they had a secretory function. Cajal then developed a fixative for neuroglial cells (**2**) and a specific staining method, the gold sublimate (**173**), which surpassed all previous techniques in both constancy and resolution. Using both this and a variation he had made for Bielschowsky's technique (**176**), Cajal classified the various types of astrocytes and described their development from neural tube cells. He also identified a completely new cell type, which seemed to have no cell expansions. Cajal considered it to be different from both neurons and astrocytes and named it "the third element" of the nervous system. Its analysis was Del Río Hortega's most important contribution to neurohistology, but also the most frequent source of debate among Cajal's team.

Achúcarro's interest in neuroglia was shared by his two best pupils, Del Río Hortega and de Castro. The latter undertook a vast project of exploration of the nervous system by means of the gold sublimate technique, although only his findings regarding the olfactory bulb were published.[3] Del Río Hortega made several modifications to Achúcarro's method (**145, 178, 208, 209**), and finally developed a method of his own (**179**). Some variations of his technique (**190, 197**) allowed Del Río Hortega to determine that the "third element" included two different cell types, the *microglia* (Hortega's cells) and the *oligodendroglia*. He also identified their functional significance and origin.[4]

Cajal also continued to unravel one of the most complex controversies of the time: the functional value of the neuron. Although the cell theory for the nervous system had been widely accepted, the inner structure of the neuron was still under discussion. Cajal disagreed with Apathy and Bethe about the continuity of the cells at their points of contact.

Professor Stephen Apathy from the University of Clausenburg in Hungary developed a method (**323**) to stain neurofibrils[14] in worms. Based on his observations using this technique, he proposed a theory whereby the "excitation" produced in the sensory receptors would diffuse along a neurofibrillary network.[5] Although Apathy's hypothesis did not really challenge the neuron theory, given that his method only worked in worms, Cajal contested his results, as he wished to prove that his own thesis was universally applicable (for a detailed account, see Ramón y Cajal, S. *Recollections of My Life,* Chapters 19–23).

Alfred Bethe's theories, however, presented more of a problem. He had developed a histological method (**105**), which in many animals showed the existence of a neurofibrillary network that connected the somata and expansions of the nerve cells with no discontinuity.[6] The nerve impulse could thus travel along this network without the need of Cajal's neurons. This hypothesis was basically similar to Apathy's but was more widely accepted, because it was supported not only by morphological findings, but also by certain functional observations. The most important experiments were those carried out on the common shore crab *Carcinus moenas* and the studies of the regeneration of the peripheral nerve trunks. (For a detailed account, see Bethe, A.: *Allgemeine Anatomie ünd Physiologie des Nervensystems.* G. Thieme, Leipzig, 1903.)

The *Carcinus moenas* has antennae inervated by a nerve containing both sensory and motor fibers. Connected to the nerve, but macroscopically separated, are the somata of the sensory neurons, thus the ganglion can be excised without sectioning the nerve. Bethe's experiment showed that the antenna maintained its tonicity and responded to stimulation with movement, therefore, it was supposed, as the system worked properly even after the removal of the neurons, these were not indispensable for the transmission of the nerve impulse. The transection of the nerve abolished both the tonicity and the reflexes of the antenna, thus suggesting that the key factor was the integrity of the "neurofibrils." Bethe also found, however, that twenty-four hours after the excision of the ganglion, the function and reflexes of the antennae disappeared, which led him to believe that the neurons, "[...] though not indispensable, were not completely useless, the neurons would act as energy-storage elements inserted along the nerve pathway, in a similar way that electric batteries were placed at regular intervals along the wires of the telegraph network."

Bethe's findings resulted in the revival of the polygenist theory of the nerve regeneration, a hypothesis that had been proposed in the early 1800s by Vulpian and Brown-Séquard, but abandoned after the research of Waller, Ranvier, His, and Cajal. Bethe's approach differed somewhat from that of his predecessors, as it made an anatomical and functional analysis of the distal stump of transected motor nerves. He found that in some cases the distal stump showed signs of impulse conduction several days after the transection. Given that the proximal and distal stumps had been (supposedly) kept apart, the reappearance of the function in the latter could not be due to reinnervation from the former but instead must arise from the "conducting matrix" (i.e., the neurofibrils) in the distal stump, without any intervention from the neurons. Axon segments would originate from independent, newly formed Schwann cells in the distal stump, which would eventually become aligned and later connected to each other, forming new complete axons. Finally, the segments would fuse to free terminal axonal endings in the proximal stump, thus reestablishing the anatomical and functional integrity of the nerve.

Bethe's ideas were well-received, even by adherents of the neuron doctrine such as van Gehuchten, Marinesco, or Waldeyer, who continued to agree, at least partially, with Bethe even after Cajal published a critique of the experiments and results of the neo-reticularists in 1903.[7] This prompted Cajal to search for a method that would stain the neurofibrils more precisely than that of Bethe (**125**) or Apathy (**323**) and more simply than that of Donnagio. Professor Donnagio, at the University of Modena, had shown some excellent preparations of neurofibrillary staining in the International Medical Meeting held in 1903 in Madrid but had not revealed his method (**106**). After trials with the method of Fajersztajn (**154**) and the combination of formaldehyde and photographic developers as fixatives (**155**), Cajal started to check the advantages of Simarro's method (**107**), which was inconstant but sharply stained the neurofibrils of certain large neurons. Potassium bromide or iodide was injected into the animal in order to achieve a high concentration of iodide or bromide ions inside the neuron, so that if the tissue were later immersed in silver nitrate, photosensitive silver compounds would be formed, which blackened on exposure to light and could be seen using a photographic developer. When Cajal tested this ingenious method, however, he soon proved its inconsistency; the same results were obtained whether bromides were administered or not. This raised a question of paramount importance: What was the exact nature of the substance that stained the neurofibrils?

On holiday in Italy in August of the same year, Cajal had a simple, but ingenious idea: "[...] the enigmatic substance which generated the neurofibrillar reaction must be purely and simply hot, free, silver nitrate, which can be precipitated by physical processes on the neurofibrillar skeleton modified by the action of temperature. The silver chlorides and bromides do not take any part in the reaction, but rather interfere with it. If the metallic deposit comes from silver nitrate in a colloidal medium, it is obvious that only a physical developer (pyrogallic acid or hydroquinone without alkali instead of the chemical developers rich in alkali used by Simarro) can precipitate the nitrate onto the protoplasmic structures, leaving the bromides and chlorides unchanged, which are not reduced by the new developers. In order, however, to retain the free silver nitrate eliminated in the method of Simarro, it would be necessary to immerse not the sections but the blocks of nervous tissue in the silver bath and to increase the strength of the latter markedly." He went on to develop his ideas and invented what he called "reduced silver nitrate," nowadays known as Cajal's method (**113–130**).

This new staining method perfectly demonstrates the neurofibrils and enabled Cajal to demonstrate that they were not continuous between cells. Bielschowsky (**108–111**) published similar results a month later (Bielschowsky. M.: "Die Silberimprägnation der Neurofibrillen." *Neurol. Centralbl.*, 22: 997–1006, 1903). Variations of Cajal's reduced silver impregnation method (**117, 118, 120, 122**) even differentiated somatic from axonic neurofibrils. The excellent results obtained (see **275–279**) when this technique was used in the study of nervous regeneration ruled out Bethe's polygenist hypothesis. This research, which had been started by Cajal in 1905, was published in an extensive article titled, "The mechanism of nerve degeneration and regeneration,"[8] which was immediately translated into French by the Société de Biologie de Paris (March 1905). This paper became the core of the well-known treatise, "Studies of the degeneration and regeneration of the nervous system" ("Estudios sobre la degeneracion y regeneracion del sistema nervioso"), published in 1913. It was translated into English by Raoul L. May in 1928 and has recently been republished in an annotated edition (J. DeFelipe and E.G. Jones, eds: *Cajal's Degeneration and Regeneration of the Nervous System*. Oxford University Press, 1991). Cajal's studies of neurogenesis were collected in a volume published as a homage to Cajal by several institutions in Uruguay and have been translated into English by Lloyd-Guth (*Studies on Vertebrate Neurogenesis*). Although Cajal and Bielschowsky had been instrumental in settling the discussion with Apathy and Bethe, they sparked off new reticularist theories, now led by Held and totally or partially accepted by a substantial number of scientists, such as Bielschowsky himself, Brühl, Auerbach, Wolff, and Holmgrem. Ironically, Held had been an ardent neuronist, translating Cajal's articles on the neuron doctrine into German for publication in his own journal, the *Archiv für Anatomie und Physiologie*. He also had supported the neuron theory with his own research on the free endings of the axons of the VIII cranial nerve in the brain stem ("chalices of Held") and the existence of axonic endbulbs (Endfüssen). However, after using the neurofibrillary methods he reinterpreted his own results and concluded that the neurofibrils of the axon fused in the Endfüssen, whereas those in the soma aggregated to form the *neurosomes*. According to his hypothesis, the Endfüssen of the axon of a given cell would be connected by "perforating fibrils" to the somatic neurosomes of the adjacent neuron, across the two cytoplasmic membranes (Held, H.: "Zür Kenntnis einer neurofibrillären Kontinuität im Zentralnervensystem der Wirbelthiere." *Arch. Anat. Physiol., Anat. Abt.*, 55–76, 1905).

Held's theories made Cajal review his own material, after which he concluded that the perforating neurofibrils were nothing but an artifact that may appear in weakly silver-impregnated sections after gold toning (Ramón y Cajal, S.: *Neuron Theory or Reticular Theory?* Translated by M. Ubeda Purkiss and C.A. Fox. CSIC, Madrid, 1954). In order to avoid this kind of artifact, the handbook presented here in Section II clearly states which variations of the reduced silver method can be stained (**116, 118, 123, 129, 299**) and which criteria and procedures must be used for this purpose (**125**). The explanation of which techniques can be used to stain the Endfüssen (**121 to 124, 129**) is so extensive and precise in order to demonstrate the inaccuracy of Held's observations. This controversy also prompted the development of new variations of Cajal's method (Ramón y Cajal, S.: "Formulas of the technique of reduced silver nitrate and its effect on the component factors of the neurons" "Las fórmulas del proceder del nitrato de plata reducido y sus efectos sobre los factores integrantes de las neuronas." Trab. Lab. Inv. Biol. Univ. Madrid, 8: fasc. 1º and 2º, 1910). Some of the variations (e.g., **123**) stain the Endfüssen and the perikaryal neurofibrils differently. This seemed to be sufficient to settle the controversy, as Cajal recorded in his autobiography (1923): "I deeply believe that the ideas and facts that I used to argue against Held and Apathy's propositions are currently indisputable. As a matter of fact, no one has been able to refute them so far. Hence, this is how another bitter battle in favour of the neuron theory ends. Will it be the last one? I don't think so."

Cajal was proved right when Held formulated the "Gründnetz theory," using general coloration methods (such as anilines). He proposed that the whole of the nervous system was a syncytium not only of neurons, but also all the types of glial cells (Held, H.: "Die Lehre von den Neuronen un von Neuronencytium und ihr heutiger Stand." Urban and Scwarzenberg. Berlin, 1929).

The last opposition to the neuron theory was made by other scientists such as Boeke, Stöhr, and Agdhur, who used different variations of Bielschowsky's method (**131, 305, 310**) to study the peripheral nerve endings. These methods revealed a fine network (Boeke's "Periterminale Netzwerke") that seemed to connect the cytoskeleton of the terminal branches of the motor endplate with the myofibrils of muscle cells (Boeke, J.: "Beiträge zur Kenntnis der motorischen Nervenendigungen. I. Die Form und Struktur der motorischen Endplatte der quergestreiften Muskelnfasern bei den höheren Vertebraten. II. Die akzessorischen fasern und Endplättchen." Int. Monatschr. für Anat. und Physiol., 28: 377–443, 1911).

Cajal was reaching the end of his life when these objections were made, and it was his disciples, especially de Castro, who participated in the scientific debate. The development of newer variations of the reduced silver method (**309, 314**) allowed both of them to demonstrate that Boeke's observations were based on artifacts (Cajal, S. R.: "Quelques remarques sur les plaques motrices de la langue des mammifères." Trav. Lab. Rech. Biol. Univ. Madrid, 23: 245-254, 1925; de Castro, F.: "Technique pour la colouration du systeme nerveux quand il est depourvu de ses étuis osseux et leurs resultats dans les centres nerveux et les terminaisons nerveuses peripheriques. " Trav. Lab. Rech. Biol. Univ. Madrid, 23: 428–446, 1925). However, despite de Castro working for six months in Boeke's laboratory to discuss their findings, the latter extended his theory to include the sensory nerve endings (Boeke, J.: "Die Beziehungen der Nervensystem und Bundegewebselemente and Tastezellen, die periterminale Netzwerk der motorische und sensibeln

Nervenendigungen." Z. Mikro-Anat. Forsch., 4: 69–94, 1926). Boeke's ideas on the periterminal network led Cajal to re-examine his old preparations of Grandy and Merkel's corpuscles and to study both structures with a technique specific for this material (**301**) developed by Martínez-Pérez, one of Tello's disciples. Cajal's conclusions considerably weakened the support to Boeke's theories and were published as a chapter, "Die Neuronenlehre" ("the neuron theory"), of a monumental treatise entitled Handbuch der Neurologie (O. Bumke and O. Foerster, eds. Springer, 1935) that contains a summary of all the arguments for or against the neuron theory during the previous forty years.

Cajal wrote what was to prove his last publication in his cellar, a place his coworkers had nicknamed "The Cave." This private working space included a small laboratory, a library of more than 5,000 volumes, and his office. Although he had to work at home at this time due to his advanced age, he had always liked to do so and recommended it to young scientists in his handbook, "Advice for a Young Investigator." Indeed, over time The Cave had become an emblematic place for Cajal, for it was here that his coworkers and pupils would drop by in the evenings to discuss the day's work. Other eminent visitors would visit, too, such as politicians, intellectuals, and other scientists to ask his advice and opinion. In May of 1934, he was working in The Cave with Ketty Levi on what would be his last manuscript,[15] when his eldest daughter burst in to tell them that there was a mob of demonstrators outside on the street. This was not an unusual occurrence in early-twentieth-century Spain, but was worrisome just the same, because such disturbances often turned violent. While Ketty called the Institute for help, Cajal climbed upstairs and went out onto the balcony. Someone from the crowd noticed him and the whole hoard of people stopped and broke out in thunderous applause. The apparent demonstrators were, in fact, medical students who had heard that Cajal was ill and had left their classes en masse to find out how he was. At this time Cajal had not taught students for more than twelve years and was so moved that he was unable to speak to them. He returned to The Cave and told de Castro, who had just arrived in answer to Ketty's call, that "I cannot ask anything more from life." Five months later, on October 17, 1934, Cajal died and was deeply mourned by the whole nation.

It would be interesting to know how much Cajal was affected by the new attacks on the neuron theory in those years previous to his death. Certainly, the arguments in favor of the reticularist hypothesis were much weaker, such as those concerning the peripheral endings of autonomous postganglionic fibers. The debate finally came to an end in 1950, before the development of transmission electron microscopy, when de Castro delivered the plenary lecture to the Meeting of the German Society of Pathology (de Castro, F.: "Die Normale Histologie des peripheren vegetativen Nervensystems. Das Synapsen-Problem: Anatomisch-Experimentelle Untersuchungen." Verhand. Deutsche Gessellschaft für Pathologie 34 Tagung. Wiesbaden, 1950). Using a careful experimental protocol of nerve anastomosis together with a vastly improved variation of Cajal's method, he proved that Cajal's ideas were also valid for the autonomic nervous system.

De Castro not only worked with Cajal's ideas, he also developed many independent concepts and hypotheses, scientific methods, and projects of his own (e.g., his research into the innervation of blood chemoceptors, especially the carotid body). In 1923 the carotid body was thought to be merely a chromaffin organ or "paraganglion," but its innervation was as yet not understood. Was it innervated directly by axons of central neurons, as happens in the adrenal medulla, or did these axons make a synaptic relay in a sympathetic ganglion? Furthermore, did it play a role in the vascular reflexes arising from the carotid bifurcation, as Druner had suggested? The problem was solved using a variation of Cajal`s method, which allows the staining of nerve fibers in specimens containing bone tissue (**314**). If this method is performed in small animals, such as newborn rats or mice, and the pieces are oriented in a sectioning plane as parallel as possible to the path of the corresponding cranial nerves, it is possible to follow visually the whole course of the fibers in not more than three or four slides. This was very important, because the area has numerous nerve anastomosis, and three-dimensional reconstruction methods were still rather primitive in the 1920s. This methodological approach was completed by degeneration studies of the glomus' endings after sectioning, at different levels, the nerve trunks contributing fibers to the region, something that required exceptional surgical skill. Surprisingly, the section of the glossopharyngeal nerve between the sensory ganglion and the carotid body comprised a massive degeneration of the carotid body endings, so that de Castro could state "[...] as a credible hypothesis, that the glomus caroticum is a sensory organ, the only one known up to now capable of detecting certain qualitative variations of blood, a function that, perhaps by means of a reflex action, could have repercussion on the activity of other organs" ("Sur la structure et l'innervation du sinus carotidien de l'homme et des mammiferes. Nouveaux faits sur l'innervation et la fonction du glomus caroticum, » Trab. Lab. Inv. Biol. Univ. Madrid 25:331, 1928). This was the first report of the existence of visceral chemoceptors.

De Castro's hypothesis and findings were characteristic of Cajal's team, although he was exceptionally skilled at dissection. Later, he was to develop his own, purely functional, approach. For instance, he analyzed the physiology of the carotid body using a unique and ingenious technique, and he performed several different surgical procedures on nerve trunks, sections, and anastomosis, so that the stimulation of the glomus resulted in changes in other organs, which were readily identifiable with the naked eye. He did this by "building" a new nervous circuit with an effector organ that could be easily seen macroscopically. First, he sectioned the vagus nerve proximally to the nodosal ganglion, and then he cut the cervical sympathetic trunk caudally to the stellate ganglion and sutured the free stumps together. Because the afferents to the cervical superior ganglion enter the chain caudally to the stellate ganglion, this surgery results in a complete input isolation of the cervical sympathetic system. This, in its turn, leads to the development of an ipsilateral Horner's syndrome. As the regeneration of the central processes of the vagus nerve proceeds, the superior cervical ganglion is innervated by these fibers, thus creating a reflex arc, isolated from the central nervous system. Under these conditions, the excitation of the vagal receptors would result in the discharge of the neurons in the superior cervical ganglion, causing the Horner's syndrome to disappear as long as the stimulation lasts.

The second part of the experiment could only begin once a good reinnervation of the superior cervical ganglion had taken place, a process that takes several months. A three-step procedure was then initiated: (1) the operated vagus nerve was sectioned distally to the nodosal ganglion, (2) the ipsilateral glossopharyngeal nerve was sectioned, distally to the sensory ganglion, and (3) the glossopharyngeal distal stump was anastomosed to the proximal stump of the vagus. After the regeneration period was over, the receptors normally innervated by the glossopharyngeal nerve (carotid body and sinus, taste buds, etc.), become reinnervated by the peripheral processes arising from the neurons in the nodosal ganglion. Because the central processes of these neurons project to the superior cervical ganglion, stimulation of the carotid body is reflected in changes seen in the status of the ipsilateral eye, such as the diameter of the pupil and the nictitating membrane.

This imaginative method was too slow, however, as many years are required to achieve sufficient regeneration for a consistent experimental model. Furthermore, as these were the first regeneration experiments done with a functional, as opposed to an anatomical, goal, it was necessary to prove that the behavior of the newly formed synapses, both in the superior cervical ganglion and the receptors, was similar to normal ones. This model was a forerunner of a fruitful line of research on the ganglionar synapse (see below). Unfortunately, it did not prove as useful in the study of the normal physiology of the glomus, because the quantitative evaluation of the activity of the receptor was not only indirect but also extremely imprecise. While de Castro refined his cumbersome technique over many years, Heymans, in Ghent, used a classic parabiosis preparation and electrophysiological methods and was awarded the Nobel Prize. This is yet another example of the adverse results of the poor conditions in which Spanish scientists had to work at this time. De Castro had no support from the physiologists at Madrid University, who were more interested in the newly emerging science of biochemistry. The head of his research team, Professor Negrín, spent more time in politics than on science. (A dedication rewarded with his being made the President of the II Spanish Republic!). Furthermore, Spain was suffering from social and economical problems generally, which eventually led to the civil war.

By the time the war had ended, the Histology School of Madrid and the Cajal Institute had practically disappeared. Cajal's disciples, despite their worldwide prestige, were considered unacceptable by Franco's regime. They were, like Cajal himself, agnostic, anticlerical liberals and democrats. Del Rio-Hortega went into exile, first to Oxford and afterwards to Buenos Aires; Lorente de Nó never returned to Spain; Lafora was barred from holding any public office, and Tello, who had been appointed by Cajal as his successor, was removed as Director of the Institute[16] and as full professor. De Castro, then Professor of Histology at Seville University, decided to stay in Spain and keep alive Cajal's scientific spirit. This meant that he had to waste a great deal of his time avoiding obstacles set by political and ideological adversaries as well as continuing his never ending struggle for funding for his research. Paradoxically, funds were often more readily available in the United States or Germany than in his own country.

The situation gradually improved. Cajal's Chair was divided into Histology and Pathology and de Castro and another of Cajal's disciples, Julián Sanz Ibáñez, were appointed to each specialty. The Institute now formed part of the Spanish Research Council (Consejo Superior de Investigaciones Científicas) and had more resources, both human and material. Its productivity, however, was handicapped in that scientists working there were expected to adhere to official political and religious doctrine. Fortunately, those days are long past and it is now an outstanding research center, worthy of its founder.

As can be seen, de Castro shared many of Cajal's scientific aims and also suffered from many of the same problems and setbacks. However, their backgrounds were very different indeed.

De Castro was born in Madrid into a wealthy, upper-class family. His father, a city councilor, could afford a private education for his son. In 1916, while still a medical student, he worked in Achúcarro's laboratory and continued to do so until he graduated in 1921. He then moved to Cajal's team and completed his PhD in 1923. He had three main lines of research during this time. One was to investigate axonal features and decide if they were synapses, a result of aging, or an abnormal process. He used sensory ganglia exposed to pathological conditions, and his results convinced Cajal of the absence of synapses in sensory ganglia. A second project involved the study of neuroglial cells, a favorite subject of Achúcarro, who believed that they played a key role in the pathogenesis of several mental illnesses, something he had started to work on while at Alzheimer's laboratory. This line of research was greatly enriched by the introduction of the gold-sublimate method in 1913 (**173**), which allowed a better identification of the neuroglia than previous techniques (**156, 171, 172**), including Achúcarro's own (**177**). Using this new method, Achúcarro aimed to study the glial architecture of the whole central nervous system as a base for analyzing changes in various pathological conditions. His early death in 1918 put a stop to this ambitious project, but some of his students continued with aspects of it. De Castro, for example, studied the glial architecture of the olfactory bulb and the origin and function of its astrocytes.

De Castro's third main field during these early years concerned the architecture, synaptology, and development of the sympathetic ganglia. Cajal had already taken an interest in this subject and his data, along with that of Langley, had laid down the basic pattern of organization of the autonomic nervous system. Cajal was, however, not totally satisfied with his results, as he considered a synaptic organization scheme necessary to provide a functional significance for the types of neurons he had described in the ganglia. Furthermore, some of his own results seemed to contradict the general principles of the organization of the nervous system that he had formulated. Two findings were especially elusive: the possibility that sympathetic neurons had several axons and the significance of the dendrites that ended embracing neuronal somata. In 1922, de Castro published an extensive article dealing with these subjects and in 1965 he started an electron microscopy study of the carotid body, but he died in 1967, before the paper was published.

De Castro managed to maintain a steady scientific output during his later years, despite the political and economic difficulties previously mentioned. He was an unusually intellectual and sensitive man[17] who was faced with the conflict of whether to emigrate and enhance his personal scientific career or stay and help to fulfill Cajal's dream of working toward putting Spain on an even par with more advanced neighboring countries. He willingly chose the latter, far more challenging option. This made for a difficult and often frustrating professional life; he had very little help in forming his own research group[18] and on many occasions was on the verge of solving a problem when scientists from other countries preempted him and published the answer. Furthermore, he was naturally a shy, retiring, extremely ethical man who found it difficult to work under the corrupt elite of Franco's regime. The years of working under such trying conditions took their toll, and when his beloved wife died at a young age, de Castro became very withdrawn.

Students found this gaunt, immaculately dressed man terrifying, especially as the examinations he set were extremely challenging, to say the least. However, his calm and efficient approach to problem solving together with his quiet confidence arising from a deep and mature scientific understanding, won him the respect and affection of all who knew him. Indeed—and much to the annoyance of Franco's regime—when de Castro died so many people went to his funeral, despite the heavy rain, that it was manifestly a public tribute to the last of Spain's great scientists.

SECTION TWO

Basic Histological Techniques

2

The Microscope and the Fixatives

Although the aim of this handbook is to enable the apprentice to stain the various structures of the nervous system, it is not out of place to recall some basic rules and formulae.

Thus, we shall briefly discuss some general aspects in this *First Section*, such as the *handling of the microscope,* the use of *fixatives, hardeners,* and *mordants,* the various *embedding, dissociation* and *sectioning* methods, the *procedures* for arranging the sections and gluing them onto the slides, the final *mounting* and *preservation* of the sections, and the decalcification of embryos and fetuses, etc., insomuch as they are pertinent to the study of the nervous system. In this way, we can avoid unnecessary repetition of the properties of the preferred fixative or the indispensable mordant in each staining protocol. We shall depart from this rule only in some special cases. For the sake of briefness, each fixative, mordant, or dye will receive a number that is referred to when describing a special staining or impregnation method.

The specific procedures for staining or impregnating each of the constituents of the nervous tissue (such as myelin, connective sheaths and axons of the nerve trunks, or the organelles of the neuronal **protoplasm**-neurofibrils, Nissl substance, Golgi reticular apparatus, centrosome, or nucleus) will be described in the *Second Section*. That part of the book, which is the most extensive and detailed, includes several methods and formulae developed in Spain.

MICROSCOPE

We assume the reader is aware of the theoretical and practical use of the *condensers,* the *immersion objectives,* the *camera lucida,* and other more sophisticated *drawing instruments,* such as **Eddinger's** and others. Here we shall just revise the following rules:

1. When the purpose of the study is the structure of nerves and ganglion cells, especially in impregnated sections, apochromatic immersion objectives should be used (*EN 1*) with the aperture of the Abbe condenser completely open.
2. When using dry objectives of medium-range magnification, the light beam should be reduced by means of the **iris diaphragm**.

3. Strongly-stained preparations that must be examined under high magnification need a lightbulb of 50 or more **candles**. The bulb must be made of frosted glass, at least in its lower half (*EN 2*), so that the section is illuminated with diffuse light, such as that reflected by a white cloud. The special lamps for microphotography manufactured by various firms, especially by Leitz, also can be used.
4. Top-of-the-range models of microscopes, with rotating stages capable of orthogonal movements regulated by means of screws, should be used to study only clean, mounted preparations. However, in order to try new methods and examine temporary preparations, which are not always well protected, it is preferable to use a sturdy microscope with a wide, fixed stage so that it does not matter if the instrument becomes stained with the substances used in section handling. We believe that, in order to move and scan the specimen, the experienced hand of the observer cannot be replaced by any mechanical device attached to the stage.[1]

FIXATIVES

Collection and Preparation of the Specimens

The nervous system must be fixed rapidly and carefully. Obviously all tissues change after death due to autolytic phenomena and cadaverous decay. The gray matter is especially susceptible, to the point that it is impossible to obtain good preparations of myelin and glial cells after twenty-four hours postmortem. Needless to say, the time varies with temperature. Thus, in winter, excellent results can be obtained with some fixatives more than twenty-four hours after death. On the other hand, in the summer we shall try to use brains from six- to twelve-hour-old corpses, or even those still warm. The spinal cord usually endures postmortem deterioration better than the brain.

Nevertheless, except for an initial decay that is always observed on the surface of the nervous centers, especially in the gray matter, some structures are preserved for a rather longer time, for instance, neurofibrils, cell nuclei and axons.

We should try to use blocks of tissue up to half a centimeter in thickness, although this recommendation is not valid for all the fixatives, because the degree of penetration varies considerably. Thus, in some cases, such as when using neurofibrillary methods, the poor diffusion of the fixative (alcohol, silver nitrate, uranyl nitrate, osmic acid, etc.) demands a maximum thickness of only 3 or 3.5 millimeters. Conversely, fixatives like potassium dichromate, formaldehyde, 96° alcohol, or pyridine, can sometimes be used with pieces up to 2 or 3 centimeters thick.

When all the blocks must be of equal thickness, as when serial sectioning a large specimen, we can use an ***Eddinger's macrotome*** to make tissue blocks of the brain. This advice does not apply to the brains of small animals (mice, rats, bats, birds, lizards, etc.), which can be hardened as a single piece. Even for mice, however, tissue blocks preferably should be made on two or three portions of the encephalon, especially when using neurofibrillary methods. In embryos, fixation and ***induration*** of the whole specimen is the rule.

The specimens should be kept in wide-neck flasks, with cotton wool at the bottom.

To distinguish the anterior or frontal end of a brain slice from the posterior or distal one, we can use two procedures:

1. Mark a spot on the frontal surface with carmine dissolved in ammonia.
2. Keep every slice in a different flask, indicating which is the frontal or occipital side. In these cases the pieces should, of course, be placed horizontally at the bottom of the bottle. All these precautions are most critical when trying to obtain precise images of particular areas of the brains of monkeys, dogs, and cats and, especially, of humans, such as with the Brodmann and Vogt's procedures.

Allow us to complete these commonsense rules with another piece of advice: touching the nervous tissue must be avoided as much as possible, because it is very susceptible to pressure. Careless handling of the specimens can cause many delicate methods to fail, as they require a perfectly preserved gray matter. We can avoid this problem by making the tissue.

We do not propose to comment on the bibliography of this specialty, but, for those who are interested and wish to read further, we suggest (besides our treatise *Manual de Histología y Técnica Micrográfica*) the following books: Orueta's masterful essay titled, *Microscopía*; the keen mathematical study of Castellarnau on microscope optics (*Teoría General de la imagen en el microscopio*); the *Enzyklopädie der mikroskopischen Technik*, and B. Romeis's *Taschenbuch der mikroskopischen Technik*; the treatise on neurohistological methods by Spielmeyer (*Technik der mikroskopischen Unterschung der Nervensystems*); the well-researched Portuguese book of Celestino da Costa and Roberto Chaves, *Manual de Tecnica Histologica*; Roussy and Lhermitte's *Les techniques anatomo-pathologiques du système nerveux*; the works of J. N. Langley (*Practical Histology*), Langeron (*Précis de microscopie*), Carazzi, and Levi (*Técnica Microscópica*). An important caution is not to touch the brain to avoid to alter the delicate neural structures. We therefore recommend making blocks with a razor blade while the brain is still in the base of the skull. The specimens are then carefully picked up with the razor blade or a spatula and immersed in the fixative. Naturally, all these precautions are unnecessary for some structures, such as the peripheral nerve ganglia.

Action of the Fixatives

The ideal fixative would not only coagulate the nervous mesh, making it insoluble in water and alcohol, but also preserve the fine structure of cells and fibers beautifully, without retractions, coalescences, or vacuolizations. Unfortunately, there is no ideal fixative for use in all cases; thus, it is necessary to compare the results of several and adjust the respective protocols.

Almost all of these reagents are also hardeners, because of their ability to coagulate protoplasmic proteins. Perhaps the only exception to this rule is chloral hydrate. As we shall see below, most fixatives also act as mordants, except the 100° and 96° alcohols, which do not seem to combine with tissue proteins.

Let us add that many fixatives, although able to preserve some morphological features adequately, alter or dissolve other details. Thus, a given fixative is often acceptable, or even excellent, for preserving just one (or a few) structural characteristics of the nerve cell. Osmic acid, for example, is indispensable for fixing myelin, but is of little use for preserving the texture of the protoplasm. Alcohol is one of the less aggressive fixatives for the latter, but deeply alters and even dissolves the myelin lipids. Formaldehyde preserves the glial cells of gray and white matter quite nicely but modifies the myelin and, to a certain extent, the axons, the Nissl substance, and some components of the nucleolus. Pyridine spares the neurofibrils but notably affects other protoplasmic components, and, when used in its pure state, produces vacuoles in the gray matter and also elicits intercellular coalescences in embryonic ganglionar corpuscles. However, Pyridine has contributed significantly to our understanding of the structure of nerve cells and peripheral endings, as well as the regeneration process, when it has been used by experts capable of interpreting the results.

A large variety of fixatives is necessary due to both the great delicacy of the colloidal architecture of the protoplasm and its lability when exposed to foreign agents. Furthermore, each fixative modifies the protoplasm and thus gives the cell specific staining properties, which also are influenced by any substances added to it. The fixative usually also acts as a mordant.

Let us add the following rules, related to the use of fixatives.

1. Always use a large amount of indurating liquid, if possible freshly prepared.
2. Use chemically pure reagents. To guarantee their purity, the best brands should be used (Poulenc in Paris; E. Merck, in Darmstadt; E. Haën, in Hannover; E. Schering, in Berlin; Kahlbaum, in Adlerhof, etc.). Some chemicals made in Spain can be used, such as alcohol, silver nitrate, and a few others.

1. Formaldehyde (CH_2O) Commercial formalin, or the aqueous solution of 40 per 100 formaldehyde, is one of the most fashionable *indurants* for neurological studies nowadays. Good fixation often is achieved with this, thus, the specimens can be used with the various techniques to reveal the structure of the nervous centers. It is especially recommended for the study of pathological specimens, as well as for those cases in which the type of technique has not been decided at the time of fixation.

Formalin cannot be used directly in its commercial form; it must be diluted with water to a 10 to 20 per 100.

40% formalin	10 or 15 cc
Distilled water	85 cc

Thin (4 to 6 mm) blocks are properly fixed after forty-eight hours in the fixative, although the optimal time is three to four days. Thicker pieces must be kept for a longer period in formalin, although not more than one to three months, because an excess of induration usually lowers the quality of the preparations. Formaldehyde can be used for numerous techniques, such as Bielschowsky's, Achúcarro's, Cajal's,

Weigert's, Kultschitzky's, Río-Hortega's, Nageotte's, or Agduhr's. In this way, several structures can be stained, such as myelin, Nissl substance, neurofibrils, centrosomes, **medullated and unmedullated** fibers, neuroglial and microglial cells, and connective tissue.

The amount of solution to be used will depend on the number and volume of the blocks. When whole hemispheres from humans or large mammals are to be indurated, either completely, or in slices, they should be immersed in large vessels containing 2 to 4 liters of 20 per 100 formalin solution. As we have already mentioned, however, it is preferable to use specimens that do not exceed 3 or 4 cm in thickness.

One of the great advantages of formaldehyde is that it is a good storage liquid. In fact, acceptable staining of neurofibrils, centrosomes, *fibrous glial cells*, myelinated and unmyelinated fibers, etc., can be achieved in pieces that have been kept for months, or even years, in this fixative. Basic aniline dyes, however, usually work poorly after formaldehyde fixation.

Formaldehyde-based Fixatives

2. Formaldehyde-ammonium bromide (Cajal). One of us has developed one of the best fixatives for staining glial cells:

Formaldehyde	15 cc
Ammonium bromide	2 g
Distilled water	85 cc

The pieces must remain in this solution for at least two to four days. After a brief rinse with distilled water, 20 to 30μm thick sections are cut with a freezing microtome and placed in the same fixative (see the *gold-sublimate* procedure and Cajal's modification of Bielschowsky's method). The addition of ammonium bromide, which acts as a mordant, to the formaldehyde allows the selective impregnation of the different types of glial cells *(macroglial* and *microglial* cells) as we shall see below.

3. Formaldehyde-uranyl nitrate (Cajal).

Neutral formalin	15 cc
Uranyl nitrate	1–2 g
Distilled water	85 cc

This is an excellent fixative for the subsequent staining of Golgi's reticular apparatus in all tissues. For this purpose, 2 to 3 mm thick pieces are immersed in this solution for eight to twelve hours. If the blocks are kept in the fixative for twenty-four to forty-eight hours, protoplasmic astrocytes, **gliosomes, nondendritic neuroglial cells,** and lipoid granules of neurons and neuroglial cells can be stained. (See Cajal's *uranyl-formaldehyde* method.) Because this fixative penetrates the gray matter poorly, sections near the brain surface are preferable.

4. Alcohol (C_2H_5OH) Alcohol frequently is used as a fixative for the nervous system and is especially appropriate for cytoarchitectonic studies of the nervous centers; indeed, it is indispensable for the Nissl method. Furthermore, it is also an excellent indurant for the study of neurofibrils, nerve plexuses, and the histogenesis of the nervous system (Cajal's method).

For induration, 100°, or at least 96°, alcohol must be used. The pieces should be small and be immersed for one to three or more days in the liquid, which must be changed two or three times. The extent of the fixation varies, depending on the size of the pieces and the technique to be used. For the Nissl method, 2 to 4 mm thick pieces will be sufficiently indurated in two or three days. Larger pieces, however, such as brains of small mammals (mouse, guinea-pig), sliced into two or three blocks, must be kept for six to ten days in alcohol. When whole hemispheres of dog, cat, etc. are to be used, properly oriented cuts ought to be made onto their surface, spanning from the gray matter to the beginning of the white matter, thus allowing the alcohol to penetrate more easily into the specimen. In the latter case, the induration will take ten or fifteen days at least and the liquid must be renewed several times. The pieces are then transferred to absolute alcohol to complete the dehydration.

For Cajal's method, the pieces must be thin (2 to 5 mm) and immersed in alcohol for one or two days. Hardening the specimens by means of alcohol renders excellent results in very early embryos, especially when they later must be impregnated with the reduced silver nitrate method. In this case, the pieces will be immersed in alcohol for twenty-four hours.

In summary: Alcohol is a good fixative of the nervous system when it has to be subsequently stained with basic aniline dyes or methods for the demonstration of protoplasmic granules or Nissl substance. It is also helpful in the study of neurofibrils, unmyelinated nerve plexuses, and the histogenesis of nervous tracts and centers by means of silver impregnation.

Additionally, alcohol is useful to dehydrate the sections prior to mounting and coverslipping, thus allowing the manufacture of stable preparations.

5. Müller's liquid. This is one of the first solutions to be used for fixation of nervous tissue. It is composed of:

Potassium dichromate	25 g
Sodium sulphate	10 cc
Distilled water	1000 cc

The reagents should be dissolved at room temperature, although heating speeds up the process. Large volumes of this solution are required and due to its slow diffusion rate, fixation requires a long time. For 0.5 to 1 cm thick specimens, the fixation will take twenty to thirty days; for whole brains of small mammals (mice, bats, etc.) and the spinal cord of cats and dogs, up to one to two months are necessary. For thick blocks of cerebral hemispheres either from large mammals or humans, induration will take as long as four to six months. The fixation period can be shortened to half if it is carried out at 30° or 35°C. It is very important not to overextend the induration time, because the pieces become too hard and brittle. When the specimens have been in the fixative long enough, but, for some reason, they cannot be sectioned immediately afterward, it is advisable to add some water to the solution, so that the pieces can be stored for longer.

It is necessary to renew the fixative frequently because contact with the pieces changes its nature; first, it turns black and later becomes contaminated by fungi.

Golgi and other authors suggest adding some ***thymol***, camphor, or sodium salicylate to the solution to avoid this problem. The liquid should be changed every two or three days during the first week and afterward every ten or twenty days. In very long fixations, it can be renewed every month or month and a half. Once fixed, the specimens should be rinsed in running tap water for one to three days, depending on their thickness.

Müller's liquid has a selective action on myelin: the latter is fixed and hardened and also stained varying shades of yellow. Furthermore, this fixative has the property of not retracting or distorting the pieces. It is a suitable fixative for myelin when Weigert's, Weigert-Pal's, Kultschizky's, and Marchi's staining methods are to be used. It is also apt for the demonstration of the morphology of neurons by means of the Golgi method (slow variation).

6. Formalin-Müller *(Orth's liquid)*. This fixative has two important properties: the rapid diffusion of the formalin and the mordant action of the chromium salt. It is composed of one part of formaldehyde and nine parts of liquid of Müller and should be prepared immediately before use.

40% Formaldehyde	10 cc
Müller's liquid	90 cc

As can be easily inferred, the fixation time will be shorter than with the regular Müller's fixative (about *three* or *four* times shorter). It is most important to note that this fixative must be replaced every one to three days. Specimens fixed in formalin-Müller can be stained with routine hematoxylin or carmine methods and with Weigert's procedure for myelin.

7. Regaud's liquid. It is composed of:

3 per 100 *Potash* bichromate	100 cc
Glacial acetic acid	5 cc
Formalin	20 cc

The tissue fragments must be very fresh, taken immediately after the animal is sacrificed. They should be immersed in this mixture for one to three days at room temperature and the liquid replaced when it turns dark. When fixation is complete, the pieces should be placed, without rinsing, in a 3 per 100 potassium bichromate solution for eight to ten days. Then they should be rinsed for twenty-four hours with running tap water and embedded in paraffin. According to Nageotte, this is an excellent fixative for the mitochondria of neurons and glial cells.

8. Osmic acid (OsO_4). Osmium tetroxide was introduced into practical histology by Schültze, and it has become one of the most important fixatives for nervous tissue. Because of its increasingly high price, its use is becoming more and more restricted. Nevertheless, this chemical is indispensable for some fixation procedures, such as the osmium-bichromic mixture, which has rendered the most important and beautiful findings in nervous centers.

It is commonly used in 1 or 2 per 100 aqueous solutions. Due to its poor ***diosmotic power***, the pieces immersed in this fixative must be very small (a thickness of 2 to 3 mm) and remain immersed for six to twenty-four hours.

An abundant amount of solution must be used. When fixation is complete, the pieces should be rinsed for twenty-four hours with water that must be replaced several times.

The main advantage of the osmic reagent, either by itself or associated with other substances, is that it preserves the morphology of the nerve fibers faithfully, fixing precisely the myelin and other lipids that are stained by reduction of black India ink.

The best results are achieved when using thin fragments of nervous tissue from young specimens of small animals, such as frog, guinea pig, rabbit, cat, or dog. Osmium-fixed material either can be dissociated (nerve trunks) or embedded for further sectioning; the sections then can be counterstained with fuchsin, hematoxylin, saphranin, etc.

For several reasons, special precautions are required in the handling of osmic acid: It is a powerful lipid solvent, it is a photosensitive compound and, furthermore, its vapors can be a powerful irritant, especially for the conjunctive membrane of the eye. Firstly, the flask where the solution is to be stored must be thoroughly cleaned by rinsing with ether, alcohol, and distilled water consecutively, and the flask should be air-tight. The solution is prepared as follows: osmic acid is sold in flame-closed glass vials, whose exterior surface must be carefully cleaned before use; these vials are broken with a file and immediately immersed in distilled water to avoid the sublimation or reduction of the compound. Alternatively, the vials can be heated, and, while still hot, dropped into cold distilled water, causing them to break. The solution is ready to use after six to twelve hours, and it must be stored in the dark.

During the preparation and use of this substance in the dissociation and impregnation of nerve trunks, the eyes and respiratory tract must be protected from the osmic fumes. Indeed, a long time ago Ranvier suggested placing a glass plate between the preparation and the observer when fresh nerve trunks were dissociated in a drop of osmic acid.

Fixatives with Osmic Acid

9. Osmium-bichromic mixture. The mixture of osmic acid with potash bichromate or Müller's liquid is the best fixative for the study of neuronal and glial morphology. This mixture, invented by Golgi and later modified by Cajal, is made as follows:

3 per 100 Potash bichromate   20 cc
1 per 100 Osmic acid   6 cc

Fresh pieces of nervous tissue are immersed in the mixture for one to three days. The fragments of nervous tissue should be small, 2 to 4 mm thick, and the volume of the solution abundant. For example, 30 to 35 cc of solution are used for three pieces of 4 mm thick tissue. Fixation time depends on the temperature of the solution and on the age of the animal. We prefer a temperature of 24°–26°C. Thus, in winter, we place the solution in an oven with a thermostat. At low temperatures, the induration will be longer (four to five days); in these cases, the optimal time must be determined by trial and error. Furthermore, it should be remembered that the younger the animal, the shorter the induration time (especially when working with embryos). For further details, see ***Rapid Silver Chromate Procedure.*** Finally, we have observed that the osmic-bichromic mixture is so stable that it can be stored, even in daylight, for several months. For this reason, we dissolve the osmic acid in the potash bichromate solution well in advance, thus avoiding the irritating problem of the reduction of this very expensive reagent.

10. Flemming's Liquor. This liquid is especially suitable for the analysis of the cell nucleus and its inner network and also of certain protoplasmic structures. It can be used either as a concentrated or a diluted solution. The former is made thus:

1 per 100 Chromic acid	15 cc
2 per 100 Osmic acid	4 cc
Glacial Acetic acid	1 cc

The weaker solution, preferred in many cases, is composed of:

1 per 100 Chromic acid	25 parts
1 per 100 Osmic acid	10 cc
1 per 100 Glacial Acetic acid	10 cc
Distilled water	55 cc

These fixatives yield excellent results in both embryonal and adult tissues.

Small pieces (2 to 4 mm thick) should be immersed for one or more days in the fixative then rinsed for twenty-four hours with running tap water and dehydrated in graded alcohols. Although the use of these fixatives for the study of nervous tissue is rather limited, they are particularly appropriate in the demonstration of the nuclear structure and mitosis.

11. Altmann's Liquid. This author proposed the use of a fixative for the study of the granular structure of the cells (*EN 3*) that is composed of equal volumes of:

2.5 per 100 Potassium bichromate
2 per 100 Osmic acid

Freshly excised fragments of tissue are immersed in this mixture for twenty-four hours, after which they are rinsed for one day with running tap water, dehydrated in graded alcohols, and embedded in paraffin. This fixative has been used in recent years by Nageotte for the demonstration of mitochondrial granules of neural elements.

12. Laguesse's Liquid. One of Laguesse's usual techniques for revealing mitochondrial and secretion granules is as follows:

2 per 100 Osmic acid	4 cc
1 per 100 Chromic acid	8 cc
Glacial Acetic acid	1 drop

Fixation time should be at least one day, after which the pieces are rinsed with running tap water for twelve hours, dehydrated in graded alcohols, and embedded in paraffin.

13. Cajal's Liquid with iron perchloride. Many years ago, Cajal suggested that the degenerating neural central pathways could be readily studied after fixation in the following solution:

3 per 100 Potassium bichromate	20 cc
1 per 100 Osmic acid	5 cc
Concentrated solution of Iron perchloride	1–3 cc

With this fixation the pieces become so hard that after five days they can be easily sectioned even without celloidin imbedding. Microscopically, most myelinated fibers are stained yellow. Only the thickest fibers are dark gray, probably due to some unknown chemical variation. Many black fibers are evident, especially in the spinal cord. Fat is consistently stained deep black, however, as with Marchi's method.

Cajal also has proposed a variation that does not turn the pieces as hard and brittle as the solution described above allowing celloidin imbedding. It is composed of:

3 per 100 Potassium bichromate	20 cc
1 per 100 Osmic acid	5 cc
3 per 100 Potassium ferricyanide	5 cc

The pieces are not as hard as with the previous method, and, therefore, treatment with alcohol and celloidin is possible. The fat is stained pure black against a translucent reddish-yellow background. For further details, see: ***Cajal's Procedure for the Staining of Fat in Nerve Fibers.***

14. Sublimate ($HgCl_2$). This is an excellent fixative, used dissolved either in water or in saline (0.75% NaCl). It preserves the cytoplasmic and nuclear textures (intracellular granules, chromatin, mitotic figures, etc.) fairly well and also is useful for the study of both the histogenetical and pathological processes of the nervous system. It is seldom used for the analysis of the normal texture of the neural lattice, although it is included in some formulae, such as Apathy's. Sublimate must be used in saturated solutions; because these solutions have very little diosmotic power, the specimens must not exceed 2 to 4 mm in thickness. Fixation times range from sixteen to twenty hours, after which the pieces need to be carefully rinsed with running tap water for one day in order to remove excess reagent. They then are immersed in iodinated alcohol. (This is prepared by dripping iodine-iodide solution (*EN 4*) onto 70°–90° alcohol until the latter turns the color of port wine.) This step will be repeated as many times as necessary until the liquid is no longer discolored. Finally, the blocks are dehydrated in graded alcohols and embedded in paraffin.

The treatment of the pieces with iodinated alcohol is necessary to remove the mercuric chloride crystals that are formed inside the tissue; these crystals interfere with the staining process.

Still more convenient than plain sublimate are other mixtures containing this chemical, such as:

15. Zenker's Fixative. It is composed of:

Potassium dichromate	2.5 g
Soda sulphate	1 cc
Sublimate	5 cc
Distilled water	100 cc

Immediately before use, 5 cc of acetic acid should be added to this liquid. The blocks should be left in the fixative for twelve to thirty-six hours, depending on their thickness, which should never exceed 2–5 mm. After fixation, the tissues must be rinsed for twenty-four hours with running tap water and then immersed in iodinated alcohol during one or more days; this must be replaced often.

16. Dominici's Liquid. Immediately prior to use, prepare a mixture of: Saturated aqueous solution of:

Sublimate	100 cc
Commercial formalin (40 per 100)	15 cc

Once mixed, slowly drip onto it an *officinal* iodine solution (*EN 5*) until the liquid becomes the color of port wine; if some precipitation occurs, filter before immersing the pieces. The fixation will last for six to twenty hours, depending on the thickness of the blocks. Fixation in Dominici's fluid, followed by nerve dissociation and iron hematoxylin staining, has been successfully used by Nageotte for the study of the Schwann cell protoplasm and of the connective *syncytium* of **Remak's fibers**.

17. Rabl's Mixture. Here is the composition of this mixture:

Saturated aqueous solution of sublimate	1 part
Saturated aqueous solution of picric acid	1 cc
Distilled water	1 cc

Fix for twelve hours, rinse with water for two to three hours then dehydrate in graded alcohols for about twenty-four hours. When working with embryos, it is advisable to add iodine to the absolute alcohol in order to eliminate sublimate precipitates.

Schaffer fixes in undiluted Rabl's mixture (equal parts of sublimate and picric acid solutions) for twelve to forty-eight hours. Subsequently, and without any rinsing, he immerses the blocks in alcohol added of iodine and **lithium** carbonate, in order to remove the sublimate and the picric acid. Finally, we must add that Rabl's mixture was used to advantage by Held for his work on the development of the nervous system, mainly for fixing embryos of amphibia and cyclostomata.

18. Sublimate-acetic acid. This is another of the fixatives used by Held to study the histogenesis of the nervous tissue. Its composition is as follows:

Saturated aqueous solution of sublimate	95 cc
Acetic acid	5 cc

The specimens must be left in this mixture from six to twenty-four hours, then immersed in alcohol with added tincture of iodine. This is an excellent fixative for the nuclear and protoplasmic structures.

19. Pyridine (C_5H_5N). This reagent was introduced for microscopical studies by Donaggio, who used it for staining the neurofibrils; in the last lustra[2] it has been frequently used by Held, Cajal, Tello, Bielschowsky, etc.

According to Cajal,[1] pyridine, when used for the reduced silver method, is the best fixative for the study of degeneration and neurogenesis. It has two invaluable properties for these purposes: first of all, it enhances the penetration of silver nitrate, and secondly, it improves the rapid impregnation of silver in neural sprouts and any structures damaged by toxic or traumatic agents.

The way in which pyridine is used and the postfixation treatment of the tissues are of paramount importance. Held, following Donaggio's example, originally used pure pyridine. The fixation time was twenty-four hours and afterward the pieces were rinsed for several hours with running tap water in order to remove the fixative. This procedure may render good results in early embryos though, as proven by Cajal, it is better to dilute pyridine in water up to 30, 40, or 50 per 100; in this way, it is possible to avoid the artefactual shrinkage and the formation of vacuoles and coalescences, which are the origin of some of Held's errors (*EN 6*). Tello, and eventually Held himself, used diluted pyridine. The penetration of pyridine is acceptable when fixing small brains or embryos, but large specimens must be sliced into thin slices.

A great advantage of pyridine fixation when followed by Cajal's impregnation is that it renders the background very clear, increasing the contrast between the impregnated fibers and the organs through which they travel or terminate. Now we shall describe the modus operandi:

20. We have already commented on the advantages of diluting pyridine; the solution we usually employ is the following one:

Distilled water   15 cc
Pure pyridine   35 cc

This liquid is allowed to act during twenty-four hours in the case of small blocks, and forty-eight hours for larger ones. Fixation is followed by a twelve-hour rinse with running tap water and by postfixation in 96° alcohol for another twelve hours.

Some *pyridine* derivatives, such as the *pyridine nitrate* (Donaggio) or the *trimethyl-pyridine (collidine)* suggested by de Castro, can prove good nervous tissue fixatives. The latter substance is barely miscible with water; therefore, it is mixed with pyridine (*pyridine*, 10 cc; water, 5 cc; *collidine*, 10 cc).

Fixatives Based on Hypnotic Substances

Some of these substances were introduced for microscopical studies of the nervous system by Cajal, who used them either as fixatives or as accelerators of alcoholic fixation in the reduced-silver method.

The importance of these chemicals is growing from day to day, as they confer an exquisite affinity for silver to the neural lattice of the nervous centers, ganglia, nerve trunks, and peripheral endings (sensitive, motor, or sympathetic).

The chemicals that are used for this purpose are *chloral hydrate, veronal, sulphonal, trional,* and *hedonal.*

The best results are obtained when hypnotics are used on fresh tissues, although on some occasions pieces fixed for several weeks or months in alcohol or formalin and then treated with these solutions have recovered their affinity for colloidal silver.

The fixing power of a hypnotic is higher the stronger its neurotropic activity, as has been proved by one of us (de Castro). This is why some of them are excellent fixatives, for instance, *chloral hydrate* (Cajal), *urethane* (de Castro) or some derivatives of *barbituric acid* such as *veronal*, used by Cajal. All these substances work better in solutions of water and alcohol than in only water or only alcohol (de Castro). Furthermore, the addition of alcohol prevents the tissue swelling with choral hydrate in aqueous solution.

Hypnotics, when added to the alcoholic fixatives used in Cajal's method (plain alcohol, ammoniacal alcohol), hasten the maturation of the block (reflected in the darkening of the piece after several days of silvering); Liesegang suggests that this darkening might be the beginning of the colloidal reduction of silver nitrate by the tissue.

Here are some formulae for hypnotics when used as fixatives and accelerators:

21. Formula with chloral hydrate.

Chloral hydrate	5 g^3
Alcohol	40 cc
Water	40 cc

The pieces should be immersed for twenty-four hours in this solution then treated for one day in ammoniacal alcohol (96° alcohol, 50 cc; ammonia, three to six drops). Urethane is used in a way similar to chloral hydrate (de Castro).

22. Formula with veronal (diethyl-barbituric acid).

96° Alcohol	100 cc
Veronal	1–2g

The pieces should be fixed for twenty-four hours in this liquid, after which they must be rinsed with water briefly before being immersed in silver nitrate.

Hypnotics are not the only substances that can be used for this purpose; other agents with similar properties are *pyridine, ethylamine* (several drops), *lysidine, piperazin, fibrolysin, acetal, acrolein, nicotine* and even *formalin*; the latter, besides having fixing and mordanting actions, acts as an accelerator in some formulae of Cajal's and Liesegang's methods and also in Bielschowsky's method.

3
Decalcifying Agents

Decalcifying agents are acidic substances that combine with *lime* in bone salts, teeth, *chitin*, etc., to form water-soluble compounds that can be easily removed.

Decalcificants are indispensable when serial sections are to be obtained from specimens like embryos, fetuses, or small animals, in which it is not possible to remove the bone protection of the neuraxis or of certain peripheral nerve endings (inner ear, teeth, etc.). A good example of the advantages of this treatment is the study of inner ear endings with neurofibrillary methods in newborn or young mice.

Some of the available solutions are convenient for general purpose staining methods for the nervous system, whereas others are especially appropriate when silver impregnations are to be performed.

Among the former, and besides the classic saturated solution of *picric acid* proposed by Ranvier, the following solutions are recommendable:

23. Fol's Liquid.

1 per 100 Chromic acid	70 cc
1 per 100 Nitric acid	3 cc
Water	200 cc

24. Ebner's Liquid.

Hydrochloric acid	2.5 cc
Alcohol	500 cc
Sodium chloride	2.5 g
Distilled water	100 cc

25. Nitric acid decalcification of tissues previously fixed in formalin.
This procedure has been used, with minor modifications, by Bielschowsky, Agduhr, Cajal, and Lorente de Nó.

The modus operandi used by one of us (Cajal) is as follows:

1. Immerse the spine, skull, etc. of newborn or young small animals (such as mice) in 12–20 per 100 formalin. This fixative requires one to three days to be effective, depending on the size of the blocks.

2. Once the fixation is finished, the pieces are transferred to the following solution:

   Nitric acid   4 cc
   Water   100 cc

3. Rinse with running tap water for twenty-four hours in order to remove the nitric acid.
4. Treat the pieces for twenty-four hours with 80 per 100 pyridine or with ammoniacal alcohol (96° alcohol, 100 cc.; five drops of ammonia).
5. Rinse again for twelve hours if pyridine has been used; when alcohol has been used, a brief rinse (for a few minutes) is sufficient.

26. Bielschowsky–Agduhr formula.
1. Fixation of tissue samples in 20 per 100 formaldehyde for seven days.
2. Decalcification in 5 per 100 nitric acid for one or more days, depending on the size of the specimens.
3. Rinse with running tap water for ten to twenty days. (The procedure continues according to the Bielschowsky–Agdurh method, to be described later.)

27. Heidenhain's fixative and decalcifying solution.

Sublimate concentrated solution   100 parts
Trichloroacetic acid   2 cc
Acetic acid   1 cc

Da Costa recommended the decalcifying action of this liquid on larvae of amphibia. It is also useful for softening the chitin of the exoskeleton of insects as well as the shell of small crustacea.

The liquid acts on the pieces from twenty-four hours to several days, depending on the size of the specimens. A solution made by adding trichloroacetic acid to water has proved useful to us when used on the crayfish *Astacus* (*EN 7*).

Although other decalcificants are available, the methods described above are sufficient for cytological studies. However, others (see below) must be used when the pieces are to be silver-impregnated by Cajal's method.

28. Nitric acid-formaldehyde formula.
Often used by Cajal to study inner ear structures, it is made of:

Formaldehyde   12 cc
Water   100 cc
Nitric acid   3–5 cc

After fixation by immersion for one or more days in this solution, the pieces are transferred to pyridine for twenty-four hours.

29. De Castro's procedure with chloral hydrate.

Water   50 cc
96° Alcohol   50 cc
Chloral hydrate   50 cc
Nitric acid   3–4 cc

Chapter 3: Decalcifying Agents

After twenty-four or more hours in this solution, the specimens are rinsed with running tap water for twenty-four hours then transferred to ammoniacal alcohol for one day.

30. De Castro's procedure with urethane.

Urethane	2 g
96° Alcohol	50 cc
Water	50 cc
Nitric acid	2–3 cc

Fixation is followed by a twenty-four hour rinse with running tap water and a further day in ammoniacal alcohol. The tissue is then ready to be impregnated with silver (Cajal's method).

All the aforementioned formulae can be used in conjunction with silver methods, except for numbers **23, 24,** and **27.** Let us add that although solutions containing formaldehyde give acceptable results with both Cajal's and Bielschowsky's methods, decalcificants without formaldehyde are suitable only for the former.

De Castro's formulae (**28** and **29**) are especially recommended due to their short decalcifying period and excellent results. Other methods demand more thorough rinsing. For instance, Cajal's technique (**28**) with nitric acid and formaldehyde requires two additional days as both the nitric acid and pyridine must be removed. Agduhr's protocol needs nearly three weeks in addition to the long impregnation period needed for this variation of Bielschowsky's method.

Observations:

1. The solutions must be used in large volumes in proportion to the size of the specimens. Although 50 to 60 cc should be enough for the nervous centers of newborn mice, to decalcify the temporal bone of a rabbit the volume will exceed 100 cc.
2. Similar rules apply to the decalcification time. Thus, small pieces are completely decalcified in one or two days, whereas large ones require one or two weeks.
3. Once removed from the decalcificant solution, the pieces will be rinsed for twelve to twenty-four hours with running tap water; if the blocks are to be immersed in pyridine (as in formulae **25** and **28**), an additional twenty-four hour rinse is necessary.
4. Rinsing is followed by immersion of the specimens in the silver solutions used in Bielschowsky's method (silver nitrate and ammoniacal silver oxide) or in the silver nitrate solution for Cajal's method.
5. When the tissue is to be processed according to routine histological techniques, it is dehydrated once the nitric acid has been removed, then embedded in celloidin. However, if the specimens are impregnated *en bloc*, dehydration and embedding must take place after the reduction step. (See the reduced silver formulae below.)

4
General Dissociation Procedures

EMBEDDING TECHNIQUES AND AGENTS (CELLOIDIN, PARAFFIN AND GELATIN)

A fundamental principle of all histological techniques is to convert the tissues into a fine sheet of their constituent cells by either mechanical or chemical procedures. Ideally, in order to achieve the best possible transparency and definition, the histological preparation would consist of a single layer of well-stained entire cells. This is sometimes readily accomplished, as in the case of blood and other cell suspensions. We commonly are obliged, however, to use procedures that only partially prevent superimposition of different tissue constituents. Luckily, selective staining techniques allow the elimination of many intermingled elements, thus producing extremely limpid and clear histological preparations.

In the study of the nervous system, several procedures are now available for the demonstration of cells and fibers in such optimal conditions. These resources are: First, *chemical or mechanical dissociation*, most suitable for nerve trunks, although less so for neurons and glial cells; second, *vascular injection*, indispensable for the study of capillary vessels; and third, *sectioning* of the tissues with microtomes.

We assume that the reader is familiar with all these procedures, and hence, we shall only summarize the two most valuable ones, namely, *dissociation* and *sectioning*.

DISSOCIATION

As we have already mentioned, the different structural elements of the nervous system can be isolated either *mechanically* or *chemically*.

Mechanical dissociation. The nervous centers fixed in potash bichromate, as well as nerve trunks treated with osmic acid, Dominici's liquid, etc., can be dissociated into their constituent elements by *mechanical means*. These procedures are carried out by placing the specimens on a glass slide against a black or white background (depending on the color of the samples) so that the smallest tissue fragments can be readily distinguished. Dissociation should be performed on pieces placed in a drop of glycerin (unless semidesiccation is required, as in the case of nerve trunks), using histological needles. Dissociation should be continued until the tissue is broken down into almost invisible fragments. In many cases, these procedures are more easily carried out under a dissection microscope.

A common method among histologists in the past, mechanical dissociation has been used recently by Perroncito, Nageotte, and Cajal for the study of both stained and unstained fixed nerve fibers. One of us (de Castro) also has studied the sympathetic nervous system by this means, peeling off the tissues surrounding the sympathetic ganglia and obtaining superb preparations of whole chains of ganglia with their *rami* stained with methylene blue. However, mechanical dissociation of the nervous centers, so fashionable in Ranvier's time, is now almost obsolete, having been replaced by modern sectioning and staining techniques.

Chemical dissociation. In some cases, we also can use chemical procedures to isolate anatomical structures by virtue of the ability of some reagents to dissolve the intercellular cement. Thus, when a nerve trunk is exposed to the action of **one-third alcohol**, the nerve fibers appear slightly separated from each other, so that they can be easily isolated mechanically. Other reagents that can be used for this purpose are: 40 per 100 potash, 30 per 100 nitric acid, Schieffedecker's liquid (20 parts of water, 10 of glycerin and 1 part of methyl alcohol), and Landois's liquid (neutral ammonia bichromate saturated solution, 5 parts; sodium sulfate saturated solution, 5 parts; potassium phosphate saturated solution, 8 parts; water, 100 parts). As a rule, dissociation is performed with the aid of fine needles, and it must be continued until the fibers or cells are completely or partially isolated. Finally, let us stress that good results by means of dissociation are only achieved with patience, time, and dexterity.

SECTIONING

This is the most common method for the study of the nervous system. It requires the use of microtomes either with or without prior embedding of the specimens in substances capable of becoming very hard. Given that the microtomy and embedding procedures are widely known from general technique textbooks, we shall only recall some indispensable sectioning techniques for nervous system structures.

There are two main procedures for sectioning the nervous system: for unembedded material, by means of the *freezing microtome,* and for embedded specimens, in either *paraffin* or *celloidin*.

FROZEN SECTION PROCEDURE

This method entails hardening the specimens by the cooling effect of fast volatilization of ethyl chloride, ether, or pressurized liquid carbonic acid.

The fragments of nervous tissue to be frozen should previously be fixed in formaldehyde or in some other mild fixative (sublimate-based fixatives, Orth's liquid, Weigert's fixative for glial cells, Cajal's formalin-bromide, etc.). There are a number of commercially available microtomes, though the most commonly used is the Leitz (Wetzlar) microtome, which uses carbonic acid. The specimens are sectioned as follows:

1. Formaldehyde-fixed specimens not thicker than 0.5 to 1 cm are immersed in water anywhere from some minutes to several hours. This step should be omitted in two of Cajal's methods, namely, the reduced-silver impregnation and the gold-sublimate technique for the demonstration of the neuroglia. In both cases the specimens are kept immersed in the fixative until they are transferred to the microtome and the sections are later replaced in the same fixative.
2. Drip some water onto the microtome freezing stage and then place the block of tissue on top.
3. Let the carbonic gas flow out by exerting gentle pressure with one fingertip on the specimen, so that its inferior surface flattens against the microtome stage. Once the tissue starts to harden, its upper face should be cut off with the sliding knife until the block has an even surface ready for sectioning. The tissue will have to be frozen further to the point when thin sections can be obtained. Underfreezing the tissue will result in incomplete, severed sections, whereas overfreezing can produce ice crystals inside the specimen that will splinter the sections. When cutting the tissue, the sections pile up on the edge of the knife, from where they are removed in groups of 15 or 20 by means of a finger, a brush, or a histological needle. The sections are placed either in water or, preferably, in the same fixative.

Observations. The thickness of the sections depends on the staining technique that is subsequently to be applied. As a rule, the sections will not exceed 15 to 20 μm in thickness, although they can be 30 to 35 μm thick for Cajal's reduced-silver impregnation and gold-sublimate method. Excess fixative should be removed by washing with distilled water before transferring the sections to the staining solutions. Although frozen sections are usually obtained from formaldehyde-fixed tissues, they also can be cut from fresh organs (except in the case of the central nervous system) or from tissues fixed by other means; if the fixative is an alcohol-based solution, the specimens must be previously hydrated for 12 to 24 hours.

Freeze sectioning cannot be performed on very hard organs (such as tendons) or in specimens subjected to a strong induration with reagents such as chromic acid, osmium-bichromic mixture, Flemming's liquor, or osmic acid. The most valuable aspect of frozen sectioning is that embedding is not necessary, thus shortening the procedure. Consequently, well-stained sections can be obtained two or three days after fixation has ended. Freeze sectioning is necessary for the following methods: Bielschowsky's and its variations, Río-Hortega's, Nageotte's, Liesegang's, and Cajal's (gold-sublimate).

When the blocks of tissue have cracks or cavities, as in the case of the cerebellum, they must be coated with 10–12 per 100 gelatin. Once this has solidified, the specimens are immersed in formaldehyde for about one hour. This technique also offers good results when used on blocks that are to be stained with Spielmeyer's (for staining the myelin), Bielschowsky's, Liesegang's, or Schulze's methods.

CELLOIDIN AND COLLODION EMBEDDING

These embedding methods were developed by Duval, who first used thick collodion, which solidifies when immersed in 36° alcohol. Now, celloidin is preferred;

this substance is a type of amber-colored, dry collodion, which can be dissolved slowly in a solution of equal parts of 65° ethyl ether and absolute alcohol. This is the method of choice for neurological techniques because it does not shrink the tissue, as opposed to paraffin embedding. The advantages of celloidin are: (1) the possibility of obtaining moderately thick sections with ease; these are required in several histological methods, and (2) it allows the sectioning of large specimens. Furthermore, the handling and orientation of the blocks of tissue are relatively simple with celloidin embedding.

Celloidin embedding is necessary for Cajal's (reduced-silver nitrate), Marchi's, Nissl's, Weigert's, and Kultschitzky's procedures, among others. The blocks must be dehydrated in alcohol prior to celloidin embedding. The usual procedure is as follows:

1. The fixed specimens, always thinner than 0.5 cm, are immersed in graded alcohols beginning with 70° alcohol. The duration of each dehydration step will depend on the size and number of the pieces. The whole dehydration usually lasts for one or two days. Obviously, the pieces that were initially fixed in 95° alcohol will be transferred directly to absolute alcohol.
2. The specimens are transferred to a mixture of equal parts of 65° ethyl ether and absolute alcohol for twenty-four hours.
3. Afterward, the tissue is immersed for twenty-four to forty-eight hours in a 2 per 100 solution of celloidin.
4. The blocks of tissue are then soaked in 8 per 100 celloidin for two or more days. The celloidin solution should have the consistency of thick syrup.
5. Once the specimen has been removed from the celloidin, it is placed on a clean, dry wooden or cork cube for some minutes, thus allowing the surrounding celloidin to air-dry.
6. These cubes are then introduced into a wide-neck flask filled with 50–60 per 100 alcohol, where they will be kept for twenty-four hours.
7. The cube with the tissue block is immobilized with the microtome stage clamp, then the specimen is sectioned, taking care that the microtome knife is always wetted with 50° alcohol.
8. The sections are placed together in water or 90° alcohol. They must be kept in 90° alcohol if the staining is to be delayed for more than two hours.

Observations: This method can be applied to any kind of tissue, even the hardest ones, once they are decalcified.

If the pieces are very small (3 to 4 mm thick) the embedding time can be shortened and the whole procedure carried out in 12 to 14 hours, as the first step in alcohol-ether and even the first celloidin solution can be dispensed with.

When working with tissues that are especially difficult to embed, the method of choice will be Apathy's, which uses water-free celloidin solutions. For this purpose, the commercially available celloidin tablets are fragmented into small pieces and either dried at room temperature or oven-dried at 30°, until they shrink and become very hard. These pieces are then dissolved in a 50/50 solution of absolute alcohol and ethyl ether until a syrupy consistency is achieved (Solution III), after which one part of this mixture is diluted in two parts of alcohol-ether solution to obtain a thin celloidin solution (Solution II). Solution II is further diluted with a similar amount of an absolute alcohol and ethyl ether solution (Solution I). The embedding protocol is as follows: the pieces are first immersed in Solution I for one day, transferred to Solution II for another twenty-four hours and kept for two additional days in Solution III. Thereafter, when the specimens are ready to be sectioned, they are mounted on cork or wooden blocks and hardened in diluted alcohol. This procedure allows rather thin sections (10 to 15 µm) to be obtained without damaging the tissue.

Although not as refined as Apathy's method, the general technique of celloidin embedding also permits the tissues to be cut into very thin sections, providing that the microtome knife is extremely sharp. The neurobiologist must get used to sharpening the knives with the grindstone previous to cutting large, thin sections.

PARAFFIN EMBEDDING

This method is more useful for general purpose techniques than for the study of the nervous system, where thick sections are preferable in order to follow nerve fibers and dendrites over long distances. Nevertheless, it can be used to obtain thin sections to study the neurogenesis and tumors of the brain and spinal cord and whenever pictures are to be taken from preparations stained by the methods of Nissl, Weigert-Pal, or Cajal. The paraffin-embedded material becomes very hard, so that rather thin sections (3 to 5 µm) can be obtained. The protocol for paraffin embedding is as follows:

1. The pieces, once properly fixed and dehydrated, are immersed in a mixture of equal parts of alcohol and chloroform. The chloroform is added onto the alcohol using a pipette whose tip is placed at the bottom of the flask, so that the chloroform forms a distinct, separate layer at the lower half of the well. Once the specimens sink to the bottom, they can be transferred to:
2. Pure chloroform, where they remain for six to twenty-four hours.
3. The sections are then transferred to a concentrated solution of paraffin in chloroform for six to twenty-four hours.
4. The specimens are then transferred to liquid paraffin, which has been warmed slightly above the melting point. The pieces are immersed in this liquid between eight hours and three days, depending on their size.
5. The pieces are then rapidly cooled so that the embedding medium solidifies as very fine crystals. (A slow solidification results in gross crystals that can damage the tissues.) The cooling procedure can be carried out using **Leuckat frames**, with which a rectangular mold can be built up with the dimensions required by the specimen; this mold is rubbed with glycerin or olive oil to ease the detachment of the solid paraffin block. Once liquid paraffin has been poured into the mold, the specimen is carefully placed inside it and positioned with the help of fine needles. After a short time, the surface of the liquid paraffin solidifies, forming a thin film; then the mold must be rapidly

immersed in cold water, which completes the hardening process. The small paraffin block thus formed is pasted onto a larger paraffin cube by means of a hot scalpel and then covered by an additional, thin (3 to 4 mm thick) layer of paraffin.

6. The block is mounted on the microtome stage and its sides trimmed until it is the size of a cube of sugar. It is placed with one of its edges parallel to the edge of the microtome knife, a position that permits the making of serial sections.
7. When the tissue has been stained *en bloc* the resulting sections are mounted on glass slides, rinsed with turpentine oil or xylene to remove the paraffi, and covered with Canada **balsam**. The staining of single sections will be considered below.

Cedarwood oil, introduced by Bolles Lée, is widely used nowadays instead of chloroform to clarify the pieces as it does not shrink the tissue. The pieces are then immersed in paraffin.

Observations: (A) Chloroform and the solution of paraffin in chloroform are used to facilitate the penetration of paraffin in the tissue. However, any paraffin solvent can be used for this purpose, including turpentine essence, oil of cloves, cedarwood oil, bergamot oil, xylene, petroleum, and toluene. All these solvents are used in the same way as chloroform.

(B) Paraffin sections are sometimes prone to curl, thus impeding serial sectioning. There are several ways to prevent this problem. Here are a few:

The rolling-up of the sections can be mechanically prevented by placing a wide, flexible brush over the upper surface of the block that is being sectioned. An alternative procedure is to trim the paraffin block into a triangular prism, with one of the angles of the upper surface facing the knife. The triangular shape of the sections thus formed facilitates their unrolling by heating when placed on a glass slide.

Another trick to avoid the curling of the sections is to wet the surface of the block with a drop of lukewarm water by means of the brush; sections deposited on warm water unroll easily. This procedure is especially useful in winter and when using hard paraffin with a melting point over 55°C. For some small specimens, we have obtained good results covering the blocks with alternate layers of hard and soft paraffin. Similar results are accomplished by covering the surface of the block with soft melted paraffin just before sectioning (Strasser).

Nevertheless, the very best method is to use paraffin waxes with different melting points, depending on the room temperature. Thus, for the torrid heat of summer, a paraffin with a melting point of 55°C is recommended, whereas in the coldest winter days (10° to 12°C), it must have a melting point of about 45°C. When working in intermediate temperatures (18° to 22°C), paraffins with a melting point of 48° to 50°C are preferred. In the latter case, mixtures of hard and soft paraffins also can be used advantageously.

(C) To obtain better series of sections, relatively soft paraffins are used, and the blocks sectioned with Minot or Cambridge microtomes.

GELATIN EMBEDDING

Nicholas Gaskell and other authors have developed a gelatin-embedding procedure suitable for tissues that are very hard or that are sensitive to alcohol or essences. Here are the technical details:

1. Fix in 10 per 100 formaldehyde.
2. Rinse the pieces in running tap water for twenty-four hours.
3. Immerse the specimens in a diluted (12 per 100) gelatin solution for twenty-four hours.
4. Transfer the pieces to a concentrated (25 per 100) gelatin solution during one more day.
5. Pour some gelatin into a small well, place the block inside it, and then let it cool to room temperature.
6. Take out the specimen with the surrounding hard gelatin, and immerse it in 10 per 100 formaldehyde for twenty-four hours in order to render the block insoluble.
7. Rinse the block for twelve hours with running tap water.
8. Cut frozen sections. This procedure is especially useful for embedding specimens to be stained with Sudan III or Hexheimer's method (see staining of lipids, below). Sections can be kept for some days in water with a little formaldehyde before staining.

SUPERFICIAL PARAFFIN IMBEDDING

In this method the specimen is attached to a paraffin cube by coating it with a layer of melted paraffin with the aid of a hot scalpel. This method is used either when the specimens are hard enough to be sectioned or when we need to cut some sections before embedding to assess the quality of the impregnation. This is our preferred method for *en bloc* impregnation with the Golgi and reduced-silver methods.

It is also useful for Nissl staining and, instead of paraffin, Arabic gum can be used to glue the tissue blocks to a cork cube. Then the cube with the tissue attached to it is immersed for 12 hours in 96° alcohol before sectioning. The sections are placed in alcohol.

Some specimens do not need to be even superficially imbedded in paraffin, such as those fixed with 20 per 100 acetone in alcohol, pure acetone, 12% formalin in 96° alcohol, or 3% pyrogallic acid in 96° alcohol. In these cases the pieces can be directly fixed to the microtome stage, providing they are large enough. However, paraffin imbedding is always preferable, given that it is very easy to spoil the specimen by crushing it with the microtome holder, even when the tissue is surrounded by fine sheets of either cork or alder pith *(Alnus sp.)*.

Handling and Mounting Serial Sections

SECTIONS OF CELLOIDIN-EMBEDDED MATERIAL

31. The sections can be organized by placing them in a row of numbered porcelain wells such as those used for watercolor painting. All the staining, rinsing, dehydration, and clarifying steps can be performed with each section kept in a different well. Once stained, dehydrated, and clarified, the sections are mounted onto glass slides and coverslipped with Canada balsam.

When each section can be placed on an individual slide (either because there are few of them or they are very large), they can be mounted without any special attaching procedure. However, if the sections are numerous or very small and several of them must be mounted serially onto a single slide, they may move when coverslipping. To avoid this problem, Cajal proposed the following trick: once clarified and arranged on the glass slide, the sections are wetted with diluted Canada balsam; after fifteen minutes the layer of balsam is almost dry and the preparation can then be covered with thick balsam and coverslipped. The pressure exerted by the coverslip will not be enough to displace the sections because the fresh balsam cannot dissolve the dry one.

An acceptable alternative method for bulk stained tissue is to transfer the sections, as they are cut, to the glass slide, keeping them moist with 80% alcohol. They are then dehydrated in absolute alcohol (on the slide itself), and clarified in origanum essence, which can be removed with xylene. Coverslipping does not move the sections, for the absolute alcohol melts the celloidin, thus sticking the sections to the slide. The essences (origanum vulgare, creosote, carbol-xylol, etc., but not the clove essence, which dissolves the celloidin) increase the stickiness of the sections by solidifying the celloidin.

It also is easy to avoid disarray of celloidin-embedded tissue sections, providing they are soaked in alcohol. The celloidin, melted by the alcohol in which the sections are placed, helps to attach the section to the slide. In this case, the sections are fixed to the slide by covering them with a strip of blotting paper and exerting a strong, regular pressure on it.

An alternative technique is to place the sections on a glass slide previously coated with a thin layer of dry 2% celloidin. For this purpose, the sections must be soaked in alcohol. For very large series of sections, however, other variations are preferable, namely:

32. Weigert's methods. These procedures allow the treatment of many sections simultaneously.

1. As the sections are cut, they are placed in order and soaked in 70% alcohol over a sheet of toilet paper.
2. The paper, with the sections facing down, is placed on a collodionized glass plate (such as the ones used by photographers for print glazing). The paper is pressed against the plate and the sections stick to the collodion. The toilet paper is then peeled off.
3. The glass plate and the sections (which must be kept moist) are coated with an additional layer of liquid collodion, which is then allowed to evaporate for several minutes.
4. Before the collodion has completely dried, the plates are immersed in water so that the sections become detached, but are kept together embedded in a thin solid layer of collodion. The sections thus prepared can be easily handled as a single set during staining, dehydration, and other histological procedures. Clarifying must be performed with creosote, because it does not dissolve the celloidin. This technique is especially useful for staining complete brain or spinal cord series by Weigert's, Weigert-Pal's, and Kultschitzky's methods.

33. Another procedure, described by Weigert and especially suitable for Nissl staining, uses paper.

1. Cut circles or squares of blotting paper to the size of a small well and number them consecutively.
2. A section is placed on the first piece of paper, soaked in alcohol, at the bottom of the well. Then the section is covered with the next piece of paper with the following section on it and this procedure is repeated with all the sections, until the series is complete. Staining with anilines can be performed by pouring the solutions into the well.
3. Once stained, the sections are dehydrated and clarified, after which the paper is peeled off and the sections mounted onto glass slides.

34. Obrégia's procedure.

1. Spread a thick sucrose or sugar solution onto glass slides with a small brush and allow it to dry.
2. Place the sections in order on toilet paper strips soaked in 70% alcohol.
3. The paper strips, with the sections facing down, are placed onto the glass slides, pressed, and then the paper is peeled off. The sections will remain stuck to the slides.
4. After most of the alcohol has evaporated, pour a decidedly thick celloidin or collodion solution over the sections. The excess of collodion is drained and the remaining is allowed to solidify. The slides are now transferred

to water so that the sugar is dissolved and the collodion film with the sections in it floats free.

35. Olt's method. This author proposed a procedure for the organization of series of frozen, celloidin, or paraffin sections, based on the observation that formalin-treated gelatin becomes insoluble. This is the modus operandi:

1. Prepare a 5%–10% gelatin solution in a water bath; once dissolved, remove the impurities by adding an egg white, as done in bacteriology to thin the culture media. In order to avoid the growth of fungi, 10 cc of 5% phenol must be added to the solution. (Other antiseptics, such as sodium salicylate, or thymol, can also be used.)
2. The hot, liquid gelatin is poured onto the glass slides or spread with a finger. Once coagulated, the sections are arranged in series on the slide, either using a fine brush or as described in Weigert's and Obrégia's methods.
3. Blot the sections with filter paper so that they remain perfectly flat and stuck to the gelatin; then immerse the slides in 10% formalin for five to ten minutes in order to harden the gelatin. Similar results are obtained by exposing the slides to formaldehyde vapors. Rinse with water, stain (if not already done), dehydrate, and coverslip.

After this treatment, the embedding media, such as celloidin or paraffin, can be removed without causing the sections to fall off the slide. This procedure is recommended for series of sections of the brain or medulla of small mammals, which are to be stained by the Nissl method, especially if Gothard's liquid is used in the differentiation step. (For more details, see the section on *Methods for the Staining of Nissl Bodies*).

36. Apathy's procedure.

1. The sections are arranged in series on a glass slide, so that the celloidin surrounding each section is in contact with that of the adjacent ones; the sections are then soaked in 90% alcohol.
2. Blot the sections with blotting paper and suspend them over a well filled with ether with the sections facing down. In this way, the ether vapors will melt the celloidin just enough for the sections to become glued to one another. They should not be exposed to ether vapors for more than one or two minutes or the celloidin may become too thin and the sections could move.
3. Allow the ether to evaporate briefly and then treat the slides with absolute alcohol, a procedure that results in the sticking of the sections to the glass slide. If the sections have been stained previously, they can be clarified with xylene (which does not dissolve the celloidin) and coverslipped with Canada balsam. If the sections have not been stained previously, they can be stored in 70% alcohol. If the sections are not surrounded by enough celloidin, it is preferable to carry out Weigert's method with collodion.

SECTIONS OF PARAFFIN-EMBEDDED MATERIAL

Series of paraffin sections are readily obtained with either Minot-type or rocking (Reichert) microtomes, provided that the paraffin is sufficiently firm. These sections are stuck to the slide by means of the following liquid:

37. Schallibaum's Liquid.

> Regular collodion   1
> Oil of cloves   3

The glass slide must be coated with a very thin layer of this mixture, which hardens quickly without drying completely. Once the sections are stuck to the slide, transfer it to a 50° to 60°C bain-marie, in which the essence evaporates after thirty minutes and the collodion layer becomes very hard.

When the tissue has been bulk-stained, the paraffin is removed with either turpentine or xylene. Coverslip with Canada balsam.

38. Sticking the sections by capillarity. Carefully place the sections with their anterior surface upward in a warm (45°C) water bath. When they are placed in the water they stretch and any wrinkles disappear. Then a slide is immersed in the water and slipped under the desired section/s. When the slide is pulled out of the water, the sections are kept in place with a fine needle. Drain off excess water and put the slides into an oven at 37°C for twelve hours so that the remaining water evaporates.

39. Method with sealing wax. Make a saturated solution of sealing wax in 40% alcohol. After several days, when the *vermillion* precipitates, the supernatant is removed and allowed to evaporate. This results in the precipitation of pure, colorless sealing wax. This substance is dissolved at a 10% concentration in creosote; the solution thus obtained can be used in the same way as Schallibaum's liquid. The creosote disappears when the slides are placed in an oven and thus only the sealing wax remains, sticking the sections, which must be stained prior to mounting (see bulk staining below), because the alcohol used to dehydrate slide-mounted sections would dissolve the sealing wax.

40. Procedure with albumin. Mix equal parts of albumin and glycerin. The resulting solution is used to coat the slides on which the sections should be arranged. The slides are then placed in the oven (at 60°C), where the sections are stuck to the slide by the solidification of the albumin. The layer of albumin must be extremely thin; otherwise, it could increase the background staining.

41. Japanese method. This is carried out by placing the sections in a water bath and then picking them up with an albumin-coated slide. Although there is background staining due to the albumin, it has the advantage of sticking the sections better, for which reason it is so widely used.

6
General Staining Methods

SOME REMARKS ON THE STAINING PROCESS

The staining of histological preparations or dissociated tissues, like the industrial coloring of fabrics, is based on the attraction of the dyes to some of the constituents of organic tissues. In the case of biological specimens, these constituents are the nucleus, protoplasm, and extracellular matrix. The more differentiated a tissue is, the greater the number of intraprotoplasmic organelles it contains and the wider the spectrum of procedures needed to demonstrate them. This is the case with the nervous tissue, whose cells, because of their great morphological and chemical complexity, have led to the development of numerous cytological methods.

The explanation of why a dye has an affinity for a given structure is a controversial matter among histologists. Some authors (Una, Pappenheim, etc.) have proposed that it must be a chemical process by which the stained substance would combine with the dye to form salt-like compounds. On the other hand, it also has been suggested (Möllendorf) that the process could be of a physical nature and thus variables such as absorption, permeability, and porousness of the specimen, as well as the diffusion capability of the dye, would be of capital importance. Some even hypothesize that colloid-chemical phenomena may play a crucial role in the staining process (Bechholdt and Liesegang). Indisputably, the latter proposal applies to procedures such as supravital colorations and metallic impregnations, as we shall discuss later. Most of the routine histological techniques, however, are not carried out on live colloids (protoplasmic and nuclear *hydrosols* and soft structural *gels*), but on colloids that have been precipitated or coagulated by fixatives. The latter are usually insoluble and stable and thus many of the principles of colloidal chemistry are not applicable to the staining process.

The possibility that so many intimate mechanisms may play a role in the staining of biological specimens, together with the ever-changing physiological states of living cells, preclude the formulation of a general theory of staining. In any case, such a theory would not be able to explain every situation, as stated by Heidenhain. For this reason, the chemical nature of a given tissue structure, as inferred from its staining affinities, must be proposed with caution. Thus, it is advisable not to consider a given dye as a reagent in a strict sense, but rather as a tool to dissect the different parts of the cell optically. Only biochemistry will, in time, provide the scientific basis to explain the staining process and to discard methodological empiricisms. In the meantime, we agree with other authors in considering that five factors may be involved in the staining process: (1) the action of mordants and fixatives that alter the physical state of the tissues; (2) the permeability and absorptive power of the cell protoplasm; (3) the presence of protein membranes and lipoid envelopes; (4) the chemical composition and physical properties of the dyes (diffusivity, ionic strength, temperature, concentration, etc.), and (5) the structure and composition of the cells. Obviously, these are rather vague premises, but the present state of knowledge in this field does not allow the formulation of a more adventurous theory, except for a few examples in which the chemical basis is well known.

Now we must classify staining according to the way in which it is carried out and explain the meaning of some technical terms.

Substantive and adjective staining. If the staining is direct, that is, without the previous use of *mordants*, it is called *substantive* staining. Some examples of this are the carmines (*alluminous carmine*, etc.), *Böhmer's or Ehrlich's hematoxylin*, and *methylene blue supravital coloration*.

Adjective staining is that in which the tissues are treated, either prior to or after staining, with mordants, which bind to some tissue components, rendering them especially receptive to a given dye.

In summary, only two elements are involved in *substantive coloration*, namely, the *dye* and the *tissue*. In the *adjective* coloration, however, there are three: the *tissue*, the *dye*, and the *mordant*. The action of the mordant as an intermediate link between tissue and dye has been compared by Weigert to the role of the blood factor termed *amboceptor*, which has the ability to link the cells to the *complement*. (Consult bacteriology textbooks for the phenomena of immunity, bacteriolysis, and cytolysis.) Needless to say, in the staining process the *complement* is represented by the dye.

Mordants. We shall mention some of the most widely used ones in histology, which are also used in the textile industry. These are *tannin, sublimate, chromic acid* and *bichromates; picric acid* and *copper salts* (especially acetate and sulfate); *regular alum* and *iron-ammonia alum; uranyl nitrate, chrome fluoride* and compounds containing *iodine* and *bromine* (such as Gram's liquid, ammonium bromide, etc.); *metallic oxides, vanadium salts, phosphomolybdic acid, ammonium molybdate, trichloroacetic acid*, etc. Some substances can improve the staining, although they cannot be considered as mordants; these include some alcohols, *formaldehyde, chloral hydrate*, and *pyridine*.

Differentiation of overstained tissues. The combination of the mordant with the dye and the cells results in the formation of compounds known as *lacquers*, which are insoluble in water, alcohol, and ether. They can be dissolved, however, by some substances, such as sodium sulfite, potassium ferricyanide, some acids, and even some mordants. Examples of procedures that take advantage of this property include *Weigert's method*, in which the excess of dye is removed by means of potassium ferricyanide or sodium sulfite, and *Heidenhain's procedure*, in which the overstaining is reduced by means of iron alum. The selective lightening of background staining is called *differentiation*.

Progressive and regressive staining. Progressive staining is that in which the dye is used at low concentrations, so that several hours, or even a day, are needed to stain the susceptible tissue components. Thus, it is a slow *substantive* or *direct* staining. Examples of this include the diluted hematoxylin method and some methods with carmines.

Regressive staining, which is used very often nowadays, is one in which the tissue is stained in excess, and then subjected to differentiation. Some of the most commonly used differentiating agents are alcohol, aniline oil, creosote, and various acids.

It is convenient to check the degree of differentiation of these preparations microscopically. A widely known technique of this kind is the *Nissl method*. It is worth mentioning that monitoring under the microscope is most useful in adjective staining.

Staining and impregnation. Thus *staining* can be defined as the result of the use of dyes with a special affinity for certain histological structures. This process does not include the chemical transformation of the dye, although subtle variations of the original color may occasionally occur, a phenomenon known as *metachromasia*. Substances that fall into this category are *carmine, hematoxylin, methylene blue, thionine, toluidine blue, fuchsin, safranin*, etc.

Impregnation is the demonstration of tissue components through the degradation of the reagent (e.g., its reduction). This staining procedure is becoming more and more important because of the striking contrast that it renders of the finest histological structures. Examples of compounds used for impregnation are *osmic acid* (reduced in presence of fats), *salts of silver, gold, mercury, platinum*, and *metallic oxides* (especially ammoniacal silver oxide). We shall discuss these substances in depth below when dealing with the impregnation methods for the nervous system.

SOURCES AND COMPOSITION OF DYES

Countless dyes are used to demonstrate histological structures, either in substantive or adjective staining. Furthermore, the list of available dyes grows every day due to the progress of organic chemistry.

Except for metallic impregnation, the various routine histological stains can yield bright and highly contrasted colorations, which span the whole visible light spectrum. Some of these agents are obtained from animal or plant cells. This is the case with carmine (extracted from the cochineal, *Coccus cacti*), *hematoxylin* (obtained from logwood), *indigo, alizarin*, etc. Most dyes are aromatic substances and are synthetically obtained.

There is a close relationship between the staining ability of a given compound and its atomic structure. Witt has reported that the dying molecule always contains an atomic group termed *chromatophore*, such as: the *azo* (N = N), the *nitrous* (NO) and, especially, the *quinonic*. In addition, in order to become bona fide stains, the hydrogen atoms of the benzene ring of these compounds must be replaced by certain radicals called *auxochromes*. These confer either an acidic or a basic nature to the substance and are *amino, hydroxyl, sulfonyl, dimethylamine*, etc. (Consult organic chemistry textbooks, especially those related to the staining industry.)[1] Dyes are somewhat whimsically classified as *basic, acidic*, and *neutral*; the former stain the nuclear chromatin, the acidic ones the protoplasm, and the neutral dyes cytoplasmic granules, which are usually known as neutrophilic.

This classification, proposed by Ehrlich, does not always hold true when applied to cellular chemistry. Fixatives and mordants often modify the acidophilic or basophilic nature of a given cellular constituent. Furthermore, many cell organelles have similar affinities toward acidic and basic dyes. This is the case with the neuronal *nucleolus* that is intensely stained by the basic anilines, carmine, and hematoxylin, but which does not repel some acidic dyes, such as the acid fuchsin. Another example would be nuclear chromatin, in which acidic and basic regions can be observed (*oxy*- and *basichromatin*, according to Heidenhain).

Natural dyes are the basis of a number of methods used in the early days of histology. We shall omit here the chemical properties and atomic structure of these compounds, and just cite the methods still employed in which they are chief components. These substances are *carmine* and *hematoxylin*. Bearing in mind the scope of this treatise, the next chapter will deal with the general methods used for staining the nervous centers.

7

Formulae for Carmine and Hematoxylin

Substantive and Adjective Coloration with Aniline Stains

BICHROMIC AND TRICHROMIC METHODS

Carmines. armine can be dissolved in ammonia, as recommended by the histologists of the first half of the nineteenth century; however, this practice is not used anymore because the *chromatin (nuclein)* may swell or be extracted. The formulae preferred nowadays are those in which carmine is associated with neutral or slightly alkaline substances. Only one of them is worth discussing: *Orth's carmine with lithium carbonate*, because it can be easily combined with other stains.

Here are the most common carmine recipes:

42. Grenacher's carmine.

Carmine	2 g
5 per 100 Alum	100 cc

The components are mixed, boiled for one hour, and filtered. The sections are stained in this liquid for one to twenty-four hours; overstaining is infrequent. Carmine turns a purplish color and stains preferentially the nuclear chromatin and mitotic structures.

43. Grenacher's boracic carmine.

Carmine	2–3 g
4 per 100 Borax	100 cc

Mix the two components, boil gently for half an hour, and then add the same volume of 70° alcohol; allow the liquid to settle for twenty-four hours and then filter.

44. Czokor's cochineal. Commercially available carmine can be replaced by cochineal (*EN 8*). The Czokor's procedure yields good results, staining the nuclear chromatin a purple-violet color.

Powdered cochineal	7 g
Calcined alum	7 cc
Water	700 cc

Boil until the volume is reduced by half; filter and use as in other carmine techniques. An advantage of this dye is that it does not overstain the tissue.

45. Orth's lithium carmine. Alkaline carmine solutions render an even staining, with little selectivity for any tissue component. However, when a section diffusely stained by alkaline carmine is treated with an alcoholic solution of hydrochloric acid, the background disappears and the nuclei are clearly shown.

Orth's solution is as follows:

Carmine lacquer	2.5 g
Saturated solution of lithium carbonate	100 cc

The sections are stained for several minutes in this solution and then rinsed, first in a 1 per 100 solution of hydrochloric acid in alcohol (for one minute or less) and afterward in distilled water.

46. Hematoxylin. This dye is a yellowish powder obtained from the bark of the logwood tree (*EN 9*). It is more soluble in alcohol or in aluminous liquids than in water, so it is usually dissolved in mixtures of alum, water, and alcohol. It stains the nuclear chromatin, the birefringent material of the muscle tissue, and the mucin of goblet cells a violet-blue color.

Hematoxylin is one of the most powerful dyes; it colors even those tissues that have been immersed for a long time in chromic acid or in mixtures of chrome and osmium. The staining solution must be allowed to mature (*EN 10*) for one or two weeks before use, and it must be discarded after two or three months. The only exception to this rule is Ehrlich's formula, which remains stable for a year.

47. Ammoniacal hematein. This dye is prepared by dissolving 1 gram of hematoxylin in 20 mL of warm distilled water. When completely dissolved, 1 cc of ammonia (specific weight, 0.875) is added. The resulting liquid must be placed in a shallow container until the water evaporates; the solid residue obtained in this way is *ammoniacal hematein*.[1] It must be used as a 2% solution in alcohol containing 5% alum for histological staining.

48. Böhmer's hematoxylin. The staining solution is prepared mixing two liquids:

Liquid 1:

Hematoxylin	1 g
Alcohol	12 cc

Liquid 2:

Alum	10 g
Distilled water	320 cc

The mixture must be kept for two weeks in an open, wide-neck flask in order to attain the suitable ripening, which is indicated by the deep violet color of the reagent. Old solutions with a reddish tonality are useless.

When only small amounts of the stain are necessary, a small volume of Liquid 2 can be placed on a watch glass, then two or three drops of Liquid 1 are added. Allow a ripening period of one week.

49. Ehrlich's hematoxylin.

Hematoxylin	2g
Absolute alcohol	100 cc
Acetic acid	6 cc
Glycerin	100 cc
Distilled water	100 cc
Alum	in excess

Once prepared, the reagent must be exposed to daylight until it turns red. This is a rather stable mixture that stains the nuclei nicely.

50. Delafield's hematoxylin.
This reagent is prepared by mixing 400 cc of a saturated solution (9%–10%) of ammoniacal alum [$(SO_4)_2AlNH_4$] and an alcoholic solution of hematoxylin (hematoxylin, 4 g; alcohol, 25 cc). This mixture should be kept in an unstoppered flask for three or four days in daylight to enhance oxidation. Once this period is over, filter the solution and add 100 cc of methyl alcohol (CH_3OH) and 100 cc of glycerin. Allow it to mature in an open flask until the solution turns dark (about two months), and then keep it in a tightly closed bottle. As a rule, it must be diluted in water before use.

We shall comment on other hematoxylin-based methods below, when dealing with the nervous system. Some formulae, such as Heidenhain's, will be discussed when talking about the staining of celloidin-embedded tissues.

51. Eosin.
Commercially available as *primrose*, it is a potassium salt of a brominated pteleine and was introduced as a histological stain by Renaut. Normally used at a 0.5 to 1 per 100 concentration it colors the cell protoplasm, the connective tissue fibers, and the erythrocytes pink. It can be used as a counterstain for hematoxylin, thus rendering a double coloration that is most helpful.

52. Methylene blue and other anilines.
Nuclear staining can be achieved using any of the basic aniline dyes, such as *methylene blue, fuchsin, gentian violet, dahlia violet, safranin,* **vesuvine***, aniline violet, toluidine blue, cresyl violet,* etc. All these substances can be used either at a low concentration in an aqueous solution with the addition of a few drops of acetic acid, or at a high concentration in mixtures of alcohol and water.

The application of these dyes for the Nissl method and for the procedures to stain glial cells or protoplasmic granules will be discussed in the second part of this book. Here it suffices to note that most of them are used as *adjective stains*, so the sections need to be treated by a mordant before staining and then bleached.

DOUBLE AND TRIPLE STAINS

Instead of staining the sections with only carmine or hematoxylin, it is possible to use double or triple colorations. Generally speaking, these methods use acidic and basic dyes, either simultaneously or sequentially. Such polychromatic tinctures can be applied to both frozen and embedded material, although the best results are obtained in the latter case.

53. Hematoxylin and eosin stain.

1. Transfer floating sections from water to a porcelain well containing a small amount of Böhmer's, Ehrlich's, or Delafield's hematoxylin. Agitate for two to ten minutes in order to obtain an even coloration but be careful to avoid folding of the sections. In some cases hematoxylin can be diluted in twice its volume of distilled water, slowing the staining process and making monitoring easier.
2. Rinse the sections with plenty of water.
3. Immerse them for several minutes in a 1 per 200 eosin solution.
4. Dehydrate in alcohol, clarify in oil of cloves, and mount in Canada balsam.

54. Heidenhain's iron hematoxylin. This author recommends this procedure in order to stain the nuclei in black and the centrosomes in gray. The best results are obtained when the material is fixed in liquids containing sublimate.

1. Paraffin sections not thicker than 5 μm and mounted on plain glass slides are immersed for several hours in a 2 or 3 per 100 aqueous solution of iron alum. Square glass jars with lateral grooves (*EN 11*) are the most suitable containers for this purpose.
2. Rinse briefly with distilled water in order to eliminate the excess mordant.
3. Immerse the slides in a solution of hematoxylin (hematoxylin, 1 g; alcohol, 10 cc; water, 90 cc) from thirty minutes to several hours. The hematoxylin solution must be prepared three or four weeks in advance and must have a yellow or reddish color; just before use, it should be diluted in half its volume of water. The demonstration of centrosomes needs a staining period of six to twelve hours; nuclei are very easily stained.
4. Differentiate in the mordant solution until the black color of the sections turns to pale gray.
5. Rinse with distilled water in order to remove the mordant completely.
6. Dehydrate, clarify, and mount in balsam.

Nuclei appear black or deep gray, whereas protoplasm is shown in various shades of gray, depending on the duration of exposure to the mordant. Sometimes the *glial fibers* are also stained, especially in some pathological material.

The sections treated by this method can be counterstained with Van Gieson's picrofuchsin, thus yielding splendid red colorations of the connective tissue fibers. For this purpose the sections are immersed in this reagent after the rinse following decoloration. Other dyes, such as the chromotropes, also can be used for background staining of the tissue.

MODIFICATIONS OF THE IRON-HEMATOXYLIN. METHODS FOR THE STAINING OF MITOCHONDRIA

The filaments discovered by Benda, named *mitochondria* and **chondriomites,** have been thoroughly studied by Meves and other histologists with Heidenhain's iron-hematoxylin procedure, which is more constant and reliable than Benda's primitive method.

55. Meves' Procedure for staining the mitochondria (1908). Meves fixes small tissue fragments in Flemming's liquid, embeds the blocks in paraffin and stains the sections with well-ripened Heidenhain's hematoxylin. The mitochondria are shown in deep black.

Regaud and Mawas (1909) fix the specimens in a mixture of formalin and dichromate (**7**) for twenty-four hours and then immerse them in 3% dichromate for four to ten days. Once this period is over, the pieces are rinsed with running tap water for several hours, embedded, and sectioned; the sections are then stained with Heidenhain's hematoxylin.

The mitochondria also are shown by Del Río-Hortega's first variation of Achúcarro's method[2] and by our method with uranyl nitrate. See *Procedures for Staining the Golgi Apparatus, Centrosome, and Mitochondria* for further details.

56. Mallory's hematoxylin with phosphomolybdic acid.

1. Immerse tissue sections for one minute in the following liquid:

   Water   100 cc
   Phosphomolybdic acid   10 g

2. Rinse briefly with tap water.
3. Stain for twenty to sixty minutes in:

   10 per 100 phosphomolybdic acid   10 cc
   Hematoxylin   1.75 g
   Water   200 cc
   Phenol   5 g

This solution must be prepared four or five weeks in advance, and it must be kept in the dark.

4. Rinse the sections with 50 per 100 alcohol for ten to sixty minutes, changing the alcohol two or three times.
5. Graded alcohols, xylene, etc. Nuclei, axons, and glial cells are nicely stained; collagen fibers are shown in blue.

57. Mallory's hematoxylin with phosphotungstic acid.

1. Fix in Zenker's fluid (**15**), embed in paraffin or celloidin, cut thin sections, and immerse these in iodinated alcohol (0.5 per 100) in order to remove the sublimate crystals.
2. Rinse thoroughly in 95° alcohol to wash away the iodine completely.
3. Place the sections for five to twenty minutes in a fresh 0.25 per 100 aqueous solution of potassium permanganate.
4. Rinse with water.

5. Immerse the sections for five to ten minutes in a 5 per 100 aqueous solution of oxalic acid.
6. Rinse several times with water.
7. Stain for twelve to twenty-four hours in the following liquid:

Hematoxylin	0.1 g
Distilled water	100 cc
Phosphotungstic acid	2 g

To prepare this reagent, the hematoxylin first must be dissolved in a small volume of warm water; after cooling, the rest of the water and the acid are added. The ripening takes several weeks, although it can be quickened by adding 10 cc of 0.25 per 100 potassium permanganate to the solution. Hematein can be used instead of **hematoxylin;** in such a case, the amount of permanganate must be reduced to 5 cc.

8. Dehydrate briefly in alcohol, clarify in *origanum vulgare* oil and xylene, and mount in Canada balsam.

This method shows glial cells in blue, nerve fibers in pale pink, and connective tissue in a dark pink; ***tonofibrils,*** myofibrils, and fibrin are also stained.

If the tissues have been fixed in formalin, immerse the sections in Zenker's liquid for fifteen to twenty minutes, rinse them two or three times with water, then follow the protocol from Step 3 onward.

58. Altmann's method for staining the bioblasts (or intraprotoplasmic granules).

1. Fixation in Altmann's liquid (**11**).
2. Rinse for several hours with running tap water.
3. Dehydrate in alcohol and embed in paraffin.
4. Fix the sections to glass slides with albumin or with Schallibaum liquid, deparaffinize with xylene and soak in alcohol.
5. Drip onto the sections a few drops of a mixture containing 20 g of acid fuchsin in 100 cc of an aqueous saturated solution of aniline. Heat the slide until vapors begin to appear.
6. Let the sections cool and differentiate them in picric acid (1 part of a saturated alcoholic solution of picric acid; 2 parts of water). This step must be carried out at 37°C.
7. Dehydrate in alcohol, clarify in xylene, etc.

Some authors, such as Schridde, have reported better results if the tissue is immersed in a mixture of formalin and Müller's liquid (formalin, 1; Müller, 9) for twenty-four hours prior to osmium fixation.

When used to optimum effect, this method shows all the primitive granules of the neuron (*neurosomes* of Held, etc.) in a bright red color against a yellow background.

59. Van Gieson's Triple Stain. Sections deeply stained with hematoxylin are placed in a mixture of picric acid and acid fuchsin (saturated solution of picric acid, 100 cc; acid fuchsin, 0.1g). After a few minutes in this reagent, they are dehydrated in

Chapter 7: Carmine and Hematoxylin

alcohol, clarified in oil of cloves, and mounted in d'Ammar resin. Nuclei are stained in violet, epithelium in yellow, and connective bundles in red.

60. Romanowski's method. The staining reagent for this method is prepared by mixing equal volumes of 0.2 per 100 solutions of methylene blue and eosin. The resulting precipitate, known as *methylene blue eosinate*, is soluble in warm water.

The solution is heated with a flame and the sections immersed in it for some minutes; after rinsing with water, the sections are immersed in alcohol until the excess of blue staining is removed.

The methylene blue eosinate is decomposed inside the tissue, staining the nuclei in blue and conjunctive bundles in red. The chief use of this method is to stain blood smears, although it also can be applied successfully to the study of the nervous system.

61. Cajal's triple stain with fuchsin (magenta), picric acid, and indigo-carmine.

1. The sections are immersed for five to ten minutes in an almost saturated solution of ***magenta red (red fuchsin)***. This stain can be replaced by Ziehl's carbol fuchsin, and by safranin or vesuvine, which usually render better results.
2. Rinse briefly with plenty of water to remove excess staining.
3. Stain for five to ten minutes in the following solution:

Saturated solution of Picric acid	100 cc
Indigo-carmine	0.25 g

4. Briefly rinse the sections in a small porcelain well containing distilled water to which two or three drops of acetic acid have been added.
5. Rinse with tap water for half a minute in order to remove excess picric acid.
6. Remove the excess of magenta red by immersing the sections in absolute alcohol until they turn violet.
7. Clarify in xylene or bergamot oil.
8. Mount in Canada balsam dissolved in xylene.

Nuclei are strongly stained bright red, the protoplasm is rendered pale-green or yellowish, and the connective tissue bundles are shown in deep blue.

62. Calleja's Variation. Calleja has modified this method in order to stain the nuclei and connective meshwork. The procedure is as follows:

1. Stain the sections, obtained either from embedded or frozen material, for a few minutes in Orth's carmine or in boracic carmine.
2. Differentiate in a 2 per 100 solution of hydrochloric acid in 96° alcohol until the only structures that remain stained are the nuclei.
3. Rinse thoroughly with water and follow the former method from Step 3 onward. The main advantage of this procedure is that an excess of alcohol cannot bleach the nuclei, which will remain stained in red.

63. Gallego's Variation. The well-known, superb results rendered by Cajal's trichromic method on embedded material are not so easily obtained with floating sections. In this case, the nuclei are poorly stained, and the collagen bundles are not shown in a pure blue color but instead appear greenish. These problems are not fully solved by the modifications proposed by Calleja, Vialeton (with safranin) or Podwyssotzky (with Ziehl's fuchsin).

Gallego has obtained substantial advantages when using the following technique:

1. Fix in formalin and cut thin sections with the freezing microtome.
2. Stain in fuchsin to which has been added a few drops of acetic acid.
3. Rinse with water.
4. Immerse the sections in formalin with acetic acid.
5. Rinse with water.
6. Stain with picro-indigo carmine for one minute. This stain is prepared by mixing 1 part of a 1 per 100 solution of indigo carmine with 2 parts of a saturated solution of picric acid in water.
7. Rinse with water.
8. Dehydrate, clarify, etc.

Nuclei are stained violet; the cartilaginous matrix, mucins, and the mast cells' protoplasmic granules acquire a deep-violet color. The cytoplasm and muscle fibers are pale green and the collagen bundles a blue or greenish-blue color.

64. Pappenheim's method. This method associates the stains of May-Grünwald (methylene-blue eosinate dissolved in methyl alcohol) and Giemsa (azur and eosin also dissolved in methyl alcohol). Both tinctures can be obtained from the usual dealers of micrographical products.

This method is mainly used on blood smears, but it also renders interesting results for the study of the nervous system.

1. Fix in Orth's liquid (**6**).
2. Rinse for twenty-four hours with running tap water.
3. Embed in paraffin and cut thin sections.
4. Deparaffinize the sections and transfer them to water. Dilute the May-Grünwald reagent in three or four times its volume and stain for twenty minutes at 37°C.
5. Immerse the sections for forty minutes at 37°C in the Giemsa liquid diluted in water (15 drops in 10 cc of distilled water).
6. Rinse briefly with distilled water.
7. Differentiate in diluted acetic acid (distilled water, 50 cc; acetic acid, 2 to 5 drops).
8. Rinse again with distilled water.
9. Dry the sections by pressing them with filter paper.
10. Dehydrate in a 50/50 mixture of acetone and absolute alcohol, clarify in xylene, and mount in Canada balsam.

The nuclei are stained blue, whereas the cytoplasm appears several different colors, depending on the content of acidophilic, basophilic, or neutrophilic substances.

65. Coloration with Mallory's anilines method.

1. Fix in Zenker's solution (**15**) if possible.
2. Embed in paraffin or celloidin.
3. Stain for five to ten minutes (depending on the type of tissue) in a 0.5 per 100 solution of acid fuchsin.
4. Rinse briefly with water and immerse the sections for three minutes in 1 per 100 phosphomolybdic acid.
5. Rinse two or three times with water.
6. Stain for two to twenty minutes in:

Water-soluble aniline blue (*Wasserblau*)	0.5 g
Orange G (from Grübler) (*EN 12*)	2.5 cc
Oxalic acid	2 cc
Distilled water	100 cc

The components of this reagent must be dissolved in warm water and the solution must be filtered after cooling.

7. Rinse again with water.
8. Differentiate in 96° alcohol, dehydrate, clarify in xylene, and mount in Canada balsam.

This method can be simplified by immersing the sections, once they have been stained in fuchsin, in the following liquid:

Water-soluble aniline blue (*Wasserblau*)	0.5 g
Orange G (Grübler)	2 cc
1 per 100 phosphomolybdic acid	100 cc

After the sections are stained, they are briefly rinsed, dehydrated, and mounted.

66. "Azan" method of Professor M. Heidenhain, from Tübingen.

The *Badische Anilin und Sodafabrik* company of *Ludwigshafen* manufactured two acidic aniline dyes that were termed *Azocarmine B* and *Azocarmine G* because they stained the tissues in a range of colors similar to that of carmine. The dye originally used for the "Azan" method was *Azocarmine G*, a red paste. At present, however, the factory produces only *Azocarmine G.X.*, which is a red powder with a fivefold dying strength compared with *Azocarmine G*. *Azocarmine G.X.* is used in 0.2 per 100 aqueous solutions acidified with glacial acetic acid. Tissue staining must be carried out at 55°C because the solution becomes turbid at room temperature due to crystallization of the dye.

The *Azocarmine* solution stains all tissue components in bright red, so that the sections need to be differentiated. This is achieved by immersing the slides in 96° alcohol containing 0.1 per 100 aniline or any other achromatic alkali, such as pyridine. The differentiation process must be monitored often under the microscope and halted with acidified alcohol when the cytoplasm becomes light-red. This step usually takes some time, although it can be sped up by adding some drops of water to the anilinic alcohol.

Once a suitable degree of differentiation has been achieved, the sections are immersed in 5 per 100 phosphotungstic acid (*Phosphowolframsäure*) so that connective tissue fibers are completely bleached and can be stained by the *Wasserblau* solution.

Modus operandi:

1. Fix the tissues in formalin or, better, in Zenker's fixative. Embed in paraffin and cut sections as thin as possible.
2. Stain for one hour at 55°C in the *Azocarmine G.X.* solution.
3. Differentiate in anilinic alcohol.
4. Stop the differentiation by rinsing the sections briefly with 96° alcohol to which a few drops of acetic acid have been added.
5. Immerse the slides for two hours in 5 per 100 phosphotungstic acid.
6. Rinse with distilled water.
7. Stain for two hours in Mallory's anilines solution as modified by Heidenhain; the composition of this reagent is:

Wasserblau (Grübler)	0.5 g
Orange G (Grübler)	2 cc
Acetic acid	8 cc
Distilled water	100 cc

8. Rinse briefly with distilled water.
9. Alcohol, xylene, and Canada balsam.

Collagen fibers are distinctly stained in deep blue and nuclear chromatin in bright red, whereas the protoplasm exhibits a range of colors from pale orange to russet violet.[3]

8

Section Mounting and Preservation

In a similar fashion to the technique used in general histology, nervous system sections, once stained, rinsed, dehydrated, and clarified, must be mounted in a preserving transparent medium that does not alter the coloration.

No mounting medium can be universally applied to every kind of preparation; in some cases alcohol and clarifying substances may be harmful to the sections, whereas in others they are indispensable. Thus there are two types of preserving media, which are explained below.

MOUNTING SECTIONS THAT REQUIRE PREVIOUS DEHYDRATION AND CLARIFICATION

67. Canada balsam and d'Ammar resin. The most popular mounting medium at present is dry Canada balsam, which is dissolved in xylene until it forms a syrupy solution. D'Ammar resin (obtained from the *Dammaria orientalis* in the Molucca islands), dissolved at a high concentration in either xylene or benzine, is especially recommended for Golgi's, Ehrlich's, Cajal's, and Nissl's methods, among others, because it is more neutral than Canada balsam. When weak solutions are used, bubbles appear between the sections and the coverslip, due to evaporation of the solvent.

Before the sections are embedded in the mounting medium, they must be dehydrated in absolute alcohol and clarified in bergamot, oil of cloves, cedar or origanum essence, xylene, or carbol-xylol. The clarifying agent must be carefully chosen. *When etching the celloidin around the section is not a problem, oil of cloves must be used*, because it clarifies the sections rapidly, without producing any shrinkage. Exceptions to this rule are some aniline methods, as the staining is spoiled by oil of cloves. For the silver nitrate method (Cajal), *origanum v.* essence and carbol-xylol are preferable because they do not oxidize the colloidal silver precipitate.

Clove essence may be used on celloidin-embedded specimens as long as the preparations are homogeneous and do not consist of separate portions. However, whenever the celloidin that holds the sections together must not be removed, the best clarifying agent is creosote, because it has three valuable properties: (1) it does not produce wrinkles in the sections, (2) the clarifying process is very fast, and (3) it does not dissolve the celloidin. In these cases, the most widely used solution is a mixture of carbol-xylol and creosote (phenol 20 cc, xylene 70 cc, creosote 10 cc).

Aniline-stained sections must be clarified with those essences that do not decolor the staining, such as bergamot, turpentine, carbol-xylol (phenol 25 cc, xylene 75 cc), and xylene. The use of the latter by itself requires perfect dehydration in absolute alcohol. Nissl's original method for the coloration of neurons' chromatic granules used colophony dissolved in xylene: The section on the slide was covered by the colophony solution, and then the xylene was evaporated by gently heating the slide. Lastly, the sections were coverslipped once the colophony had thickened.

For the sake of clarity, here is the protocol for mounting the preparations with balsam:

1. Dehydrate the sections by passing them through a series of porcelain wells containing 96° or, better still, absolute alcohol.
2. Rapidly immerse the sections in the clarifying agent (clove essence, creosote, bergamot, etc.).
3. After a few minutes, when the sections are almost transparent (opaque spots are due to the presence of water in the tissue), transfer them to a glass slide.
4. The excess essence is removed by tilting the slides, or by pressing the sections with clean blotting paper to soak up the fluid. They are then briefly immersed in xylene.
5. Drain the excess xylene and coverslip with balsam or d'Ammar resin dissolved in xylene.

68. Mounting in d'Ammar resin without a coverslip (encrustation procedure). The preparations obtained with some methods must not be coverslipped, because the stains can be spoiled due to the slow drying of d'Ammar resin. This fact is especially relevant for Golgi's, Golgi-Cox's, Ehrlich-Dogiel's, or Marchi's methods. In all these cases, desiccation of the mounting medium can be sped up by leaving the preparation uncovered.

For this mounting technique, weak solutions of d'Ammar resin in xylene must be used, because concentrated ones will dry before reaching the deepest portions of the section. The sections, once dehydrated and clarified with xylene, are placed on a glass slide, blotted with blotting paper and lubricated with d'Ammar resin. After five or ten minutes, the resin will be almost completely dry; if any section is not completely coated, a second and even a third layer of resin should be added, so that all the sections are embedded in resin. When the mounting medium is completely dried, the cells and fibers will appear to be encrusted in glass.

69. Mounting in cedarwood oil. This mounting medium has been recommended by Dominici for sections colored with blue aniline basic dyes, which fade rapidly when mounted with Canada balsam. Preparations stained with methylene blue, thionine, Unna's polychrome blue, Nissl's method, etc., can be conserved perfectly for a long time when mounted in regular cedarwood oil (immersion oil) (*EN 13*). The mounting technique is the same as with Canada balsam or d'Ammar resin, though it is advisable to hasten the desiccation of the medium by placing the slides

Chapter 8: Section Mounting and Preservation

in an oven at 37°C for three or four days. Cedarwood oil has the refraction index of glass, thus conferring great transparency to the tissues.

SECTION MOUNTING WITHOUT DEHYDRATION AND CLARIFICATION

70. Glycerin. Glycerin is recommended as the mounting medium in those few research methods that involve the use of stains that cannot be dehydrated, such as Sudan III, scarlet red, or Ehrlich's method with fixation in ammonium picrate. Nevertheless, this mounting medium is falling out of use, because the preparations deteriorate with time.

The procedure for mounting in glycerin is as follows:

1. Immerse the stained sections in a 1:1 mixture of glycerin and water.
2. Transfer the sections to a glass slide, drain off excess liquid, and cover them with a drop of glycerin; cover with a coverslip without exerting any pressure.
3. Blot the margins of the glass slide and seal the margins of the coverslip either with paraffin and sealing wax or with *Jews' pitch*. Details of these procedures can be found in the general treatises on histological techniques.

71. Apáthy's liquid. This liquid gives better results than glycerin. It is composed of:

Cane sugar	50 g
Distilled water	50 cc
Clean Arabic gum	50 g

To prepare this mounting medium, place the sugar and the Arabic gum in 100 cc of distilled water and heat gently until completely dissolved. When cold, filter and heat again until the volume is reduced to half; add 0.5–1cc of formalin to prevent contamination by fungi.

The sections, arranged on the glass slide, are wiped with blotting paper, covered with a drop of Apáthy's liquid, and coverslipped. Sealing of the coverslip is not necessary.

SECTION THREE

Special Techniques

9

Methods for the Demonstration of Neuronal Morphology

Golgi's Procedures and Their Variations

Golgi developed two methods for studying neuronal morphology: the black reaction, using silver chromate, and the gray reaction, with mercuric chloride.

The black reaction method is the technique most widely used by modern neurologists. It involves the induration of the neural tissues in either potash dichromate or Müller's fluid and their subsequent exposure to the action of silver nitrate. The latter reagent produces the accumulation of an opaque brick-red silver chromate precipitate in only some tissue components. This precipitate is laid down inside the protoplasm of some neurons, so that the nerve fibers and dendrites can be readily identified against a clear, translucent background.

The gray reaction method involves the fixation of the specimens in Müller's fluid (5) and subsequent treatment with a pure sublimate solution. A gray or black metallic precipitate is thus formed on some neurons, which are visible against a transparent, pale-yellow background.

The black reaction method is more commonly used and has proved especially useful in revealing the texture of the gray matter. The gray reaction method has been used to check the findings obtained with the black reaction method and also to achieve good impregnations of some neurons and axonal endings that are resistant to the black reaction. There are two variations of the silver chromate method, *rapid* and *slow*.

In the *slow variation*, which was preferred by Golgi for the study of the brain and the cerebellum, the specimens are indurated in Müller's liquid or potash bichromate for one or two months prior to their immersion in silver nitrate. The *rapid variation*, commonly used by Cajal, Kölliker, Van Gehutchen, Von Lenhossék, Retzius, Tartuferi, P. Ramón, and Held, among others, uses a mixture of potash bichromate and osmic acid as the fixative (9). This allows the shortening of the induration stage to two to six days. Furthermore, impregnation is more delicate and extensive. This method also was developed by Golgi and produces its best results in embryos and young animals.

72. Slow silver chromate procedure. This variation involves two separate steps:

1. Induration of pieces of nervous tissue in potash bichromate.
2. Immersion of the indurated blocks in a silver nitrate solution.

Induration in bichromate. This is the key step in the method and care must be taken that the pieces acquire the right degree of induration so that the second reagent can work properly. The pieces are immersed in either Müller's liquid (**5**) or in a 5% bichromate solution. This step will take 15 to 40 or more days, depending on the temperature of the surroundings. The specimens must be fresh, obtained immediately after sacrifice if possible, although good results also can be obtained in tissues dissected within the first twenty-four hours postmortem. The blocks must be smaller than half a centimeter in thickness and immersed in a relatively large volume of fixative. To make the induration faster and more uniform, the concentration of potash bichromate is gradually increased from 2.5 to 5%. Nevertheless, it is advisable to replace the induration fluid frequently, either with the same solution or at progressively higher concentrations. The extent of the induration depends on the temperature of the induration fluid: in the heat of the summer, fifteen to twenty days would be sufficient, whereas in winter, this step can last up to fifty days. The problems arising from variations in room temperature can be solved by using an oven with a thermostat set at 20° to 26°C[1] (*EN 14*).

Immersion in silver nitrate. After a brief rinse with either a 0.50 per 100 silver nitrate solution or tap water (for only a few seconds), the pieces are immersed for twenty-four to thirty hours in a 0.50–0.70 per 100 silver nitrate bath. The blocks can be kept for several days before sectioning in the same solution without worsening the quality of the impregnation. Prior to sectioning, the specimens will be dehydrated in 96° or absolute alcohol and embedded superficially in paraffin (see Section I, Chapter 3). The dehydration, clarification, and mounting of the sections are those explained for the rapid Golgi method.

73. Rapid silver chromate procedure. Here we shall include the minor variations of the original Golgi method developed by us and other authors.

1. Start by trimming down the nervous tissue with a pair of scissors or a straight razor blade into four-millimeter thick slices. These blocks are immersed for 24, 48, or 56 hours in the *osmium-bichromate mixture* (**9**).

The amount of induration liquid must be proportional to the number of slices. Thus, 30 cc will be used for three 4-millimeter thick blocks, that is, almost 10 cc per piece.

Although it is not relevant whether the pieces are exposed to light during the induration step, the temperature at which induration takes place plays a crucial role. The most suitable temperature is about 20° to 26°C; nevertheless, good results also are achieved at 8° or 9°C, providing that the pieces remain in the induration solution for a longer time.

2. Once removed from the indurating solution, the pieces are rinsed briefly with either distilled water or 0.75 per 100 silver nitrate. They are then transferred to a large volume of 0.50 to 0.75 per 100 silver nitrate solution for one to several days. We usually remove the pieces from the silver solution after 36 hours.

When impregnating pieces of almost mature brain or spinal cord, Cajal adds *one* or *two* drops of formic acid (CH_2O_2) per 300 cc of the silver nitrate solution as it seems to give a greater transparency to the background and, moreover, facilitates the axonal impregnation. Formic acid is not appropriate, however, for tissues that prove difficult to impregnate, such as those from the early embryonic stages; we never use it in these cases.

The influence of light and temperature during the silvering step is negligible. We usually carry out the impregnation in daylight, at room temperature; nevertheless, it is advisable to perform this step in the dark if the specimens are not to be sectioned for several days, otherwise irregular precipitates will appear in the sections, as reported by Van Gehutchen.

3. The pieces are cut in thick sections, in order to be able to follow complete neuronal expansions within a single section. The tissue slices are mounted on a cube of cork or paraffin, and then coated with the latter substance. The cube is then fixed to the microtome stage.

Here is our procedure: The surface of the tissue slab is first dehydrated in 95° or absolute alcohol for five to twenty minutes, after which it is dried with blotting paper and transferred to the paraffin cube. We then insert a hot scalpel briefly between the tissue slab and the paraffin cube, thus melting its upper surface and resulting in the attachment of the specimen to the underlying paraffin cube. Needless to say, this procedure must be carried out very quickly, in order to avoid excessive desiccation of the specimen. The tissue is then dipped in 95% alcohol and fixed to the microtome stage; the knife edge must be repeatedly wetted with alcohol during sectioning.

4. The sections are dehydrated in three or four baths of 96° alcohol; dehydration should not take more than half an hour, otherwise the finest fibrils may be decolorized by the alcohol.
5. Once dehydrated, the sections are clarified for two to five minutes in oil of cloves and then mounted on glass slides.
6. The sections are then wiped gently with filter paper and the remaining oil of cloves removed with xylene (two or three changes are needed).
7. Excess xylene is drained off by placing the glass slide in a vertical position and covering the sections using d'Ammar resin without a coverslip. The resin is allowed to dry with the slide placed horizontally and protected from dust. After ten to fifteen minutes, this first layer of resin, which will now be dry, should be covered with a second layer and, if necessary, a third, until the surface of the section is completely coated with the resin. (For more details, see paragraph **68**.)

It is important to emphasize that both slow desiccation of the resin and coverslipping can spoil the staining. According to Sanasca, this is due to the existence of diffusion streams that remove the silver precipitate from the impregnated neurons.

Because the preparations cannot be covered, special care is necessary when storing them to ensure that they are protected from dust and light. Unfortunately, even when appropriate precautions are taken, conservation is far from optimal: After three or four years, the background darkens and the silver chromate shows some diffusion around the impregnated cells. Nevertheless, darkening of the background can be compensated for optically by using a more powerful illumination with the microscope. Thus, the preparation may still be useful, though perhaps not as beautiful and limpid as when first mounted. As a general rule, the thicker a section is, the sooner it will turn dark; sections of medium thickness (80–100 micrometers) will remain completely unaltered for six or more years.

N. Holmgrem mounts the sections on coverslips: Once the mounting medium is dry, the shorter borders of the coverslip are glued to toothpicks, which are then glued onto a glass slide. This ingenious trick is a modification of Golgi's classic procedure using a fenestrated wooden or glass slide. Both techniques, however, render very fragile preparations, although those mounted by Golgi's procedure are less prone to breakage, because the entire perimeter of the coverslip is attached to the slide. Furthermore, this last procedure allows us to examine the section with the microscope on both sides; such an advantage may be critical when studying very thick sections.

Finally, let us mention that one of us (Cajal) uses glass slides with a large hole in them in order to mount Golgi-impregnated sections. This is easy and effective because unlike the wooden slides used by Golgi (*EN 15*), the glass slides do not bend.

Poljak has recently recommended placing coverslips over Golgi-impregnated sections once the resin has hardened. The way to do this is as follows: Arrange the sections on the glass slide, cover them with a thin resin solution as usual, and place the slides in the oven (40°C) for two or three days. When the resin is dry, spread a thick solution of balsam over it, warm the slide until the balsam becomes more fluid, and cover with the coverslip. According to Poljak, this method allows for a good conservation of the preparations. It also is easier to remove the cedarwood oil after studying the specimens under an oil immersion objective. Poljak adds that sections mounted in this way were still unaltered after one year. Nevertheless, some of the preparations mounted in the classic way by one of us (Cajal) remain unaltered after as many as thirty years (*EN 16*). As previously stated, the main rules to achieve a good conservation of the impregnation are: (a) rinse thoroughly in alcohol; (b) remove the oil of cloves completely; (c) cover the sections with a layer of resin as thin as possible; and (d) keep the slides protected from dust and in a cool place, especially in summer.

Several procedures are known to make Golgi impregnations indelible, such as Greppin's with hydrobromic acid and Obregia's with gold chloride. These methods preserve the staining of the somata and thick dendritic branches but the delicate fibrils are more or less (or even completely) bleached.

74. Cajal's double impregnation procedure.

1. Follow Steps 1 and 2 of the rapid Golgi method (**73**). Remove the pieces from the silver solution, wipe them with filter paper,[2] and immerse them for one or two days in a solution made of:

Potash bichromate	6–7 g
Distilled water	100 cc
1 per 100 osmic acid	30–35 cc

The volume of osmic acid may be reduced if the specimens become too brittle. The osmium-bichromate mixture used for the first induration may still be useful, providing it contains enough osmic acid. If not, some drops of 1 per 100 osmic acid can be added.

2. Wipe the pieces gently and immerse them for twenty-four hours in 0.50–0.75 per 100 silver nitrate, as in the first impregnation. Follow the rapid Golgi method from Step 3 onward.

With successful impregnation, the nerve cells and fibers are clearly stained against a pale yellow background. The perikarya and thick dendrites are stained black, the cylinder-axes brown or reddish-brown and their finer collaterals yellow to red. Glial cells are either deep red or black.

The biggest advantage of the Golgi method is its ability to impregnate just a few cells so clearly that they look as if they had been painted. Furthermore, the background is very transparent, which can be of great help in the microscopic examination of very thick sections, because the processes of a given cell can be traced for quite long distances. When the cell body has a small volume of cytoplasm the nucleus is visible and is a coffee color, surrounded by a narrow rim of black cytoplasm.

Finally, it should be pointed out that the silver chromate is not located on the cell surface, as proposed by Sehrwald and Rossbach, but inside the protoplasm.

75. Rules for using the rapid silver chromate method. To complete the technical details given above, we offer guidelines for the use of Golgi's method, which, if followed exactly, will prevent fruitless trial and error.

1. The rapid Golgi method gives consistent results in almost-myelinated nervous centers. If the animal is too young or the myelination is complete, the impregnations are very variable.
2. It must be kept in mind that all nerve centers are not equally well impregnated.

Based on numerous trials, we classified the nerve centers according to the constancy of their impregnation. The specimens that are more consistently stained and are, therefore, the best choice for beginners are:

(A) *Ammon's horn* from eight- to fifteen-day-old rabbits, *brains* of fifteen- to twenty-day-old rabbits or cats, and the *spinal cord* from chick embryos of five to fourteen days incubation. Good impregnations of other organs also can be achieved by determining the ideal volume of the fixative and the extent of the induration period. We shall discuss now some details of the *cerebral cortex*.

The optimal age of the animal for the best results depends on the species. For *mice*, it is between eight and thirty days. In the early postnatal period, the neurons are so immature that it is not possible to obtain good impregnations. For *rabbits*, it is between ten and twenty days. Gyrencephalic mammals must be used twenty-five or thirty days after birth. The neurons of mouse, rat, and rabbit embryos are stained rather unpredictably, but epithelial cells, blood vessels, and nerve fibers are readily stained, providing that the induration does not exceed two or three days.

The extent of the induration period not only depends on the animal species, but also on which elements of the nervous tissue are to be impregnated. Hence, cells of the molecular layer of the rabbit, cat, and human require five to six days, whereas the collateral fibers in the white matter need six to seven days induration.

When the aim of the study is the most superficial portion of the brain, care must be taken to avoid the deposition of silver chromate crystals on the surface of the specimens. This can be accomplished by retaining the *pia mater* or by covering the piece with a thin layer of gelatin or blood from the same animal. This procedure also gives good results for the impregnation of nerve fibers of the heart and retina of small mammals (Cajal).

(B) The *olfactory bulb* of young rabbits and dogs, as well as the *cerebellum* of young mammals (eight-day-old guinea pigs and one-month-old rats and rabbits) also can be used, but the results obtained are more variable than those discussed above.

(C) The *sympathetic ganglia, olfactory mucous, sympathetic* and *auditory endings,* and the *retina* are rather difficult to stain.

The main problem when impregnating the deep layers of the retina is the accumulation of silver chromate crystals on its surface. This can be solved by coating the retina with either a thin layer of celloidin or thin fresh tissues, such as peritoneum, prior to immersion in the silver nitrate bath.

The easiest and most reliable procedure, however, is that named by Cajal as the *rolling method*. After removing the vitreous humor, the retina must be sectioned around the optic papilla. The choroid is then carefully separated with a fine brush and the retina gently rolled up. This will produce a firm, multilayered cylinder, which is coated with 2% celloidin to prevent it from unrolling. As soon as the celloidin is dry, the specimen is immersed in the osmium-bichromic bath. The rolled-up retina is indurated and sectioned as a compact mass. Microscopically, the retina appears sectioned in all directions, parallel, perpendicular, and oblique. If these precautions are taken, silver precipitates will occur only on the outer layer of the cylinder. An additional advantage is that excess induration is avoided due to the increased thickness of the piece. In fact, irrespective of the length of induration, some portions of the specimen will always show the right degree of induration. Using this ingenious method, Cajal discovered the nerve fibers of the *outer plexiform layer*, the origin of the

Chapter 9: Golgi's Procedures

optic nerve fibers, the *neuroglial elements* in the optic fiber layer, the dendritic arbors of *ganglion cells* and *spongioblasts* (*EN 17*). Needless to say, this procedure can be used with double and triple impregnations.

This method is especially valuable in mammals, although it also works in other vertebrates. In medium-sized retinas (e.g., rabbit, dog), a single cylinder suffices; in large mammals (e.g., horse, bull, lamb), the retina is cut into two or three pieces to avoid incomplete impregnations of the innermost portions of the cylinder.

3. Regardless of the age of the animal, the choice of the animal species is an important issue. The size of the organ, its spatial relationship with other organs and some as yet unknown chemical properties, can either favor or hamper the impregnation. For instance, retinae from birds and large reptiles stain better than those from batrachians, fish, and mammals.[3]

The cerebral cortex of eight-day-old rabbits stains better than that of rats, guinea pigs, mice, or dogs of an equivalent developmental stage. The spinal cord in chicks has more affinity for the silver chromate than that of reptile and mammal embryos. The optical lobe of birds stains better than the **quadrigeminal tubercles**.

4. Early developmental stages need shorter induration periods than later ones. For example, for the spinal cord of chick embryos of five to six days incubation, twenty-four hours of induration is sufficient, but if the embryo is fourteen to –fifteen days old, a three-day induration is necessary to obtain good impregnations. The cerebellum of the newborn rabbit will be properly fixed after twenty-four hours in the osmium-bichromate mixture, but this period must be prolonged for up to two or three days in a one-month-old animal.
5. The irregular precipitates of silver chromate that often appear on the surface of the pieces can be avoided if the specimen is covered with a small portion of the surrounding tissues; for example, the early chick embryo spinal cord can be immersed in the fixative while still attached to the spine.
6. The sections obtained from *underindurated* specimens show an even red background with incompletely impregnated cells and fibers. *Overinduration,* however, results in sections with a pale yellow background and no stained cells, though some fibers may be revealed.
7. *Slight overinduration* can be recognized when fibers are stained but there are no identifiable cells. This problem can be solved with a second or even a third impregnation, as is common practice when studying the sympathetic ganglia, retina, gut plexuses, auditory nerve endings, etc.
8. Many variables have to be determined by trial and error when the Golgi method is applied to a given area of the nervous system, the most important of these being the induration time. In order to establish the optimal induration period, all the other parameters are maintained while the length of induration is varied. We usually cut several slices of the material to be studied and apply a different induration period to each one (e.g., twenty-four, thirty-six, or forty-eight hours; three days or four days, etc.). The overindurated specimens are impregnated two or even

three times. In this way, adjustments can be made promptly. Nevertheless, it is necessary to bear in mind that the success of the method depends mainly on the experience and perseverance of the person performing it. The beginner should not expect brilliant results in material difficult to impregnate until he has had several weeks of careful practice. This is true of the gold chloride method, which is hard and inconstant for the novice and yet has proved an easy and reliable method for some experienced workers, such as Ranvier, Loewitt, Retzius, Golgi, and Ruffini.

Before the beginner becomes discouraged and discards the Golgi method, he should bear two important things in mind: Firstly, silver chromate initially stains only a few neurons in a given section, but after several months of perseverance a splendid coloration of the most elusive cells will unexpectedly appear. Secondly, any research carried out with the Golgi method requires a large number of preparations so that the fragmentary data contained in each of them can be assembled coherently to obtain a complete picture of the organization and neuronal types of the region analyzed. Furthermore, it must be kept in mind that the only way of being sure that a new histological finding is not an artifact is to show it repeatedly in different sections. As a matter of fact, most of the criticism that several authors have made about the silver chromate method is due to their lack of expertise with this procedure; only after having examined a fairly large number of slides is it possible to distinguish the sharply stained neuronal processes from random precipitates.

To avoid misinterpretations, a comparison of the results of the Golgi stain with those of other methods (Weigert-Pal, Ehrlich, Nissl, or the neurofibrillary ones) from the same area of the nervous system is recommended. Slides stained by Nissl-type techniques are most useful as a complement of the silver chromate procedure, because they allow a precise assessment of the topography of the impregnated cells and of the characteristics of their neighboring elements; furthermore, these aniline methods can be used to ascertain which neurons have not been impregnated, thus indicating that our Golgi study is not complete and that new trials are necessary.

76. Combined method. This procedure is not very popular with neurologists. It combines some of the advantages of the *slow* and *rapid procedures*, thus making it possible to stain some neurons and nerve fibers that do not show up when only one of the procedures is used. Here is the modus operandi:

1. Indurate small fragments of nervous tissue two to four days at 20°–26°C in 2.5–3 per 100 potash bichromate.
2. Immerse the pieces without rinsing for three to five days in the osmium-bichromate mixture (**9**) at 25°C.
3. Rinse the specimens briefly with either water or a weak silver solution and impregnate them in a 0.75 per 100 silver nitrate solution during twenty-four to thirty-six hours.
4. Section and mount as usual for the rapid Golgi method.

Cajal demonstrated that the *combined method* is better than either the *rapid* or *slow* techniques alone for staining the short-axon neurons of the human cerebral cortex. This method helped him analyze the many classes of cells with short, profusely branched axons in the cortical projection areas of human, dog, and cat brains.

77. Rapid indirect silver chromate method. This method was originally developed by Golgi for the demonstration of the neuron reticular apparatus; however, as Pensa and one of us (de Castro) have proved, it also renders good results in the visualization of nerve endings in some glands. Basically, the technique consists of overindurating the pieces in the osmium-bichromate mixture and subsequently subjecting them to the action of a copper acetate or sulfate bath. This "refreshing step," as termed by Golgi, is necessary to stain the nerve cells and fibers.

The details of the procedure are as follows:

1. Fix the pieces for eight to fifteen days in osmium-bichromate mixture (**9**).
2. Immerse the blocks in a solution of equal parts of 2–3 per 100 potash bichromate and 4–5 per 100 copper sulfate. The time needed for this step depends on the degree of overinduration of the specimens, but the type of tissue and the age of the animal must also be taken into account. As a general rule, twelve to twenty-four hours in the bichromate-copper liquid should be enough for pieces indurated for eight to ten days. The refreshing action is sped up by increasing the amount of copper sulfate. When the specimens have been kept for a long time in the osmic acid mixture, they must be treated with plain copper sulfate solution and then reindurated in potash bichromate or in a osmium-bichromate mixture.
3. Transfer the pieces directly to 0.75 per 100 silver nitrate for twenty-four to thirty-six hours.
4. Dehydrate, section, and mount as for the rapid method.

78. Juschtschenko's modification of the silver chromate method. This author added osmic acid to the silver bath in order to stain the sympathetic ganglion cells. The procedure is as follows:

1. Fix very small fragments of sympathetic ganglia for one to seven days in the osmium-bichromate mixture.
2. Briefly rinse the pieces with distilled water and wipe them with filter paper.
3. Immerse the specimens for two or three days in the following osmium and silver solution:

Silver nitrate	2–3 g
Distilled water	5–75 cc
1 per 100 osmic acid[4]	25–50 cc

4. Section, mount, etc., as usual.

The results of this procedure depend on the extent of the fixation period: The dendrites and perikarya of ganglion cells appear after short fixations (two to three days), whereas axons require a fixation of five to seven days.

The greatest disadvantage of Juschtschenko's procedure, apart from its elevated cost due to the use of large amounts of osmium, is the formation of large precipitates within the tissue due to the high concentration of silver nitrate. Furthermore, the addition of osmic acid to the silver bath reduces the low penetration of the silver even more. This is especially noticeable when trying to use the method on samples of the central nervous system when the central portion of the block is barely stained even with minute pieces. Nevertheless, Juschtschenko's method reveals some elements that otherwise require a double impregnation (**74**). Using this technique, one of us (de Castro) has been able to stain the sympathetic nerve endings in the intestines, pancreas, and salivary glands. He did, however, use a lower concentration of silver nitrate than in the original procedure (1 per 100) in order to avoid precipitate formation. The specimens of nervous tissue must not remain in the osmium-silver solution for more than two or three days. If a longer storage time is necessary, they must be transferred to a plain 0.50 to 0.75 per 100 silver nitrate solution.

79. Timofejew's modification of the Golgi method. This author suggests using the following variation to stain the nerve endings of the male genitalia.

1. Immerse tissue fragments of 1cm in length for six to seven days at 25°C in:

    5 per 100 potash bichromate   2 parts
    1 per 100 osmic acid   1 part

2. Impregnate for two or three days in a 400 cc solution consisting of 1 per 100 silver nitrate solution to which has been added 1 drop of formic acid (CH_2O_2) and some grains of sodium sulfate (Na_2SO_4).

Lawrentjew obtained pleasing results using this formula to stain the nerve endings and ganglia of the female urethra.

80. Replacing the osmic acid with formalin in the Golgi procedure. Several authors have proposed replacing osmic acid with formalin in the rapid Golgi method (Kopsch, Strong, During, Lachi, Kenyon, Sánchez y Sánchez, Fich, etc.). The formulae recommended by these authors differ in the bichromate concentration and in the volume of formalin, but none of these variations render such clear and delicate impregnations as those obtained when using the osmium-bichromate mixture.

The formalin-bichromate procedures are recommended for the study of the central nervous system of adult and young vertebrates. They usually fail in embryos, however, because the fixatives used are unable to harden the specimens properly. These methods render better results in invertebrates, showing the neural arborizations nicely, although the perikarya seem to be difficult to impregnate. Nevertheless, good staining of the somata is sometimes obtained in crustaceans and insects (Kenyon, Sánchez, and Cajal).

81. Kopsch's formula. Immediately before use prepare a mixture of:

3.5 per 100 potash bichromate   40 cc
Formalin   10 cc

Cut thin slices of tissue and place them for twenty-four hours in a large volume of this liquid; use about 50 cc for three to four fragments, always thinner

Chapter 9: Golgi's Procedures

than 5 mm. If larger pieces are used, the fixative must be replaced after the first twelve hours.

Once the fixation period is over, immerse the specimens for two to six days in 3.5 per 100 potash bichromate; impregnate in 0.75 per 100 silver nitrate as in the regular Golgi method.

82. Strong's formula. The fixative is made of:

3.5 per 100 potash bichromate   100 vols.
Formalin   2.5–5 cc

The nervous organs must be indurated for several days in this liquid then transferred to 1 per 100 silver nitrate. The author also suggests removing the pieces from the fixative after one or two days and immersing them for twelve to twenty-four hours in:

3.5 per 100 potash bichromate   2 parts
Formalin   1 part

The pieces are then directly placed in the silver bath.[5]

83. During's formula. This author proposes a double impregnation procedure.

Nervous tissue fragments thinner than 5 mm are immersed for three days in a liquid made of equal parts of 3 per 100 potash bichromate and 6 per 100 formalin. The pieces are then blotted with filter paper and impregnated in 0.75 per 100 silver nitrate. Afterward they are returned to the formalin–bichromate mixture for two days and reimpregnated in the silver nitrate solution to which one drop of formic acid has been added.

84. Sánchez's formula for invertebrates.

1. Fix thin slices for three to five days in:

   3–5 per 100 potash bichromate   50–100 cc
   Formalin   5–10 cc

   Renew the fixative every twelve hours.
2. Rinse with 0.5 per 100 silver nitrate for about one minute.
3. Immerse the pieces for two or three days in 0.75 per 100 silver nitrate.
4. Repeat Steps 1 and 2.
5. Dehydrate in absolute alcohol, embed in celloidin, cut sections, and mount them without a coverslip.

85. Golgi's method with mercuric bichloride. This method has two steps, similar to the silver chromate procedure: the pieces are first indurated in potassium bichromate and then impregnated in mercuric bichloride. This last reagent is reduced into metallic mercury that precipitates on some nerve cells and fibers. As previously stated, the stained elements appear black when observed against a bright field but have a grayish tinge under reflected light.

Below is the *modus faciendi*, including the last modifications introduced by Golgi.

1. Indurate fresh brain tissue fragments in 2–3 per 100 potash bichromate. The fixation period ranges from three to four weeks to several months. It is advisable not to use very thick pieces, but if the specimens are large, Golgi recommends injecting the fixative prior to immersion in order to obtain an even distribution of the reagent inside the tissue.
2. Immerse the specimens in 0.5–1 per 100 mercuric bichloride. Because the sublimate diffuses very slowly inside the tissue, this step takes between eight days and two months, depending on the thickness of the slab. The liquid must be replaced several times.
3. Dehydrate for twenty minutes in 96% alcohol and embed in celloidin; superficial paraffin embedding also can be used. Cut the sections the same thickness as in the silver chromate method.
4. Rinse the sections with distilled water and immerse them for several minutes in 5 per 100 sodium *hyposulfite* or bisulfite. The photographic toners and developers, such as the following ones render the best results:

Water	500 cc
Sodium hyposulfite	125 g
Ammonium sulfocyanide	10 cc
Alum	5 cc
1 per 100 gold chloride	20 cc
Lead acetate	5 g

5. Rinse again in distilled water, dehydrate, clarify, and mount in d'Ammar resin as in the silver chromate methods.

86. Cox's method. This author has improved the previous method and used it successfully to study the brain cortex. Cajal has obtained magnificent results with this technique in his analysis of the cerebellum and Ammon's horn, confirming and completing the data obtained with the silver chromate.

Here is the modus operandi:

1. Immerse fresh, thin fragments of nervous tissue in the following liquid:

5 per 100 potash bichromate	20 cc
5 per 100 mercuric bichloride	20 cc
Distilled water	30–40 cc
Strongly alkaline, 5 per 100 potash chromate	16 cc

The specimens must be fixed in this mixture for at least one month in summer and two or three months in winter. Large specimens and whole brains of adult rabbit, cat, monkey, etc. need at least six months induration.

2. Rinse the pieces for one hour in 90° alcohol in order to remove the excess of sublimate that precipitates as crystalline needles.
3. Cut sections as for the silver chromate method; rapid celloidin embedding can be used in some cases.
4. Rinse the sections thoroughly with water.
5. Immerse the sections in an alkaline solution until they become dark brown or black; 5 per 100 solutions of sodium hydroxide, potash, sodium carbonate, soda bisulfite or *soda hyposulfite* can be used for this purpose. One of us (Cajal) adds a few drops of 40 per 100 soda or potash to a porcelain well full of water. Sometimes we dissolve a few crystals of soda hyposulfite directly in the well, thus obtaining a 5–10 per 100 solution. Cajal, however, prefers to darken the sections in a saturated solution of sodium sulfite because it is less aggressive.
6. Rinse with a large volume of water for some minutes in order to remove excess alkali.
7. Rinse thoroughly with alcohol to remove any remaining sublimate, clarify with oil of cloves and xylene, and mount without a coverslip using either d'Ammar resin or the sandarac varnish recommended by Cox. The composition of this mounting medium is:

Sandarac (*EN 18*)	75 g
Camphor	15 cc
Pure turpentine essence	30 cc
Lavender essence	22.5 cc
Absolute alcohol	75 cc
Castor oil	5–10 drops

The last rinse with alcohol is indispensable to remove any trace of sublimate that might later precipitate as crystalline rods. Mounting in sandarac resin can be carried out after immersing the sections in an essence and it does not require clarifying in xylene. Embedded in sandarac, the sections can be preserved for a long time and are both more transparent and less prone to cracking than those mounted with d'Ammar resin.

Cox's technique, like the silver chromate method, renders better results in young animals than in old ones. In young animals, the full length of the axon and its collaterals are shown, and this technique enables impregnation of many short axon cells that are not revealed by the standard Golgi method. In a similar way to the silver chromate method, this technique in adult animals reveals only the perikarya and the dendritic arbors and the axonal impregnation is restricted to the short, unmyelinated initial segment. Our best preparations with Cox's procedure have been obtained from the cerebral cortex, cerebellum, and Ammon's horn of rabbit, cat, and dog sacrificed twenty to thirty days after birth. The sections usually show a large number of neurons that are stained gray to black against a pale yellow or colorless background and superficial precipitates are almost nonexistent. Very good results also can be obtained after impregnating the brain of small mammals *in toto*, such as newborn guinea pigs or one-month-old mice and rats. An additional advantage is the possibility of counterstaining the nuclei with hematoxylin or Grenacher's carmine.

Cox's method is frequently used to confirm the findings made with Golgi's technique. The former is better for the study of neuronal somata or thick fibers, while the fine collaterals and the delicate terminal branches of the axonal arborizations are better demonstrated by the latter.

10

Continuation of the Methods for Demonstrating the Morphology of Neurons

EHRLICH'S METHYLENE BLUE AND ITS VARIATIONS (*EN 19*)

87. In 1885, Ehrlich developed one of the most useful neurological techniques: a procedure based on the use of methylene blue, which reveals neuron morphology, especially the terminal arborizations of the cylinder-axes of the peripheral nervous system.

The method consists of the injection of a solution of methylene blue dissolved in saline into the circulatory system of a living or newly sacrificed animal. After a short time, thin slices of brain tissue are dissected and exposed to the atmosphere when they become an intense blue color. Ehrlich discovered that nerve cells are specifically stained only when the reaction takes place in an alkaline medium and the tissues are then saturated with oxygen. Aronson has suggested a satisfactory explanation for this: Reducing agents are formed in the tissues immediately after death, some of which are capable of inserting two hydrogen atoms in the methylene blue molecule transforming it into a colorless base. If this methylene blue leukobase is subjected to a powerful oxidant, such as atmospheric oxygen, it recuperates its original blue color, thus revealing the cells that previously had metabolized the dye. In the living animal, the tissues are fully oxygenated and the reduction of methylene blue does not take place, although it happens immediately after death. This is the reason why Dogiel advises against using methylene blue as a vital stain *stricto sensu*; after innumerable trials this author has concluded that the best results are obtained when the dye is injected into the animal immediately after it has been bled. It must be borne in mind that methylene blue is a very neurotropic substance with a high affinity for nervous cells that become more intensely stained than cells from other tissues.

Finally, we should add that the Ehrlich-Dogiel method has the disadvantage of staining only neurons located in the superficial areas of the block; deeper regions are poorly oxygenated and are colorless or only very faintly stained. Nevertheless, the reaction can take place in the absence of air, as in the case of Meyer's variation, discussed below. To differentiate between both types of reactions, Cajal calls the Ehrlich-Dogiel method *aerobic* and Meyer's reaction *anaerobic*.

88. There are several types of methylene blue that can be used for staining the nervous system; the more recommendable ones are the Methylene Blue B.X. (*Methylenblau nach S. Meyer*) and the Ehrlich's Methylene Blue (*Methylenblau rectif. nach Ehrlich*), both sold by Grübler from Leipzig.

The dye must be dissolved in saline (0.75–0.80 per 100 sodium chloride in distilled water). Usually, as proposed by Dogiel, a 1 per 100 stock solution is prepared, which is further diluted for use to a fourth, a sixth, an eighth, etc., in saline (*EN 20*). The solutions must be warmed prior to use in order to dissolve the methylene blue precipitate that is formed at the bottom of the flask. They must be injected at a temperature of 37°–38°C.

All the methylene blue solutions must be kept in very clean, neutral glass flasks (*EN 21*); Dogiel recommends filling the vessels with either hydrochloric or nitric acid, then washing them with plenty of water and rinsing them successively with alcohol, distilled water, and saline. Methylene blue also can be dissolved in Ringer-Locke's or Tyrode's liquids and even in the animal's own blood serum, although such solutions do not give better results than plain saline and are troublesome to prepare and actually rather unstable. Nevertheless, one of us (de Castro) has found some improvement in the results after the addition of Cl_2Ca to the solution of methylene blue in saline; just enough should be added to make the solution slightly hypertonic. It seems that calcium helps to prevent the swelling of dendrites and axons produced by the harmful action of sodium and oxygen.

The procedures to stain neurons with methylene blue are: (a) vascular injection; (b) lubrication; (c) dye diffusion; and (d) in vivo subcutaneous injection.

89. Intravascular injection procedure. Ehrlich's original method for staining both the central and peripheral nervous tissue is described below, including some modifications introduced by Cajal and Dogiel.

1. The animal is sacrificed and bled. Immediately afterward, the circulatory system is rinsed with saline at 37°C. A half to a quarter methylene blue solution (or a quarter to a sixth according to Dogiel), previously warmed to the body temperature of the animal (or at room temperature for cold-blooded animals) is then injected into the main artery of the organ to be studied. It is important fill the blood vessels (including capillaries) as completely as possible; consequently, large volumes of dye must be used and should be administered in two or three injections at five- to ten-minute intervals.

2. Twenty or thirty minutes after the last injection, the organ is removed thus: (a) if the organ is very tiny and thin it must be placed in a Petri dish and sprinkled from time to time with a sixth to an eighth methylene blue solution. The dish should be covered to avoid desiccation and kept at 37° or at room temperature. (Keeping the tissues at a temperature close to the animal's own does not seem to offer any advantage over carrying out the process at room temperature.); (b) If the organ is large it should be carefully cut into 2–3 mm sections using a straight sharp razor blade. The sections are then placed for thirty to ninety minutes in a Petri dish,

Chapter 10: Morphology of Neurons

preferably with cotton or glass wool placed in the base so that the tissues are kept moist by (but not soaked in) the staining liquid. The dish is kept either in the oven or at room temperature.

3. Once the organs turn a deep blue color after thirty or ninety minutes, the oxygenation step is complete. The organs must then be transferred to the fixative. During oxygenation and until the color reappears, the tissues are moistened every ten or fifteen minutes with weak methylene blue solutions, to avoid desiccation. The sections are dipped either in saline or in very diluted methylene blue solutions and treated by any of the methods for stabilizing the methylene blue staining, such as the ammonium picrate (**94**), or molybdate (**95**), or the combined picrate–molybdate procedure (**99**).

90. Methylene blue staining is much more variable in the cerebral cortex than in the peripheral nerve endings. Nevertheless, according to Cajal, good results can be obtained in the cerebral cortex, especially in its *molecular layer*, if the following rules are observed (*EN 22*):

1. Intravascular injection of methylene blue must be performed immediately after death. This technique may not be sufficient to stain the whole cell; usually only the myelinated fibers of the molecular layer and the terminal apical dendrites of the pyramidal cells are shown.
2. The lubrication procedure (**91**) is necessary for the demonstration of short axon neurons in the molecular layer. The brain must be exposed, cut into large blocks, placed in a moist chamber and put into the oven. There, using a thin brush, the molecular layer is painted with methylene blue every ten or twelve minutes. During this procedure, the pia mater must not be peeled off.
3. After ninety minutes, once the tissue has acquired a deep blue color, it is immersed in the fixative. If ammonium picrate is used, this step must last only four to six hours, in order to prevent the softening of the brain. Afterward, the specimens are immersed in ammonium molybdate and formalin (**99**).
4. The more intensely stained areas must be selected for sectioning, because these are where the Cajal's cells (*EN 23*) and the short axon neurons have the best coloration. Remove the pia and cut thick, tangential sections by hand.
5. Dehydrate in absolute alcohol, clarify in bergamot and xylene, and mount in d'Ammar resin or in neutral Canada balsam without a coverslip. The staining never extends beyond the inferior limit of the molecular layer; therefore, pyramidal cells are not shown.

91. Direct staining by lubrication. This procedure was developed by Dogiel for the demonstration of the gut nerve plexuses and ganglia. The main steps are as follows:

1. Remove the organs to be studied from a newly sacrificed animal and, if necessary, cut them into 1–2 mm thick sections with a razor blade. If the specimen either contains muscle tissue or is very small, as is the case with

the gut, skeletal muscles, bladder, etc., the sections must be spread over a cork sheet and fixed to it either with pins or quills. The samples are then placed in a Petri dish with some cotton in the bottom, and moistened every ten to fifteen minutes with a half to a tenth methylene blue (**88**) applied with a fine paint brush. The staining procedure must be carried out at 37°C in a moist chamber.
2. Staining is completed when the pieces become deep blue (one to two hours); if the organ is transparent or the slices are very thin, the process must be carried out with the aid of a microscope. When the desired degree of staining has been achieved, the pieces are briefly rinsed with saline and fixed either in picrate or in molybdate.

92. Dye diffusion method. Cajal[1] has proposed an anaerobic technique for staining the nervous system with methylene blue, which readily reveals the pyramidal neurons and the dendritic spines. The *modus faciendi* is as follows:

1. Immediately after the animal (a cat or a rabbit) has been sacrificed and without removing the brain from the skull or removing the pia mater, 2–3 mm thick slices of cortex are cut with a straight razor blade.
2. The cut surfaces are exposed to methylene blue either by painting them with a very fine brush soaked in a saturated solution of the dye or, preferably, by sprinkling them with methylene blue powder (the B.X. variety). The pieces of gray matter can be kept in place, covered by the top of the skull.
3. After thirty to forty-five minutes, the slices are carefully removed from the skull, briefly rinsed in saline, and transferred to Bethe's fixative (**97**) for two to three hours. Afterward, they are rinsed thoroughly with water, indurated in formalin (as proposed by Cajal), sectioned, dehydrated, clarified, and mounted without a coverslip.[1]

93. Procedure of the in vivo subcutaneous injections. Meyer has recently proposed a variation of the methylene blue method that does not require the exposure of the pieces to air. Although complete coloration of the neurons is not achieved with this procedure, it may be useful when studying the cytoarchitecture of the cerebral and cerebellar cortex. Here is the modus operandi:

1. First, 5%–6% methylene blue (Methylenblau B.X. nach S. Meyer, from Grübler) is injected subcutaneously using a Pravaz's syringe (*EN 24*). The methylene blue injection must be repeated every one or two hours until the animal is poisoned to death. It is advisable to lengthen the procedure by injecting only small volumes of methylene blue at the start, to avoid the animal having seizures and dying too soon. Small volumes must be given in each dose (e.g., 8–10 cc for rabbit, cat, and rat). For the newborn guinea pig, Meyer suggests injecting 2 cc of a saturated methylene blue solution every fifteen minutes.
2. When the animal has died, the brain is removed immediately, sectioned in small fragments, and fixed in the ammonium molybdate mixture recommended by Bethe (**96**).

Chapter 10: Morphology of Neurons

This technique stains the cells and fibers of the nervous centers intensely, although the distal dendritic branches, dendritic spines, axon collaterals, and terminal arborizations are not revealed, with the exception of Held's acoustic baskets in the nucleus of the trapezoid body. Although Meyer claims that axonal collaterals and bifurcations are stained in the brain, cerebellum, and spinal cord, our results (Cajal) do not confirm this. We do not deny that this procedure stains the thick collaterals, but it shows neither the constrictions present at the axonal branching points nor the thin unmyelinated fibers. Because of these disadvantages, this method should be regarded as less valuable than Ehrlich's procedure.

FIXATION, SECTIONING, AND MOUNTING TECHNIQUES FOR METHYLENE BLUE STAINED MATERIAL

Two substances can be used to fix the pieces colored by Ehrlich-Dogiel's supravital staining method, namely, *ammonium picrate* and *molybdate*.

94. Fixation in ammonium picrate. Dogiel recommended this chemical, which should be used in solutions that have been saturated at room temperature. It reacts with methylene blue to form a deep violet precipitate that is very soluble in water and alcohol, less so in glycerin, and almost insoluble in mixtures of glycerin and ammonium picrate.

When nerves and neurons are sufficiently stained by methylene blue, the pieces are immersed in the ammonium picrate solution for two, six, twelve, or eighteen hours, depending on their thickness and on the operations to be carried out later. The rule of thumb for thin slices is to end the fixation after two or four hours, when the tissue becomes transparent. Then complementary colorations with picrocarmine can be performed. If the myelin sheaths are to be studied, 1–2 cc of 2% osmic acid can be added to every 100 cc of picrate, as suggested by Dogiel. The indurating solution must be abundant, compared with the number of specimens to be fixed.

Once indurated and perfectly transparent, the sections are placed on a glass slide, blotted with blotting paper, and coverslipped using a 1 to 1 mixture of anhydrous glycerin and ammonium picrate as the mounting medium. In order to obtain permanent preparations, the coverslip must be cemented with paraffin, sealing wax, or Jews' pitch. Regardless of which is used, the maximum life of the preparations is one or two years. Thick or opaque slices must be teased apart by means of fine tweezers, scissors, or a razor blade.

Alternative mounting media are Apáthy's liquid (**71**) with sucrose or levulose; both must be prepared using a solution of ammonium picrate instead of water. They are prepared with 1 or 2 parts of water and 1 part of concentrated ammonium picrate solution. Apáthy has proposed that an ammonium picrate-fixed preparation can be made absolutely stable by mounting it with Canada balsam or d'Ammar resin. The method is as follows: the section is placed on a glass slide kept warm in the oven, after which a transparent gelatin solution (2 parts of gelatin and 5 parts of water, to which 2–3 drops of a saturated solution of ammonium picrate have been added) is poured onto the section. This step requires four to five minutes to allow the gelatin to penetrate the tissue. A coverslip is gently pressed upon the section and, once cold, carefully removed with the section stuck to it. After air-drying, a layer of d'Ammar resin is spread over a new glass slide onto which the section with the attached coverslip will then be placed. The tissue is thus very transparent, and the cell staining is notably stable.

95. Fixation in ammonium molybdate. This substance was proposed by Bethe as a fixative for methylene-blue-stained tissues. It reacts with the dye forming a compound that is insoluble both in water and in alcohol, thus allowing the embedding of the pieces in celloidin; furthermore, fixation in molybdate enhances the contrast of the sections, because the bright blue color of methylene blue turns darker after this step.

Ammonium molybdate can be used in various ways, which will be discussed in the following paragraphs.

96. The original Bethe's procedure, which is also used by Szymonovicz, is as follows:

1. The methylene-blue-stained pieces are immersed for four to twenty-four hours in a mixture of:

Ammonium molybdate	10 g
Distilled water	100 cc
Hydrogen peroxide	10 cc
Hydrochloric acid	X drops

The length of the fixation depends on the type of tissue and on the thickness of the piece. In all cases, however, it is advisable to carry out the fixation at 0°–2°C; thus, the flask containing the piece must either be surrounded with ice or placed in the ice-chest.

2. Once removed from the fixative, the pieces are rinsed for thirty minutes to two hours (depending on the volume of the specimens) with either distilled or tap water; the water must be replaced several times.
3. Dehydrate the pieces in ice-cold absolute alcohol for thirty minutes to six hours; dehydration should be as short as possible and the alcohol must be replaced frequently (every five, ten, and fifteen minutes at the start) to avoid using an alcohol solution with a large amount of water in it.
4. Clarify in oil of cloves or, preferably, in xylene, and mount in Canada balsam. If thin sections are needed, the material can be embedded in paraffin. Nuclear counterstaining can be performed with Grenacher's carmine (**42**) or with Czokor's cochineal (**44**).

97. Cajal recommends Bethe's fixation procedure for the brain, cerebellum, and spinal cord, but hydrogen peroxide must not be added to the fixative, as it affords no advantages.

Ammonium molybdate	10 g
Distilled water	100 cc
Hydrochloric acid	X drops

According to Cajal, fixation is accomplished in two or three hours and can be carried out at room temperature (except in summer).

Once the fixation is complete, the pieces are rinsed with water for thirty to sixty minutes (several changes) and indurated during three or four hours in the following mixture:

Formalin	40 cc
Distilled water	60 cc
1 per 100 platinum chloride	5 cc

Finally, the pieces are briefly rinsed with water, immersed for some minutes in an alcohol solution of platinum chloride (platinum chloride, 1 g; absolute alcohol, 300 cc)[2] and either embedded in paraffin or mounted and sectioned as described for the Golgi method (see **73**, Step 3). The latter procedure is advisable for small specimens, such as retina, peripheral ganglia, frog's brain, or spinal cord; large blocks (mammals' brain, skin, etc.) can be transferred to the freezing microtome directly after rinsing. The sections, which should be fairly thick (thirty–forty thousandths of a millimeter), are clarified in either xylene or in essence of bergamot and mounted in d'Ammar resin without a coverslip.

Notes: Platinum chloride has the property of rendering methylene blue almost insoluble, although it cannot be used immediately after staining because it produces coarse methylene blue precipitates. It has, however, the invaluable advantage of avoiding dye extraction by water, formalin, alcohol, glycerin, etc. In fact, the only reliable way to ensure that no stain will be lost during dehydration is to use alcohol-platinum, because even the ice-cold dehydration in plain alcohol recommended by Bethe and Meyer results in some bleaching of the sections. The last step in alcohol can be carried out using absolute ethanol, as long as it is performed quickly and at a low temperature.

In order to prevent decomposition of the platinum salt by the alcohol, the solution used must be fresh. The best way to proceed is to add two or three drops of 1% aqueous platinum chloride solution to the alcohol-filled porcelain well containing the sections. In this way, we can avoid using ice to prevent the bleaching action of alcohol, as recommended by Bethe and Mayer.

98. Dogiel has proposed a simpler technique to fix the stain with ammonium molybdate; this procedure renders similar results to the aforementioned ones but uses neither hydrochloric acid nor hydrogen peroxide. According to this author, the methylene-blue-stained pieces are fixed for six to eighteen hours in 5–8 per 100 ammonium molybdate. The ammonium molybdate solution frequently has a milky color, in which case it must be filtered before use. Large volumes of fixative must be used (100–200 cc for a 2–8 mm thick piece). Fixation time is extended for thicker specimens.

When the fixation period is over, the pieces are rinsed for one or two hours and dehydrated in absolute alcohol; dehydration must be as short as possible, because the alcohol partially removes the dye. The pieces are clarified in xylene and mounted in Canada balsam. If sectioning is necessary, the specimens are transferred from absolute alcohol to a 5–6 per 100 celloidin solution. One to three hours later, the blocks are removed from the celloidin, mounted in a piece of cork, immersed in 70° alcohol, and sectioned; if sectioning cannot be performed immediately, the specimens, still attached to the cork, can be kept for two or three days in water, as suggested by Markovitin. The sections can be counterstained with alum carmine.

One of us (de Castro) prefers to embed the molybdate-fixed specimens in paraffin rather than in celloidin; he suggests clarifying the specimens, once dehydrated, in cedarwood oil, because this agent neither alters the staining nor shrinks the tissue. Furthermore, cedarwood oil can be used to store the pieces for long periods prior to embedding; this substance is also the best mounting medium for methylene blue preparations, which then can be coverslipped without bleaching the dye. (See **69** for more details about the use of cedarwood oil as a mounting medium.)

Comments: When working on tissues that are prone to retraction, such as muscle, tendons, intestines, stomach, or bladder, it is advisable to extend and pin the specimen onto a piece of cork or cardboard prior to fixation. Needles or sea urchin spikes can be used for this purpose. After removing the pieces from the alcohol, they are detached from the cork or cardboard sheet and transferred to a final absolute alcohol bath. From this step onward, the procedure continues as usual.

For the purpose of staining the myelin sheath, Dogiel suggests immersing the methylene-blue-stained pieces in a mixture of osmic acid and ammonium molybdate:

5–8 per 100 ammonium molybdate	20 cc
1 per 100 osmic acid	1–5 cc

The specimens must stay in this reagent for fifteen to thirty minutes, until they turn dark.

99. Combined fixation with picrate and molybdate. This procedure has been proposed by Cajal, and also is recommended by Bethe, Dogiel, and Smirnow. Cajal's *modus faciendi* is as follows:

The pieces, once colored, are immersed for less than six hours in a saturated solution of ammonium picrate; they are then blotted with filter paper, and, without rinsing, placed for six to twelve hours in Bethe's fixative (**96**) that has been previously saturated with methylene blue. Finally, the specimens are rinsed with tap water for one to one and a half hours to remove the excess of molybdate then indurated for twelve hours in the following mixture:

Formalin	40 cc
Distilled water	60 cc
Saturated solution of ammonium picrate	20 cc

Some drops of platinum chloride also can be added to this liquid to enhance fixation and to prevent practically any bleaching of the dye. Fixation also can be achieved with absolute alcohol, but in this case Bethe advises carrying it out at 0°C and adding methylene blue and molybdate to saturation to the alcohol, otherwise some decoloration can be expected. We prefer formalin to alcohol, however, because the former produces a more complete induration.

Once fixation is complete, the specimens are dipped in the aforementioned saturated solution of molybdate and methylene blue in absolute alcohol then blotted with filter paper. They then are mounted on paraffin blocks and sectioned (see more details about this sectioning procedure in **73**, Step 3); the sections are mounted in d'Ammar resin without coverslipping, after being dehydrated in absolute alcohol, and clarified in either xylene or bergamot. Mounting the sections without a coverslip allows the preparation to be examined microscopically under oil, regardless of its thickness. Furthermore, staining seems more stable in this preparation than in preparations that are coverslipped and mounted with balsam.

100. Rules for the use of methylene blue for impregnating central nervous system cells. (*EN 25*) There are three main procedures for staining cells of the central nervous system with methylene blue: (1) by means of in vivo subcutaneous injections (Meyer's method) that produce very pale neurons unsuitable for the study of the cellular expansions; (2) by Ehrlich-Dogiel's method, which involves the lubrication of exposed specimens with a tenth of a gram per cent methylene blue solution; (3) using Cajal's diffusion method, in which the action of the air on the dye is not necessary. In this method, the stain, either powdered or in a saturated solution, is deposited on the surfaces of blocks of nervous tissue, not thicker than two or three millimeters.

The results obtained with each one of these methods are notably different. *Dogiel's method* (**90**) only colors the superficial cells of the cerebral and cerebellar cortices. Thus, in the avian and mammalian cerebellum, it is common to visualize the small stellate cells of the molecular layer that show strongly varicose dendrites.[3] From time to time, a parallel fiber is also stained. In the mammalian cerebral cortex, the somata and proximal dendrites of multipolar cells are stained; occasionally a Golgi cell or a polymorph neuron also can be observed. The pyramidal cells are seldom demonstrated; on these rare occasions, the staining is incomplete. In the olfactory bulb, only some olfactory fibers can be seen, although a tufted peripheral fiber sometimes can be stained. In the medulla and spinal cord, it is possible to impregnate the fibers of the white matter and their collaterals regularly, but dendritic spines are never shown.

Cajal's dye diffusion method (**92**) yields better results than the previous one for the study of cells located in deep layers. Regrettably, this procedure is rather variable and numerous trials are necessary to obtain deeply and completely stained cortical pyramids.

The most beautiful and demonstrative results are obtained in the brain. When thin slices of cortex are painted on both sides with the stain, the undersurface of the section is decorated with blue patches formed by groups of strongly stained pyramidal cells. All the morphological details revealed by the silver chromate method are then demonstrated in these preparations.

After numerous trials, we have come to believe that the best procedure for coloring the nervous centers with methylene blue is the *Ehrlich original intravascular injection method*. It is the most reliable of the methylene blue techniques and can be used on almost any kind of material. The basis of this procedure is to inject methylene blue concentrated solutions repeatedly until the nervous centers are intensely colored. Then the blocks are hand cut into large slices that are exposed to the air in an oven for forty-five minutes to two hours.

The time of exposition of the pieces to air will depend on the results desired; dendrites and unmyelinated fibers are stained after just thirty or forty-five minutes of exposure to oxygen, whereas one or two hours are needed to stain the myelinated fibers with their bifurcations and collaterals. Oxygenation is readily achieved in the stationary atmosphere inside the oven, albeit sometimes it may be useful to use a humid air current such as that produced by the ***Roux's apparatus***.

For this method to succeed, it is most important to control the concentration of the methylene blue solution. Practice has convinced us (Cajal) that the only way to avoid having to paint the pieces directly with the dye (Dogiel's method, **91**) is to use *room temperature saturated solutions of methylene blue*. This reagent must be injected into the aorta or into the carotid artery at a high enough pressure to render the nervous centers an intense blue color. Because special care must be taken to avoid the rupture of the blood vessels, we usually make two or three injections, leaving a short interval (some minutes) between them; in this way, the dye delivered in one injection has enough time to diffuse before a new volume of reagent is administered. Nevertheless, the injection must be performed carefully, because the chemistry of the cell can be altered so rapidly as to make the Ehrlich reaction impossible. Besides, an excess of the dye in the nervous tissue always results in the formation of crystalline precipitates in the presence of the fixative. Thus, optimal conditions can be determined only by trial and error, because they change with the age and species of the animal. Generally speaking, a medium-intensity blue coloration of the tongue and the conjunctiva indicates that the nervous centers have received a suitable dose of methylene blue to produce a nice staining.

Because the reagent is rapidly reduced within the gray matter, when the skull is opened it is common that the brain and cerebellum appear only faintly stained. The exposure to air restores the blue color so that, after cuts are made, the grooves will turn pale blue.

Another important factor to be considered is the size of the animal. Because the reaction only occurs on the surface of the pieces (the depth of the properly stained band usually does not exceed 0.5 mm), it is advisable to use small animals, such as frogs, lizards, mice, and guinea pigs. This way, it is more probable that even the deepest cortical cells become correctly impregnated. Needless to say, this only applies to those organs that must be exposed to the action of air still intact. Thick pieces also can be stained, however, as suggested by Dogiel, by rapidly sectioning the specimens and letting them oxygenate on one side; or, if both sides of the pieces are to be stained, by placing them onto a thin gauze, so that the lower surface is not in direct contact with the bottom of the flask being used to provide a humid atmosphere. This sectioning method is not as satisfactory when performed on the spinal cord (and other specimens that are difficult to section while fresh); it is preferable to oxygenate the intact block. On the other hand, oxygenation of the pieces through cuts is indispensable in the brain, cerebellum, Ammon's horn, and medulla oblongata. The knife must be carefully sharpened and lubricated with aqueous humor or methylene blue dissolved in either blood serum or water.

Only when the injection is not complete and the specimens do not turn blue after exposure to the atmosphere, is it permissible to paint the surfaces of the block with the dye. The water in which the dye is dissolved is harmful to the coloring process, for well-stained preparations without significant background are only achieved when the dye has penetrated into the tissue from the vascular system, mixed with blood plasma.

Obtaining properly stained cells in adult specimens is tricky. Cortical pyramidal neurons and Purkinje cells are very refractory to methylene blue staining. On the other hand, brain Golgi (short axon) cells and stellate cells of the molecular layer of the cerebellum are easily demonstrated. The poor sensitivity of pyramidal and

Purkinje cells for the dye is only relative, because, for unknown reasons, pyramids and dendrites of Purkinje cells sometimes can be intensely stained.

Cells and fibers of young and newborn animals are more easily stained. The eight-day-old cat is a good specimen from which to obtain crisp colorations of dorsal root axons and their collaterals in the spinal cord, especially in its thoracic portion, where it is thinnest. The Ammon's horn of the fifteen-to-twenty-day-old rabbit and the cerebellum of the pigeon are better stained than their adult counterparts. We (Cajal) also have observed that immature cells and premyelinated fibers of fetuses of large and medium-sized mammals are more readily colored than fully developed neurons and thick, myelinated axons.[(2)]

A further advantage of working with fetuses and young animals is the thinness of the white matter and, thus, the short distances that the fibers have to travel. This fact is crucial, given that this method only stains the most superficial portion of each block. This property has allowed us to study in detail the course and termination of some collaterals in the Rolando's gelatinous substance.

In some cases, we also use the reaction proposed by Meyer (**93**). In this procedure, the animals do not have to be poisoned by subcutaneous injections and Ehrlich's method is sufficient, as long as the nervous centers are saturated with methylene blue by means of arterial injections of the dye in newly sacrificed animals. This is done using highly concentrated solutions and allowing five to ten minutes between injections. After the last injection, the specimens are left untouched for two hours before the nervous centers are dissected and treated with Bethe's fixative. In this way, the staining is absolutely constant and the results are better than with Meyer's method, because all the cell corpuscles in the medulla are stained, as well as the cortical pyramidal cells, etc.

101. Kreibich's procedure with rongalite (*Rongaliteweiss*). This substance, which was introduced as a histological dye by Unna, has been proposed by Kreibich for staining the unmyelinated nerve fibers and the terminal arborizations of axons. It has been successfully used by Glaser and Müller to study the neural endings, ganglia, and neural plexuses of the guts. This procedure is described below:

1. Inject either subcutaneously or in the peritoneum 0.2–1 per 100 rongalite (Grübler).
2. After ten to sixty minutes, the organs to be studied are excised from the animal and exposed to air until they turn deep blue; large specimens must be cut into 2–3 mm thick slices with a straight razor blade. In some cases, it may be useful to immerse small pieces of fresh tissue in the rongalite solution itself.
3. Immerse the pieces for one or two hours in 5%–6% ammonium molybdate.

Rinse thoroughly with water, dehydrate in alcohol, clarify in xylene or, even better, in cedarwood oil, and embed in paraffin.

Methods to Study the Structure of the Nerve Cell

Just as we have explained the procedures for demonstrating the morphology of the neuron (Golgi's, Cox's, and Ehrlich's methods), we shall now describe the techniques that show the structure of the cell body. Its components are the cell membrane, nucleus, Nissl substance, neurofibrils, Golgi apparatus, **plastosomes,** and centrosomes, as well as other organelles.

NISSL CHROMATIC BODIES

102. The Nissl substance can be demonstrated by several methods; one of the first, developed by Nissl himself, is as follows:

1. Fix small cubes of brain tissue for five days in 96° alcohol, placing some cotton in the bottom of the flask to avoid any misshaping of the pieces.
2. Cut thin sections (5 to 10 µm) without embedding the tissue: stick the blocks to a wooden cube with gum arabic and immerse them in 36° alcohol in order to solidify the glue. Use a sliding microtome, being careful to wet the knife and the block continuously with 96° alcohol.
3. Stain the sections in:

B.X. Methylene blue[1]	3.75 g
Venice soap	175 cc
Distilled water	1000 cc

    Immerse the sections in this liquid, heating with a flame until it begins to boil.

4. Transfer the sections to a porcelain well containing an abundant volume of the following differentiating solution:

Aniline oil (Höchster)	10 cc
96° Alcohol	90 cc

The sections must remain in the solution until no blue stain diffuses from the sections.

5. Mount the sections on glass slides and cover them with essence of *cajuput*; after some seconds, blot the sections and pour benzine over them.
6. Drain off the excess of benzine and cover the sections with a saturated solution of colophony in xylol.
7. Warm the slides until the colophony thickens and coverslip exerting moderate pressure.

The Nissl method shows the *nuclei* and *nucleoli* nicely and especially the *chromatic bodies* of the neuron. Regrettably, this method does not stain the dendrites, except for those of the largest neurons and even then only the initial trunks that contain chromatic bodies are demonstrated. The strict rules that Nissl dictated must be faithfully observed in order to obtain what he called *equivalent images* (EN 26); such a goal cannot be achieved using procedures that include alcohol fixation, because the position of the nucleus and the chromatic bodies changes, due to water extraction by the alcohol. However, these alterations or those caused by heat or sectioning (when cutting 5 to 10 μm thick sections, the knife scratches and distorts the superficial portion of the neurons) are never so marked that they can be misinterpreted as pathological changes.

The method of Nissl has been simplified by Von Lenhossék and Spielmeyer, among others. Nowadays, other dyes are preferred for this staining procedure (e.g., *thionine, cresyl violet, toluidine blue, Unna's polychrome methylene blue*) Also, the introduction of celloidin embedding permits the making of serial sections.

103. Simplified procedure. The original procedure by Nissl has been simplified by several authors. In our laboratory we use the following technique, developed by Roussy and Lhermitte:

1. Stain floating sections for six to twenty-four hours at room temperature in a 1 per 100 thionine or toluidine blue solution; use Grübler's dyes tested by Hollborn.
2. Rinse for a few minutes with water.
3. Immerse the sections for five minutes in 95° alcohol.
4. Differentiate in Gothard's liquid:

Absolute alcohol	75 cc
Xylol	25 cc
Creosote	25 cc
Essence of cajuput	20 cc

This mixture must be poured into three wells and the sections passed through each consecutively. During this step the degree of differentiation must be monitored with the microscope.

5. Pass the sections through three dishes containing absolute alcohol in order to clarify the background.
6. Immerse the sections consecutively in two wells containing xylol.
7. Mount the sections on glass slides and cover them with neutral Canada balsam or d'Ammar resin.

104. Observations on the Nissl method. The best fixative for the Nissl method is 95°–96° alcohol. The alcohol must be renewed several times during the first twelve hours of fixation. On the second day the pieces are transferred to absolute alcohol. Sublimate mixtures, such as Dominici's liquid, also can be used, although the results are not as good and constant as those yielded by alcohol.

Although Nissl explicitly recommended not embedding the tissue, celloidin embedding renders excellent results and allows serial sections to be obtained easily. Paraffin embedding, on the other hand, is not advisable. The sections remain immersed in the staining solutions for at least six hours at room temperature. Longer staining periods do not impair the quality of the staining.

The differentiation is carried out by passing the sections through three or four wells containing Gothard's liquid; it must be monitored under the microscope until the desired coloration is achieved. Once differentiated, the sections are immersed in absolute alcohol until the background is completely bleached, after which the alcohol must be removed completely from the sections with xylene, otherwise the staining will fade after some time (this step lasts at least fifteen minutes). The preparations must be covered with d'Ammar resin or colophony or, even better, with thick cedarwood oil.

METHODS FOR STAINING THE NEUROFIBRILS

The methods suitable for the demonstration of the internal network of neurons are usually classified as *staining* and *impregnation* techniques; we shall begin with the former.

105. Bethe's method. This method is scarcely used nowadays because of its inconstancy and also because impregnation methods render better results. Nevertheless, it is worthwhile mentioning because this procedure was the first serious attempt to stain neurofibrils selectively in vertebrates. Apáthy's method, which is unreliable, will be discussed when dealing with the procedures for the study of the invertebrate nervous system (see Chapter 19).

1. Cut fresh brain slices, not thicker than 4–10 mm.
2. Immerse the slices for twenty-four hours in a 3 to 7.5 per 100 solution of nitric acid (sw, 1.40).
3. Transfer the specimens immediately into 95° alcohol and leave them for one day in this reagent.
4. Treat the specimens for twenty-four hours in:

Ammonia (sw 0.95)	1 part
Distilled water	3 parts
96° Alcohol	8 cc

5. Rinse for two to six hours with 96° alcohol and immerse the blocks during twenty-four hours in the following solution:

Hydrochloric acid (sw 1.18)	1 part
Distilled water	3 parts
96° Alcohol	8–12 cc

6. Treat the pieces for three to six hours in 96° alcohol.
7. Rinse with distilled water (two to six hours).
8. Immerse for twenty-four hours in 4 per 100 ammonium molybdate, which acts as a mordant.
9. Dehydrate and embed in paraffin.
10. Cut thin sections (5–8 μm) and stick them to the slides with albumin. The sections cannot be placed in water because the molybdate will be washed out. The temperature at which this step is carried out must not exceed 20°C.
11. Dip the slides in alcohol and immerse them in distilled water. Wipe the undersurface of the slide and pour 1–2 cc of distilled water on the section, then place them in the oven (60°C) for two to ten minutes. The timing of the latter step is critical for the success of this method but has to be determined in each individual case by trial and error. Drain the water off the slides and stain for ten minutes at the same temperature in:

| Toluidine blue | 1 g |
| Water | 3000 cc |

12. Rinse with water until the excess of color is removed.
13. Absolute alcohol, xylol, and Canada balsam.

Results: Neurofibrils are nicely shown when the method is well done. However, this imaginative procedure also stains the Golgi lattice and, even worse, a labyrinthine system of extracellular trabeculae throughout the whole of the gray and white matter. The images are thus rather puzzling because they suggest the existence of a network spanning the whole of the nervous system (*EN 27*). Because of the confusing images rendered by this technique, it has been replaced by Donnagio's method and by impregnation procedures.

106. Donnagio's method.

1. Fix small fragments of brain tissue, not exceeding 5 mm in thickness, in pure pyridine for five to six days; the best results are obtained in medulla and spinal cord.
2. Rinse thoroughly for one day in order to remove the fixative.
3. Immerse the pieces for a further day in a freshly prepared 4 per 100 solution of ammonium molybdate to which has been added four drops of hydrochloric acid.
4. Rinse briefly with water (two to four minutes), dehydrate in graded alcohols (no more than four hours for the whole dehydration), embed in paraffin, and cut sections as thin as possible.
5. Attach the sections to the slides without any glue and immerse them in water for less than a minute.
6. Stain in a 1 per 10.000 thionine solution until the gray matter acquires a pinkish violet color (five to thirty minutes).
7. At this point, the sections can be dehydrated and covered, although the author suggests treating them again with molybdate.
8. Dip the slide in water, in alcohol, and again in water; immerse it in the molybdate solution (see Step 3) for fifteen minutes.
9. Rinse, dehydrate, and mount.

Chapter 11: Structure of the Nerve Cell

This technique renders beautiful colorations in giant neurons (motoneurons, etc.), but may fail in the small cells of the brain. Neurofibrils are distinctly and selectively stained, because thionine is bound neither to the Golgi network nor to the ground substance.

SILVER IMPREGNATION METHODS

These procedures are preferable to those using anilines, because they render sharper and more limpid images; furthermore, they are easier and more constant. Three of these methods are known to date: Simarro's, Bielschowsky's, and our own technique (Cajal), which has plenty of variations.

107. Simarro's method. This renowned psychiatrist deserves the credit for being the first scientist to stain the neurofibrils by reducing haloid silver salts with photographic developers.

1. The first step is to poison the animal with daily subcutaneous injections of potassium bromide or chloride; as a rule, eight to fifteen injections (0.5 g each) should suffice. Sacrifice the animal and select fragments of medulla or spinal cord. From this step onward the method must be carried out in the darkroom using, at the most, only a photographic red lamp. The second step comprises the immersion of the pieces for four to fifteen days in 1 per 100 silver nitrate, so that silver bromides (or chlorides) are generated inside the nerve cells.
2. Transfer the pieces to alcohol and allow them to harden for one to two days in the dark.
3. Embed in celloidin and assemble the sections on a tray with water under a red light.

Expose the tray containing the sections to daylight until they acquire a yellowish color.

4. Immerse the sections in any of the photographic developers currently available (mixture of sulfite, pyrogallic acid, and either ammonia or potassium carbonate).
5. Rinse, clarify, and mount.

Neurofibrils are usually impregnated in a pale-brown color; too deeply stained sections can be softened by immersion in Gram's liquid and then bleached in sodium hyposulfite. The method works satisfactorily for large and medium-sized neurons of the spinal cord but fails to stain cells in the brain, cerebellum, and ganglia; in addition to this inconvenience, the axons are not impregnated and the superficial neurons appear encrusted with aggregates. This procedure produces an artifact known as ***Frohman's striae***.

108. Historical notes on Bielschowsky's method. Bielschowsky's method is a useful modification of Fajersztajn's procedure,[1] an old and almost forgotten technique, which rendered excellent impregnations of cylinder axes in nervous centers (**153**). Fajersztajn deserves the credit for introducing the impregnation of frozen sections with ammoniacal silver oxide followed by their reduction in formalin. He also should be acknowledged as a precursor of Gros, given that he was also the first to use ammoniacal silver nitrate. Finally, allow us to claim it as a remote antecedent of our old method (Cajal, 1881) for staining motor end plates. In this procedure, that yielded only partial impregnations, silver reduction was accomplished not by means of formaldehyde (this reagent was seldom used at that time for histological purposes) but by exposing the sections to daylight.[2]

Here is the modus operandi to impregnate neurofibrils with Bielschowsky's method in the nervous centers.

109. Bielschowsky's standard method (1903).

1. Fix brain slices, less than 1 cm thick, in 15%–20% neutral formalin; fixation must last at least twenty days.
2. Rinse the pieces for twelve hours with running tap water and immerse them for another twelve hours in distilled water.
3. Cut frozen sections and place them in distilled water; the sections must never exceed 15 μm in thickness.
4. Briefly rinse with distilled water and immerse the sections in a 2–3 per 100 solution of silver nitrate for twenty-four or forty-eight hours.
5. Dip the sections in distilled water and place them in a well containing ammoniacal silver oxide until they turn pale brown (ten to twenty-five minutes, depending on the thickness of the section).

The ammoniacal silver oxide solution is the basis of Bielschowsky's method; it is prepared by dripping five drops of 40 per 100 caustic potash onto 5 cc of 10 per 100 silver nitrate. The resulting precipitate is dissolved by dripping ammonia slowly into the solution; once the complete dissolution is achieved, add 25 cc of distilled water.

6. Rinse with distilled water and reduce in 20 per 100 formalin. The sections can be now mounted, although it is preferable to tone them with gold, which reinforces impregnation and gives the preparation a pleasanter color. Gold-toning can be achieved by immersing the sections for twenty to twenty-five minutes in:

    | Distilled water | 10 cc |
    | 1 per 100 yellow gold chloride | 2–3 drops |
    | Acetic acid | 2–3 cc |

7. Rinse briefly with water and fix the gold-toning (*EN 28*) by immersing the sections for thirty seconds in 5 per 100 sodium hyposulfite to which a few drops of a concentrated solution of sodium bisulfite have been added.
8. Rinse thoroughly with water to remove the hyposulfite, dehydrate, clarify in carbol-xylol, and mount in balsam.

If the reaction is successful, the neurofibrils are stained violet and both myelinated and unmyelinated cylinder axes also are shown.

Chapter 11: Structure of the Nerve Cell

General remarks: Because metallic needles react with silver, the sections must be handled with bent glass rods previously washed in distilled water.

Formalin is usually somewhat acidic, therefore, it must be treated with magnesium carbonate or chalk and filtered before using; this precaution is not necessary if pure formalin (Kahlbaum, Schering) is used.

110. Previous treatment of the sections with pyridine. Bielschowsky has reported that at times it is useful to immerse the sections in pyridine for one to two days prior to Step 4. After this treatment, the specimens must be thoroughly rinsed with distilled water until the smell of pyridine disappears, and then impregnated as described above.

111. Bulk impregnation of nerve endings. As demonstrated in the past by Donnaggio, Held, and ourselves, pyridine is suitable for en bloc staining. Bielschowsky also makes use of this property in his method:

1. Fix as in Bielschowsky's standard method and immerse the specimens in Merck's pure pyridine for two or three days. The pieces must not exceed 5 mm in thickness.
2. Rinse for several hours with distilled water.
3. Immerse for three to five days at 37°C in 3 per 100 silver nitrate.
4. Rinse briefly and impregnate for twenty-four hours in ammoniacal silver oxide (**109**) diluted in 3 times its volume of distilled water.
5. Rinse for two hours with distilled water and reduce in 20 per 100 formaldehyde for twelve to twenty-four hours. Rinse, dehydrate, and embed in paraffin; cut sections, mount them on slides, and gold-tone them as in the main procedure (**109**).

This technique stains neurofibrils even more selectively than the previous ones. It works well even in pieces that have been kept for years in acidic formaldehyde solutions. More details will be added when discussing the methods for demonstrating peripheral nerve endings (see Chapter 18).

112. Gros's Procedure.

1. Fix in 20 per 100 neutral formalin.
2. Cut 10–30 μm thick frozen sections and place them in distilled water.
3. Immerse the sections for five to sixty minutes (depending on the type of tissue) in 20 per 100 silver nitrate.
4. Reduce in a 20 per 100 solution of formaldehyde in tap water, replacing the formalin when milky clouds appear (*EN 29*).
5. Transfer the sections to a solution of ammoniacal silver nitrate. This next step is critical for the success of the method and must be carried out as follows: drip ammonia onto 20 per 100 silver nitrate until no more brown precipitate is formed; continue to drip ammonia while stirring vigorously until the precipitate is completely dissolved; add one extra drop of ammonia per each milliliter of solution. Place a small volume of this reagent onto a watch glass, immerse the sections in it, and transfer the glass to the microscope stage. Allow the ammoniacal

silver nitrate to act until neurons and nerve fibers stand out clearly against an almost colorless background; if the background is not bleached sufficiently, drip more ammonia onto the watch glass (usually one to three drops per milliliter are sufficient) until only the neurons and cylinder axes remain stained.
6. Immerse the sections for one minute in:

   25° Ammonia   2 parts
   Distilled water   8 cc

7. In order to remove excess ammonia, rinse briefly with distilled water to which a few drops of acetic acid have been added.
8. Stain in 1 per 300 gold chloride until the sections acquire a violet color.
9. Fix in 5 per 100 sodium hyposulfite to which a few grains of sodium bisulfite have been added.
10. Rinse thoroughly with water. Counterstain the nuclei with Ehrlich's hematoxylin or carmine. Mount as usual or, for better results, in levulose or Heringa's medium (*EN 30*) in order to avoid shrinkage.

This method renders superb impregnations of peripheral nerve endings, of dorsal root and sympathetic ganglion neurons, and of the cells of Meissner's and Auerbach's plexuses. Lawrentjew has obtained splendid results in the autonomous nervous system by immersing fresh pieces in a special fixative (96° alcohol, 30 cc; 20 per 100 neutral formalin, 30 cc; saturated solution of arsenious acid, 30 cc), for one hour prior to formalin fixation.

113. Cajal's reduced silver nitrate method. (1903). This method is based on the same principle as Simarro's, namely, the reduction of silver salts inside the tissue. The main difference is that, in our method, silver nitrate is reduced directly by a neutral reductor without alkali and is slow acting, whereas in Simarro's procedure the silver nitrate is used to produce silver chlorides inside the tissue, which are later decomposed on exposure to light and an alkaline reductor. Our technique, developed by Cajal in 1903,[3] yields the sharpest and most delicate impregnations of the neurofibrils not only in the spinal cord but in all nervous centers and endings. Thanks to the simplicity of the method and to its remarkable results, many relevant findings have been made that have been confirmed subsequently by other silver methods.

Fundamentals of the method. In our first attempts, we tried to impregnate the pieces en bloc, by immersing them for three or more days in 1.5 per 100 silver nitrate at 37 °C, after which they were reduced in pyrogallic acid or in hydroquinone. The nervous tissue must become tanned under the effect of heat, resulting in what we call *ripening of the reaction*. The pale-brown tanning that the tissue shows after exposure to heat is possibly due, as suggested by Liesegang, to an early, incomplete reduction of silver to form tiny, invisible seeds, which would subsequently become visible under the action of pyrogallic acid, which, in turn, would make them grow by accretion. This hypothesis is, however, very controversial.[4] The action of light is harmful for this method, therefore, the silver precipitation must take place in complete darkness or under a very weak light.

We shall now explain the formulae most commonly used in our laboratory for the past twenty-five years. Bulk and section staining procedures are treated separately.

Formulae for Bulk Staining

114. Formula without fixative (1903).[2] Here is the modus operandi:

1. Immerse brain slices, not thicker than 3 mm, in 1.5–3 per 100 silver nitrate; this step must be carried out in the oven (34°–37°C) and takes three or four days. The silver nitrate solution must be about 100 cc for four to six pieces.
2. Rinse for one minute with distilled water in order to remove the superficial silver nitrate.
3. Place the pieces for twenty-four hours in this liquid:

Pyrogallic acid or Hydroquinone	1 g
Water	70–100 cc
Formalin	5–10 cc

Although formalin is not necessary for the reaction to take place, it does improve it as it hardens the tissue and enhances the fineness of the precipitate.

4. Rinse briefly, dehydrate, and embed in celloidin.

Remarks: During the impregnation step, the pieces must be observed daily and placed in the reducing pyro-formalin mixture when they show a dark brown color, similar to that of dry, dark tobacco leaves. This coloration heralds the beginning of the ripening period, as Cajal called it; if the reduction is performed before or after this moment, the tissue will be either under- or overimpregnated. Usually, three days at 37°C are sufficient.

The addition of 30–50 per 100 alcohol to the silver nitrate solution improves the staining of the axons.

This variation renders good results in the spinal cord, medulla, cerebellum, and ganglia of embryos and fetuses and also in the cortex and cerebellum of the adult rabbit; however, the best impregnations are obtained in the nervous centers of young rabbits (ten to –twenty days old). As will be discussed later, this method is suitable for invertebrates (*hirudo, alaustomum*, etc.), especially if the silver nitrate is used at a 6% concentration.

The main limitation of this technique is the poor penetration of silver nitrate, so that, except with embryos, only the more superficial sections are useful. Moreover, the axons are imperfectly stained in the adult.

115. Formula with plain ethanol.

1. Fix for twenty-four hours in 96° alcohol.
2. Dip in distilled water or, better still, blot the pieces with blotting paper.
3. Immerse them for one week in 1.5 per 100 silver nitrate in the oven (35°–37°C).

4. Reduce as in the anterior formula, embed in celloidin, and section.
5. Rinse the sections thoroughly and stain them with gold chloride (see **125**).

This technique renders excellent impregnations in the cortex, cerebellum, dorsal root- and sympathetic ganglia, peripheral nerve endings, and regenerating nerve trunks, as well as in early chick and mammalian embryos. In the cerebellum, the baskets around the Purkinje cells and the plexuses in the granular layer are beautifully stained; in the cerebral cortex, it reveals not only the nerve fibers but also the dendrites of large and medium-sized pyramidal cells.

We used this formula frequently before the World War (*EN 31*) because of its excellent results, especially in the brain, cerebellum, and ganglia. Presently, however, whether due to postwar poverty or some other unknown reason, it is almost impossible to get alcohol that is free of *acetone, aldehyde, furfural, methyl alcohol* and other contaminants. We have, therefore, completely discarded this technique. At present we prefer, especially for adult animals, to use alcohol plus an alkaline substance that acts as an *accelerator*; this practice yields a more uniform and constant reaction and shortens the impregnation period. The accelerators most commonly used are *ammonia, chloral hydrate, veronal, pyridine, nicotine, antipyrine*, etc. In the following paragraphs we shall mention the most relevant of these formulae.

116. Formula with ammoniacal alcohol.

1. Fix the specimens for twenty-four hours in:

    96° Alcohol   50 cc
    Ammonia   4 to 6 drops

2. Rinse briefly with water and immerse the pieces during five to seven days in 1.5 per 100 silver nitrate; this step must be carried out in a 37°C oven.
3. Reduce as in the previous formulae. Gold-toning is advisable.

This variation is especially recommended for demonstrating the neurofibrils of the spinal cord of young animals (ten- to twenty-day-old rabbits and kittens); it is also used for the study of nerve regeneration processes (Cajal, Perroncito, Lugaro, Tello, etc.).

The ammonia content of the fixative must be reduced to two to three drops in the case of the brain cortex, adult ganglia, and peripheral nerve endings. On the other hand, an increase in the volume of ammonia up to eight to ten drops results in an enhancement of the neurofibrils because the interfibrillar substance is partially removed; in this way, neurofibrils appear more separate and their individual analysis is thus straightforward. Beautiful preparations can be thus obtained in young cats, rabbits, and dogs.

117. Fixation with hypnotics (Cajal, 1910).

1. Fix the specimens for twenty-four hours in:

    Chloral hydrate   5–10 g
    Distilled water   50 cc

Fixation can be improved by dissolving the chloral hydrate in a mixture of water and alcohol (**21**), as suggested by de Castro, who also recommends the addition of one or two drops of ammonia to the fixative for certain purposes.

Chapter 11: Structure of the Nerve Cell

2. Rinse for a few minutes with distilled water and immerse the pieces during twenty-four hours in:

   96° Alcohol   50 cc
   Ammonia   4–6 drops

3. Blot the pieces with blotting paper and immerse them during five to six days at 35°–38°C in the 1.5 per 100 silver solution.
4. Reduce as usual.

Instead of dissolving the chloral hydrate in distilled water, it is advisable, according to de Castro (**21**), to use a mixture of water and alcohol, which renders a better fixation of the specimens.

This variation is most constant; besides which, it produces almost no shrinkage of the tissue, so that neurons are shown with their normal configuration and size.

Chloral hydrate fixation facilitates the impregnation of myelinated and unmyelinated fibers of the brain, medulla, cerebellum, and spinal cord. The baskets and the mossy fiber rosettes of the cerebellum are thus beautifully shown, as well as motor end plates, the sensitive end terminals of the skin (Martínez), and the acoustic receptor (de Castro, Tello). With this method, the surfaces of the specimens do not become overstained. The variations of de Castro and Tello will be discussed in the chapter dealing with the demonstration of the peripheral nerve endings (see Chapter 18).

Chloral hydrate can be replaced by other hypnotics (**22**), such as *urethane*, *somniféne* (de Castro) or a 2 per 100 alcoholic solution of *veronal* (Cajal).

118. De Castro's formulae with hypnotics[5] (*EN 32*). For staining the ganglia and sensitive and motor nerve endings, de Castro uses the following formulae, based on the addition of a small volume of nitric acid to the fixative in order to avoid the staining of the connective tissue; in this way, the sections show a most limpid background, being possible to color them first, and then counterstain the nuclei with carmine, hematoxylin, or basic anilines.

The procedure is as follows:

1. Fix 0.4–0.6 mm thick specimens for twenty-four hours in one of these solutions:

   (A)

   Chloral hydrate   5 g
   96° Alcohol   50 cc
   Distilled water   40–50 cc
   Nitric acid (40°) 1–2 cc

   (B)

   Ethyl urethane   2–4 g
   96° Alcohol   50 cc
   Distilled water   40–50 cc
   Nitric acid (40°) 1–2 cc

(C)

Somnifène (H. Roche)	4 cc
96° Alcohol	50 cc
Distilled water	40–50 cc
Nitric acid (40°)	1–2 cc

2. Rinse thoroughly with running tap water (for six to twelve hours) and immerse for one day in:

96° Alcohol	50 cc
36° Ammonia	2–3 drops

3. Impregnate, reduce, and stain as in the routine Cajal method.

The proportion of nitric acid varies depending on the organs to be studied. If the endings of the skin, glands, arteries, ganglia, or muscles are to be stained, the percentage of acid can be lowered to 1%. In the brain and other nervous centers, the acid can be omitted from the procedure.

119. Fixation in pyridine. As previously stated (**19, 20**), pyridine is a most penetrating fixative; when associated with Cajal's method it provides very intense impregnations, especially in embryos (Held). In adult tissues the results are not as good, because thick axons and other structures are poorly stained. The procedure is as follows:

1. Fix for twenty-four hours in 60 to 70 per 100 pyridine.
2. Rinse for twelve hours with water, which must be renewed several times; it is advisable to remove the alkali (pyridine) by rinsing the pieces with running tap water. During this step it is advisable to protect the specimens with gauze or a thin metallic fabric.
3. Immerse in 96° alcohol for eight to twelve hours.
4. Rinse briefly with distilled water to remove the superficial silver nitrate.
5. Impregnate and reduce in 1.5% silver nitrate solution for five to six days in the oven at 35°–37°C.
6. Reduce in pyrogallic acid/formalin mixture.

Besides its high diffusion and good results in embryonal material, in the adult this variation has the advantage of staining the thin unmyelinated fibers and, less frequently, the end-bulbs of Held. Its most fruitful results, however, are obtained in studies of nerve regeneration,[6] in which the silver demonstrates newly formed endings especially well. Let us add that it stains the peripheral nerve endings particularly well, although we shall comment in Chapter 18 about this property and about the combined use of pyridine with decalcifiers.

120. Formula with chloral hydrate, alcohol, and pyridine (Cajal, 1927).

1. Fix for one or two days in:

96° Alcohol	50 cc
Pyridine	15–20 cc
Chloral hydrate	3–5 g

2. Rinse for twelve hours.
3. Impregnate and reduce as in the routine Cajal method.

This variation is especially recommended for the impregnation of cerebellar structures: it stains the finest branches of the *glomeruli* of the rabbit, cat, and dog beautifully, as well as the *transverse* and *parallel fibers* of the molecular layer. The *baskets* on Purkinje's cells, on the other hand, are poorly demonstrated, perhaps due to the fact that this technique only stains the most delicate and thinnest unmyelinated fibers. Nevertheless, nice colorations of peripheral myelinated endings (both motor and sensitive) can be obtained by adding one part of water to the fixative.

121. Formula with ammoniacal formalin (Cajal, 1904).

1. Fix for twenty-four to forty-eight hours in the following liquid:

40 per 100 Formalin	25 cc
Water	100 cc
Ammonia	from 6 drops to 1 cc

2. Rinse thoroughly (twelve or more hours) in order to remove the formaldehyde completely.
3. Impregnate for three days in the oven in a 1–3 per 100 silver nitrate solution.
4. Reduce as usual.

This formula impregnates preferentially the *cerebellar* baskets, showing also the neurofibrils of many central nervous system neurons; the end-bulbs of Held are also sometimes impregnated.

122. Formalin fixation with subsequent pyridine treatment (Cajal, 1930).

1. Fix fragments of brain tissue from small mammals (mice, rats, rabbits, cats, etc.) for two or three days in 15 per 100 neutral formalin (*EN 33*). The mouse brain can be fixed *in toto*, only detaching the lateral parts of the piriform lobe.
2. Immerse the pieces, without rinsing, for one or two days in 70 per 100 pyridine.
3. Rinse with running tap water for twelve to twenty-four hours to remove the pyridine.
4. Cut 5 mm thick slices and impregnate them for three days in 1.5 per 100 silver nitrate at 37°C.
5. The specimens, which turn dark very quickly in the silver nitrate bath, are rinsed with distilled water, reduced in pyrogallic acid, and embedded in celloidin.

This technique stains the nuclei red, the perikarya yellow, and the axon terminals a brownish black color, making them appear completely independent from the cell bodies with which they are in contact.

This procedure renders splendid colorations of Held's chalices and also of the cerebellar baskets and other terminal arborizations. Later we shall comment on the application of this technique to frozen sections.

123. Formalin fixation with subsequent ammoniacal alcohol treatment.[7]

1. Fix pieces, not thicker than 4 mm, in 15 per 100 neutral formalin for one to two days.
2. Rinse for several hours in order to remove formalin.
3. Immerse for twenty-four hours in:

   96° Alcohol   50 cc
   Ammonia   5–7 drops

4. Blot the specimens with blotting paper and transfer them to 1.5% silver nitrate. The flask containing the pieces must be kept in the oven for five to six days.

Reduce as usual, in pyrogallic acid-formalin mixture for twenty-four hours. Rinse briefly, dehydrate through graded alcohols, embed in celloidin, and section. Gold-toning is advisable for pale or thin sections.

This option renders a striking demonstration of the boutons of Held's pericellular baskets, the chalices of the trapezoid body, the endings in the **ventral acoustic ganglion,** etc. The thin unmyelinated fibers of the centers are better demonstrated than the thick ones, which appear only faintly stained yellow or orange. When dealing with the cerebellum, we shall comment further on this method that has given such excellent results for the impregnation of central nerve endings.

124. Formula with pyridine-silver nitrate (Cajal).

1. Fix in 12 per 100 formalin for two days.
2. Rinse for twelve hours.
3. 36° alcohol for twenty-four hours.
4. Immerse the pieces for two or two and a half days in 2 per 100 silver nitrate plus pyridine (silver nitrate solution, 50 cc; pyridine, 5–6 drops), at 37°C.
5. Reduce as usual in pyrogallic acid-formalin.

Results: This method, which is similar to Levaditi's and Manouélian's for the syphilis microbe, stains the nerve fibers and the neurofibrils of several neuronal types distinctly and also provides clear images of Held bulbs and spinal cord fibers. The staining reaches the deep portions of the sections and, furthermore, the background is practically unstained.

125. Gold-toning of sections obtained from specimens impregnated en bloc by Cajal's method (de Castro).

Gold-toning of the sections is convenient when the impregnation is somewhat faint, given that it enhances the contrast. It is also useful when an accurate topographic analysis of the impregnated cells or endings is required, because this technique allows the nuclei to be counterstained with anilines, hematoxylin, or carmine.

Toning can be achieved in several ways (see any handbook of photographic procedures). The following method, which is rather similar to the one used in the Bielschowsky procedure, is very easy to do and reliable.

1. Thin celloidin or paraffin sections (the latter fixed to glass slides) are immersed in a 1 per 600 yellow gold chloride solution until the silver colloid has almost disappeared. In some cases, it is useful to add some acetic acid (1 drop per 10 cc of solution) (excessive toning must be carefully avoided).
2. Briefly rinse with distilled water and immerse for thirty or forty seconds in 5 per 100 sodium hyposulfite, eventually add sodium bisulfite (1 drop of a concentrated bisulfite solution for every 10 cc of hyposulfite solution).
3. Rinse for thirty minutes with running tap water. Counterstain the nuclei if desired with anilines or hematoxylin, dehydrate, clarify, and mount in Canada balsam.

After gold-toning, some sections may turn almost opaque; in such cases, they must be immersed during one or two minutes in Veratti's liquid:

Distilled water	1000 cc
Potassium permanganate	0.5–1 g
Concentrated sulfuric acid	1 cc

4. Briefly rinse with water and immerse the sections in either 5 per 100 oxalic acid or 0.1 per 100 sulfurous acid; freshly prepared Pal's differentiating solution (oxalic acid, 1 g; sodium sulfite, 1 g; water, 200 cc) can also be used. The purpose of this step is to bleach the background.

Section Staining with the Reduced Silver Nitrate Method

126. For a long time, and despite numerous attempts, we failed to stain nerve fibers with Cajal's method in floating sections. At best, only fragmentary coloration of neurofibrils was obtained, but in all cases the background contained irregular precipitates.

Liesegang has proposed a hypothesis to explain these failures; he suggests that the main problem is that sections do not have any colloidal coating. Under such conditions, silver precipitates abruptly, forming not ultramicroscopic micelles, but large aggregates that lack any affinity for nerve fibers. Consequently, Liesegang suggested reducing the sections in a liquid containing hydroquinone, silver nitrate, and a colloidal substance, such as gum arabic. Nevertheless, our own trials have shown that selective impregnations also can be obtained by using a reductor containing a large volume of formalin and a small quantity of hydroquinone. As will be described later, this technique is excellent for demonstrating the medullated and unmedullated fibers of the central nervous system.

127. Liesegang's procedure[8] with gum arabic is as follows:

1. Fix in 12 per 100 formalin and cut frozen sections.
2. Immerse in 0.75–1 per 100 silver nitrate until the sections turn brown; this step can take a few hours or several days.

3. Reduce in a liquid composed of equal parts of 5 per 100 hydroquinone, 50 per 100 gum arabic, and 1 per 100 silver nitrate. The sections will become dark brown after a few minutes.
4. Rinse thoroughly and stain.

Neurofibrils are intensely stained in the cortex, cerebellum, spinal cord, etc., although the background is rather dark, especially after gold-toning. In any case, the results are not as subtle as those obtained with the bulk-impregnation formulae.

128. The previous method has been modified by Balbuena, who recommends applying Liesegang's technique to celloidin sections obtained from pyridine-fixed material and replacing the gum arabic with some drops of tincture of *succinum*.

129. Formula with hydroquinone, suitable for the cerebellum (Cajal, 1925).[9]

1. Fix for more than three days in 12 per 100 formaldehyde.
2. Cut 30–35 μm thick frozen sections and immerse them for four to twelve hours in the following liquid:

2 per 100 Silver nitrate	10 cc
Pyridine	7–8 drops
96° Alcohol	5–6cc

The sections will turn brown during the next four hours, although this stage can be extended for up to twelve hours at no disadvantage. If the sections are yellowish or pale brown, the well containing the sections must be heated with a flame for some minutes, until the impregnation is completed.

3. Dip the sections in a porcelain well containing 96° alcohol; special care needs to be taken not to remove the silver nitrate completely, otherwise the staining is too pale and incomplete. Only two sections at a time should be placed in the well.
4. Reduce for one to three minutes in the following mixture:

Hydroquinone	0.3 g
Distilled water	70 cc
Formalin	20 cc
Acetone	15 cc

The sections must become a brown to black color; if they are paler, one or two drops of 2 per 100 silver nitrate can be added to the reducing solution.

5. Rinse thoroughly with water, tone in 1 per 500 yellow gold chloride and fix in soda hyposulfite. The sections must be handled with glass rods during these steps.
6. Rinse, mount on a slide, blot with filter paper, dehydrate in alcohol, clarify in carbol-xylol and xylol, and cover with Canada balsam or d'Ammar resin.

Chapter 11: Structure of the Nerve Cell

This technique yields superb impregnations of the cerebellar structure, especially of the mossy fibers; Held's end-bulbs and chalices also are demonstrated beautifully. Neurofibrils are not clearly shown in other axonal endings.

130. Staining of the axons in sections (*EN 34*).

1. Fix fragments of nervous tissue for one to three days in:

Chloral hydrate	5 g
Formalin	15 cc
Water	75–100 cc

2. Cut frozen sections and place them in the following liquid:

96° Alcohol	90 cc
Water	50 cc
Ammonia	5 drops

3. Immerse the sections for twelve hours in:

Silver nitrate	2 g
Water	100 cc
Pyridine	8 drops

4. Dip the sections one by one in 96° alcohol.
5. Reduce, tone, and mount as in the previous technique.

This variation is especially useful to study the cerebellum.[3]

131. Schultze and Stöhr's method. Schultze and his disciple Stöhr believe that formalin reacts with some tissue components, forming a lacquer that interferes with the neurofibril staining. They propose to remove this lacquer with caustic soda prior to silver impregnation. Although Stöhr has reported several variations of this method designed to achieve better impregnations according to the organ to be studied and the elements of the neurofibrillar apparatus to be demonstrated, the most usual modus operandi is as follows:

1. Fix fresh brain fragments in formalin for at least forty-eight hours. Cut 30 μm thick frozen sections and place them in distilled water.
2. Immerse the sections for one day in a solution of caustic soda made as follows: Take 6 to 10 parts (depending on the organ to be studied) of a solution made dissolving 4 grams of Merck's *purissimus grade* quality sodium hydroxide in 100 cc of distilled water and mix them with 50 parts of distilled water.
3. Rinse for one hour with distilled water (four changes).
4. Impregnate overnight in 2 per 100 silver nitrate.
5. Make the following mixture:

Hydroquinone	2.5 g
Commercial formalin	5 cc
Distilled water	100 cc

This solution will be diluted 1:20 in water immediately before use, and the sections reduced in it for a few seconds.

6. Tone (if desired), dehydrate, etc.

This method renders nice impregnations of both myelinated and unmyelinated fibers that stand out against an almost colorless background. The most delicate terminal arborizations, however, are often incompletely stained; hence, this procedure is not as good as our silver-pyridine-alcohol method (**129**).

Stöhr recommends changing the concentration of the soda and silver nitrate solutions according to the organ to be studied; thus, soda and silver nitrate concentrations must be increased to 10 in 50 parts and 10 in 100 parts respectively, for the brain, medulla, spinal cord, and peripheral ganglia. Yet, for the study of the cerebellum, both baths must be more diluted (2 parts of soda in 50 parts of water, and 0.25% silver nitrate solution).

IMPREGNATION OF THE GOLGI APPARATUS

132. The ***internal reticular apparatus*** of the nervous cell has some specific characteristics that have been studied by several scientists.

The original method of the "sage from Pavia" (*EN 35*) was actually a variation of his old silver chromate procedure (**77**); however, we now have more reliable and straightforward techniques, some of which we describe below:

133. Golgi–Veratti's procedure.

1. Fix nervous tissue fragments for twenty or thirty days in this liquid:

5 per 100 Potassium bichromate	20 cc
1 per 100 Solution of platinum and potassium chloride	20 cc
1 per 100 Osmic acid	10–20 cc

2. Trim the fragments down to small blocks and immerse them in:

5 per 100 Potassium bichromate	20 cc
5 per 100 Copper sulfate (or acetate)	20 cc

3. Impregnate for forty-eight hours in 1 per 100 silver nitrate.
4. Dehydrate and section as in the regular Golgi method.

The Golgi apparatus is clearly shown against a nearly colorless background.

134. Primitive method of Cajal (1908).

1. Immerse fragments of nervous or epithelial tissue (glands, intestines, etc.) for at least twenty-four hours in a 50/50 mixture of formalin and acetone; sometimes it is useful to add 1 or 2 drops of ammonia for every 100 cc of solution.

Chapter 11: Structure of the Nerve Cell

2. Rinse for four to six hours in order to remove the formalin.
3. Cut 3 mm thick slices and immerse them for twenty-four hours in:

   96° Alcohol   50 cc
   Ammonia   5–7 drops

4. Impregnate and reduce as in the routine Cajal's method (**114**).

This technique reveals the Golgi apparatus in almost all the tissues and also impregnates the pericellular reticulum membrane (**152**).

135. Golgi's method with arsenious acid (1908). This formula is more complicated than the previous ones, but it yields good results when practiced by skilled histologists, as has been shown by Golgi, Luciani, Vechi, Brugnatelli, Perroncito, E. Luna, Deineka, etc.

1. Fix for six to eight hours in a mixture of equal parts of 96° alcohol, arsenious acid, and neutral formalin (**112**).
2. Immerse in 1 per 100 silver nitrate; the impregnation period ranges from thirteen hours to several days.
3. Rinse briefly with distilled water and reduce in the following solution:

   Hydroquinone   20 g
   Formalin   50 cc
   Soda sulfite   5 g
   Distilled water 1000 cc

4. Rinse briefly with tap water, embed in either celloidin or in paraffin, and cut thin sections. Because the background often shows a grainy brown precipitate, the sections must be toned and then treated by potassium permanganate to eliminate this artifact.
5. *Toning of the sections.* After rinsing the sections, immerse them for ten to thirty minutes in a freshly prepared mixture of solutions A (10 cc) and B (3–4 drops):

Solution A[4]:

Sodium hyposulfite   3 g
Ammonia sulfocyanide   3 cc
Distilled water   100 cc

Solution B:

Gold chloride   1 g
Distilled water 100 cc

6. *Intensity reduction.* Although hyposulfite clarifies the background to some extent, an additional bleaching is frequently required; otherwise the precipitate will obscure the results. Thus, the sections must be treated

for thirty to 40 seconds with slightly modified Lumiere's photographic softener:

Potassium permanganate	0.50 g
Sulfuric acid	1 cc
Distilled water	1000 cc

7. Immerse in 1 per 100 oxalic acid, rinse thoroughly, counterstain the nuclei with carmine-alum, dehydrate, clarify, and mount.

When the method has been carried out correctly, the internal reticular apparatus is clearly shown in a violet to black color against a pale background.

136. Cajal's technique with formalin and uranyl nitrate (1912). The Golgi apparatus can be stained in invertebrates (*lumbricus*, etc.) and in young rabbit brains with the reduced silver nitrate method (**114**), as we demonstrated in 1903. We later used the formalin-acetone technique (**134**), which was only successful for certain specimens, providing indirect proof of the variable physicochemical composition of the Golgi apparatus. Thus, we finally developed the present formula, which renders constant results in all types of material. In this technique, acetone is replaced with uranyl nitrate and the sections are reduced in a slightly alkaline solution, as proposed by Golgi.

The modus operandi is as follows:

1. Fix 2–3 mm thick pieces in:

Uranyl nitrate	1–2 g
Neutral formalin	15 cc
Distilled water	100 cc

Fixation time is critical; the Golgi apparatus will be stained after a fixation period of six to nine hours. If the specimens are left in the fixative for twenty-four or forty-eight hours, neuroglial cells and gliosomes will appear instead of the internal reticular apparatus.

2. Rinse briefly with distilled water and immerse the pieces for twenty-four hours in 1.5–2 per 100 silver nitrate; the concentration of the silver solution can be reduced to 0.75–1 per 100 for very small pieces.
3. Rinse quickly with water to remove the superficial silver nitrate precipitate. Reduce for twelve to twenty-four hours in:

Hydroquinone	2 g
Formalin	6–10 cc
Water	100 cc
Anhydrous soda sulfite	0.15–0.25 g

A sufficient amount of the latter compound must be added so that the bath acquires a pale yellow color. In certain cases (adult specimens), this reagent may be omitted.

4. Rinse briefly with distilled water, embed in celloidin, etc.

Important remarks: The best preparations are those obtained from embryos or young mammals (eight-to-twenty-day-old rabbit, cat, or dog, and mammalian and bird embryos). The fixation time for embryos must not exceed six hours. In adult tissues, the Golgi network usually appears somewhat fragmented[5]; for this material, it is advisable not to use sodium sulfite in the reductor (de Castro) or to increase its formalin content, as suggested by Pendfield. Mitochondria are regularly stained in the glands.

Gold-toning can be performed, especially if the sections are to be counterstained with hematoxylin; however, it is seldom necessary, because the nuclear outline can be readily identified.

The great advantage of this technique is its constancy and simplicity; furthermore, no photographic softeners are necessary. It is, in fact, the technique preferred by many investigators. As usual in en bloc staining, however, the superficial sections should be discarded.

137. Kopsch's method. This author has visualized the *Golgi apparatus* by immersing small fragments of fresh tissue in 2 per 100 osmic acid; the reticular apparatus needs at least five days to be stained, but it should be borne in mind that overfixation will result in a complete blackening of the tissue. Once the optimal staining period has concluded, the blocks are rinsed, embedded, etc.

138. Kolatschew's modification of the method of Kopsch.

1. Fix for twenty-four hours in Champy's liquid at room temperature:

3 per 100 Potassium bichromate	7 cc
2 per 100 Osmic acid	4 cc
1 per 100 Chromic acid	7 cc

2. Rinse for twenty-four hours with running tap water or with frequently replaced distilled water.
3. Stain for three to nine days at 37°C in 1 per 100 osmic acid; the reagent must be renewed when it turns dark. The volume of osmic acid solution must be proportional to the volume of the tissue; usually, two or three small specimens not exceeding 3 mm in thickness require about 10 cc of osmic solution.
4. Rinse for thirty to sixty minutes in running tap water or in plenty of distilled water.

Embed in paraffin and cut 5–7 μm thick sections.

The Golgi apparatus is shown in a black color against a pale yellow or grayish background. If the nuclei are to be counterstained, safranin staining is the most advisable procedure.

In order to control the stain, Nassonow suggests tearing small fragments from the piece with a needle when the tissue is thoroughly blackened, from the third or fourth day onward. These fragments are then dissociated in glycerin, mounted and examined at the microscope.

139. Da Fano's modification of Cajal's uranyl-formalin method.

1. Fix small tissue fragments, thinner than 2–3 mm, at room temperature, in:

Cobalt nitrate	1 g
Formalin	15 cc
Distilled water	100 cc

   Fixation must last six to eight hours for specimens obtained from young animals and twelve to twenty-four hours in the case of adult animals.

2. Rinse briefly with distilled water and impregnate for one day in 1.5% silver nitrate; this step must be carried out in the dark and at room temperature.
3. Rinse the pieces, place them in Cajal's reducing solution with hydroquinone (**136**), etc.

Remarks: Cajal's original method (**136**) renders better results than this variation in all neural areas; Da Fano's technique is useful only in those organs, such as the liver, where the uranyl-formalin method fails to stain the reticular apparatus. Furthermore, as de Castro pointed out, the silver precipitate is coarser than in Cajal's procedure.

DEMONSTRATION OF PLASTOSOMES, CENTROSOMES, OXIDASES, AND PIGMENTARY SPHERULES

140. The techniques reported in Chapter 6 of Section One (**55, 58**) are useful to stain the plastosomes of the nervous cells.

141. Excellent results are also provided by *Alzheimer's method* with fuchsin and light green solution.
Here is the modus operandi:

1. Fix for twenty-four hours in 10% formalin.
2. Without rinsing, immerse the pieces for eight days in concentrated Flemming's liquid (**10**); add 1 or 2 drops only of glacial acetic acid.
3. Rinse for twelve hours with running tap water and embed in paraffin; cut 2–4 µm thick sections.
4. Place the sections in water and stain them for one hour (at 58°C) in a saturated solution of acid fuchsin.
5. Rinse with distilled water until the rinse water is colorless.
6. Immerse for ten to twenty seconds in:

Saturated solution of picric acid in 96° alcohol	30 cc
Distilled water	60 cc

7. Rinse again and stain for twenty to fifty minutes in a saturated light green solution diluted at 50% in water.

Chapter 11: Structure of the Nerve Cell

8. Rinse briefly with water, blot the sections with filter paper, dehydrate, clarify, and mount in balsam.

Results: This procedure stains the neuronal plastosomes and neurosomes in bright red; the glial and connective fibers in pale red; and the Nissl bodies in green; *neuroglial amoeboid cells* are also shown, in pale green.

142. Cowdry has obtained excellent plastosome staining using *Bensley's method*:

1. Fix for two to sixteen hours in the following liquid:

2.5 per 100 potassium dichromate	16 cc
2 per 100 osmic acid	4 cc
Concentrated acetic acid	1–2 drops

2. Rinse for one hour with distilled water, embed in paraffin and cut 2–4 μm thick sections.
3. Deparaffinize, hydrate, and immerse the sections for thirty seconds in 1 per 100 potassium permanganate; then bleach them for thirty more seconds in 5 per 100 oxalic acid. Rinse thoroughly with water.
4. Stain for six minutes in Altmann's acid fuchsin solution (**58**) at 60°C; fuchsin staining can be enhanced by previously immersing the sections in 2.5–3 per 100 potassium bichromate (thirty seconds).
5. Rinse with water until the rinse water becomes colorless.
6. Differentiate in 1 per 100 aqueous solution of either methyl green or toluidine blue.
7. Rinse in 96° alcohol, absolute alcohol, and toluene, and mount in Canada balsam.

Results: Plastosomes are stained pale red and the Nissl bodies appear green or blue; neurofibrils are faintly stained a brownish color.

143. Del Río-Hortega's *first variation* (**145**) of Achúcarro's method (*EN 36*) renders excellent impregnations of the plastosomes of large neurons that appear as rodlets and clear-cut granules. Del Río-Hortega's technique (**188**) for the **chondrioma** of glial cells also yields very nice images of these organelles in neurons.

144. Demonstration of the centrosomes of neurons. These organelles were first stained by von Lenhossék in the dorsal root ganglia of frogs; he used the Heidenhain's iron hematoxylin method, but this procedure does not stain these structures in highly specialized neurons. Fortunately, some silver techniques are more precise and reliable; we describe one of the best below:

145. Achúcarro's method with tannin and ammoniacal silver has been modified by Del Río-Hortega in order to stain the centrosomes of neurons and neuroglial cells; this modification is usually known as *Del Río-Hortega's first variation of Achúcarro's method*.

1. Fix for at least ten days in 10 per 100 formalin.
2. Cut frozen sections as thin as possible. The sections are immersed in 3% tannin for five minutes at 50°–55°C. This temperature is attained using

a flame placed at some distance from the well containing the sections to avoid overheating (see *EN 40*).
3. Immerse the sections in 20 cc of distilled water to which 4 drops of ammonia have been added; the sections will thus regain the original flexibility and transparency.
4. The sections are then immersed successively through three wells containing 10 cc of distilled water and 1 cc of ammoniacal silver oxide.

The latter liquid is prepared as follows: add 40 drops of 40% soda to 30 cc of 10% silver nitrate. A precipitate is formed in the solution that must be washed ten to twelve times with distilled water (at least 1 liter of water must be used). Then 50 cc of distilled water is poured onto the remaining precipitate, after which ammonia is slowly added while stirring. Care must be taken not to add more ammonia after the solution presents a strong smell of alkali. Once the precipitate is dissolved, up to 150 cc of distilled water is added and the resulting mixture is kept in a yellow flask or in the dark (see *EN 40*).

5. The sections, which should have acquired a dark yellow color, are rinsed with plenty of water.
6. The sections are then immersed in a solution of 1/500 gold chloride for twenty to thirty minutes at room temperature, or ten minutes at 40° to 45°C.
7. Fix in 5% soda hyposulfite.
8. Rinse thoroughly with water.
9. Dehydrate, clarify, and mount as usual.

This procedure, which uses formaldehyde as a reductor, stains the centrosomes of many neurons, including the cortical pyramidal cells and the granules of the cerebellum. It also intensely impregnates the protoplasmic rod found by one of us (Cajal, 1903) in the cells of the *nucleus of the trapezoid body*. Furthermore, this technique provides beautiful preparations of the fibrillary astrocytes, showing the fibers of **Ranvier-Weigert** clearer than any other method.

The centrosomes also can be stained by the method of Meves (**55**), especially in embryonic tissues.

146. Demonstration of oxidative ferments. For this purpose Marinesco recommends the use of Gräff and von Gierke's technique, which is based on the synthesis of indophenol blue inside the tissue. This procedure renders permanent staining, which cannot be achieved with the Winkler-Schültze procedure.

Here is the *modus faciendi*:

1. Fix in 10 per 100 formalin.
2. Cut 15 μm thick frozen sections and transfer them directly to a 50/50 mixture of solutions A and B; stain for about fifteen minutes (the sections will first turn violet and afterward deep blue).

Solution A:

Naphtol	0.10 g
Saline	150 cc

Solution B:

Dimethylparaphenylendiamine	0.10 g
Saline	200 cc

Both solutions must be prepared twenty-four hours in advance and kept in dark flasks; naphthol needs gentle heating in a bain-marie.

3. Rinse in saline and immerse for some minutes in diluted Gram's liquid:

Gram's liquid	10 cc
Saline	30 cc

Six drops of 1 per 100 osmic acid can be added to this solution. Gram's liquid contains 2 g of potassium iodide and 1g of iodine in 100 cc of distilled water.

4. Immerse the sections in a mixture containing 40 cc of saline and 3–4 cc of a saturated solution of lithium carbonate; the sections must remain in this liquid until they regain a blue color.
5. Counterstain with a nonacidic dye. Mount in glycerin jelly.

The protoplasm and neuronal processes exhibit numerous blue-stained granules, although it must be borne in mind that the topography of the oxidases changes in the various neuronal types. If osmium is used, lipids can be readily distinguished from oxidases, because the former are stained in brown.[10]

147. Demonstration of the pigmentary spherules of the protoplasm. Almost all neurons, especially those from old animals, contain one or more lipid spherules that show a yellow-brown color and are larger than plastosomes; their chemical composition is far from understood.

There are several methods for staining these organelles, although we only use the following ones:

1. Cut frozen sections from formalin-fixed tissues.
2. Rinse thoroughly in order to remove formalin.
3. Immerse the sections for some minutes in 1 per 300 gold chloride solution.
4. Place the sections in a large well containing some drops of acetic acid and expose them to daylight (or to the light of a powerful lightbulb) until they become a pale violet color.
5. Fix in 5 per 100 sodium hyposulfite.

The pigment stands out as a deep purple color against a pale violet background.

148. The pigmentary spherules also can be readily stained with Cajal's uranyl-formalin method (**136**), although it is necessary to lengthen the fixation period up to one or two days. (See the variation of this method to stain glial cells in **175**.) If this precaution is taken, the pigment clearly will be shown as almost bl ack against a pale yellow background, especially in the sections taken from the center of the block; at this level neither the Golgi apparatus nor the neuroglia are stained.

The pigment also can be impregnated, though more faintly, by osmic acid (use a 2 per 100 solution for three to five days). Other methods for pigment staining are reported in **231–232**.

149. Del Río-Hortega has developed a modification of his silver carbonate method in order to reveal the neuronal pigment and prepigment.

Here is the technique:

1. Fix in 10 per 100 formalin or in Cajal's formalin-bromide (**2**); there is no limit to the time of the fixation period.
2. Overexposure the pieces to ammonium bromide in Cajal's indurating solution, at 40° to 50°C.
3. Cut frozen sections and rinse them in strong ammoniacal water.
4. Immerse the sections for some minutes in 5–10 per 100 sodium sulfite.
5. Without rinsing, immerse the sections in a well containing 10 cc of silver carbonate and 3 drops of pyridine (see the preparation of the silver carbonate solution in **187**); stain at 50°C until the sections turn pale brown.
6. Rinse with water for thirty seconds.
7. Rinse again, but with 96° alcohol, for the same length of time.
8. Reduce in 1 per 100 formalin.
9. Tone with gold and fix in 5 per 100 sodium hyposulfite; gold-toning must be performed at 40°–45°C.
10. Rinse, dehydrate, clarify, and mount.

NUCLEUS AND CELL MEMBRANE

150. Coloration of the nucleus. All the general procedures for nuclear staining can be used in the nervous system. Thus, hematoxylin- or carmine-based methods are useful, although the most instructive results are obtained when using *basic anilines*.

The dyes of the latter group should be used following the same rules as for the *Nissl method* (e.g., the sections must be overstained and then differentiated with 96° alcohol or with anilinic alcohol). The recommended stains are *thionine, Unna's polychrome blue, Unna-Pappenheim's liquid, Biondi's mixture, toluidine blue*, etc.

Heidehein's procedure with *ferric hematoxylin* (**54**) also yields excellent results, especially if the sections are counterstained with acidic dyes, such as *eosin* or *erythrosine*. The former methods[6] clearly demonstrate the principal and *accessory nucleoli*, as well as the chromatic granules of the karyoplasm; the *nuclear membrane* is barely shown, except in large neurons.

Some nuclear organelles require special stains:

1. The **nucleolar spherules**, which were first partially reported by von Lenhossék and Marinesco using routine aniline methods, are vigorously revealed by the silver procedures (Simarro, Cajal, Marinesco, Athias, Tello, Collin, Lache, etc.). The most recommendable of these methods are the reduced silver nitrate techniques, especially the formulae that do not

involve fixation (**114**) or those that use ammoniacal alcohol (**116**), chloral hydrate (**117**), and pyridine (**119**); Bielschowsky's method, on the other hand, does not impregnate these structures.

2. ***Levi's perinucleolar cap.*** This organelle is shown by aniline stains, even after silver impregnation.[11] An especially useful stain is diluted *Biondi's mixture* (Levi) (14), which stains the cap with methyl green (*EN 37*); good results also are obtained using the *Unna and Pappenheim's liquid (pyronine-methyl green;* see **254**), although special care must be taken when differentiating the sections with 96° alcohol.

3. *Roncoroni's intranuclear rodlet*. This organelle sometimes is stained with the methods using basic anilines, but it is best revealed with Cajal's method (formula without fixative, **114**), especially if the silver nitrate concentration is reduced to 0.75 per 100. With this technique, we were able to demonstrate this structure even in the cerebellar granules (Cajal, 1903).

151. Demonstration of the cell membrane. The cell membrane has a very poor affinity for the usual dyes, making it almost impossible to reveal[7]; although, occasionally, some large neurons show a double outline that clearly indicates its presence.

A little cunning is needed to visualize this structure; one of the tricks we use is to fix fragments of spinal cord, acoustic nuclei, etc., in absolute alcohol, leaving them to rest undisturbed until they are embedded in celloidin. The rapid removal of water by alcohol that takes place at the periphery of the pieces shrinks the neuronal protoplasm, so that the membrane can be shown up by the Nissl method.

Another strategy is to produce a *chromatolytic reaction* in the spinal cord by tearing a nerve trunk; under these conditions, the nucleus is displaced to the cell's periphery, forming a bulge on the cell outline that only can be explained by the existence of the membrane.[8]

152. The reticular membrane of Cajal–Golgi. This membrane was first described by one of us (Cajal) using Ehrlich's method and later studied in more depth by Golgi with the silver chromate technique and by Bethe in tissues fixed in 7.5 per 100 nitric acid (see Bethe's method in **105**). Nevertheless, much controversy still exists as to this membrane being a real structure or a coagulation artifact[9] (*EN 38*).

In any case, this structure can be shown by the procedures of Ehrlich (**89**) and Donaggio (staining of the sections for several hours in a highly diluted methylene blue solution). The formalin-acetone variation of Cajal's method (**134**) also shows this network, mainly around the large short-axon neurons. Unfortunately, this procedure is rather inconstant, being only appropriate for fifteen-to-twenty-day-old cats and dogs. It often fails in the rabbit.

12

Staining of Neuronal Axons in the Centers

153. Almost all silver methods render satisfactory axonal impregnations both in the white and gray matter. Thus, here we shall merely summarize the methods described previously.

The demonstration of central axons depends on their caliber; thus, we must differentiate between (a) large and medium-sized axons, and (b) thin axons and delicate terminal arborizations.

(a) Axons from the first group are readily stained with Bielschowsky's (**109**), Cajal's (formulae with ammoniacal alcohol and chloral hydrate, **116, 117**), and Schültze's methods (**131**), as well as with Fajersztajnz's old procedure[1] with ammoniacal silver nitrate (**154**).
(b) The delicate central endings and thin axons are best shown using Cajal's method, especially the formulae with pyridine (**119**), pyridine-alcohol-chloral (**120**), formalin (**122, 123**), etc.

As a rule of thumb, those techniques that stain large axons well are not suitable for thin ones and vice versa, as if their physicochemical natures were different. This is not an invariable rule, however; there are exceptions and intermediate states. Thus, from time to time the methods recommended for thick axons (**109, 114, 116, 121**) render splendid colorations of the central axonal endings (baskets, end-bulbs, chalices, and terminal plexuses of the brain, cerebellum, medulla, and spinal cord).

The central axons also can be stained by Ehrlich's method (**89**) and other aniline-based techniques, although the results are not as uniform or accurate as with silver methods; besides, methylene blue only stains the thickest axons.

Finally, allow us to mention the Golgi method (**73, 74**), which yields splendid images of axons, axon collaterals, and axonal endings in young animals. On the other hand, the presence of myelin is an insurmountable obstacle for these methods; therefore, they must be performed in fetuses or newborn animals.

154. Fajersztajn procedure to stain axons in the centers (1901).

1. Fix in 10 per 100 formalin for some days or even months.
2. Cut thin frozen sections.

3. Rinse with distilled water in order to remove the formalin.
4. Immerse for five to twenty minutes in ammoniacal silver nitrate. This mixture is prepared by dripping ammonia onto a 2 per 100 silver nitrate solution. The solution is ready to use when the precipitate that first appears dissolves completely; care must be taken to avoid any excess ammonia. If there is an excess of ammonia (this can be detected by a strong, pungent alkaline odor), add some drops of silver solution until a small volume of insoluble precipitate is formed.
5. Without rinsing, reduce in 5 per 100 formalin. The latter process takes place almost instantaneously.
6. Rinse, tone with gold chloride or with platinum chloride, fix in sodium hyposulfite, etc.

This method stains the thick central axons nicely, especially in the cerebellum and spinal cord; however, both Bielschowsky's and Cajal's methods render more complete and delicate images.

155. For the sake of completeness, we will mention some of our old techniques[2] using ammoniacal-silver-nitrate impregnation in specimens fixed in mixtures of formalin and hydroquinone, formalin and tannin, or formalin and pyrogallic acid. We no longer use these, however; not only do they require a photographic softener (e.g., Lugol's solution, potash hypermanganate, or potassium ferricyanide), but also both Bielschowsky's method and reduced silver nitrate techniques give better results.

Myelin Staining

156. Weigert's method. This is the classic method for coloring the myelin sheaths and possibly it is the most reliable one. Many variations of the primitive procedure of Weigert exist, one of which we describe below. It was developed by Paula Mayer who worked at Edinger's laboratory.

1. Fix the tissues in 10 per 100 formalin.
2. Cut slices, not thicker than 1.5–2cm and immerse them for four to fourteen days in Weigert's first mordant (rapid mordant). This reagent is prepared as follows:

Potassium dichromate	5 g
Chrome fluoride	2.5 cc
Boiling water	100 cc

    Boil the mixture, and filter when cool.
3. Transfer the blocks directly to 70° alcohol until no color is drained off; this step must be carried out in a dark flask.
4. Embed in celloidin and cut thick sections (15–20 µm). Special care must be taken to avoid ripping the sections by using a perfectly sharpened microtome knife set at a wide angle. The edge of the knife must be wetted with 70° alcohol. Attach the sections to the slide (**32**) and place them in water.
5. Immerse the slides for twenty-four hours in Weigert's second mordant (this mordant is also used for staining glial cells, see **165**) at 37°. To prepare this reagent, place 2.5 g of chrome fluoride or chrome alum in 100 cc of water; boil until it is dissolved and immediately add 5 cc of glacial acetic acid and 5 g of neutral copper acetate. Stir the mixture thoroughly with a glass rod.
6. Rinse the sections with water or in 70° alcohol and stain for twenty-four hours in a 50/50 mixture of the following solutions:

    Solution A

Hematoxylin	1 g
96 per 100 alcohol	100 cc

Solution B

Officinal solution of iron sesquichloride[1]	4 cc
Water	96 cc

The hematoxylin solution must be allowed to ripen for at least two months[2] before use. Weigert's hematoxylin formula can be replaced by the following one:

Hematoxylin	1 g
Absolute alcohol	10 cc
Saturated solution of lithium carbonate	1 cc
Water	60 cc

7. Rinse for thirty to sixty minutes, changing the water several times.
8. Differentiate in the following liquid:

Potassium ferricyanide	5 g
Borax	4 cc
Water	200 cc

The differentiation process takes from fifteen minutes to twenty-four hours; the solution must be replaced several times. Differentiation must proceed until the white and gray matters become distinguishable. It is advisable to check the reaction under the microscope.

9. Rinse with running tap water, dehydrate in alcohol, clarify in carbol-xylol and xylol, and mount in Canada balsam.

When the differentiation is done correctly, the myelin sheaths appear blue-black against an almost colorless background. The gray matter is a yellowish color.

157. Pal's method.

1. Fix the specimens in the liquids of Müller (**5**) or Erlicki. The latter acts faster and an excellent degree of induration is achieved in a third of the time required for Müller's liquid. The composition of Erlicki's fluid is

Potassium bichromate	2.5 g
Copper sulfate	0.5 cc
Distilled water	100 cc

The fixative must be replaced every two days.

2. Dehydrate in alcohol and embed in celloidin.
3. Place the sections in Weigert's iron (or lithium) hematoxylin (**156**) for twenty-four hours at room temperature or for one hour (or less) at 37°C.
4. Rinse in tap water for one to two hours, and then immerse the sections for fifteen to thirty seconds in freshly prepared 0.25 per 100 potassium permanganate; the sections will turn brown during this step.
5. Briefly rinse the sections with water and bleach them completely (one to five minutes) with the following reagent:

Potash sulfite	1 g
Oxalic acid	1 cc
Distilled water	200 cc

This solution must be prepared immediately before use. For the sections to be bleached completely, this procedure may have to be repeated several times.

6. Rinse the sections in plenty of water.
7. Counterstain with boracic or lithium carmine (**43, 45**).
8. Rinse, dehydrate, and clarify in creosote or in bergamot oil and mount in Canada balsam.

Pal's method has the disadvantage of decolorizing the thin myelin sheaths of the gray matter; this decoloration is unavoidable in large brain sections, especially when complete differentiation is required.

158. Kulschitzky's method.

1. Fix in Müller's (**5**) or Erlicki's liquids (**157**). Formalin fixation also can be used, but the specimens need to be treated with Weigert's first mordant (**156**) for five days in the oven.
2. Dehydrate and embed in celloidin.
3. Stain the sections for twelve to twenty-four hours in this mixture:

| 10 per 100 hematoxylin in alcohol | 10 cc |
| 2 per 100 acetic acid | 90 cc |

The hematoxylin-alcohol solution must be prepared six to eight months in advance.

4. Transfer the slides directly to this differentiating solution:

| Saturated solution of lithium carbonate | 100 cc |
| 1 per 100 potassium ferricyanide | 10 cc |

The differentiation process takes place very slowly, three to four hours being necessary for the brain cortex and approximately twelve hours for the spinal cord and brain stem; this step must be monitored hourly under the microscope.

5. Rinse in abundant water.
6. Dehydrate, clarify, and mount.

This method is very popular now because of its constancy; furthermore, large brain sections are more easily stained with this procedure than with Weigert-Pal's, in which the permanganate and sulfite treatment renders the sections rather fragile.

Spielmeyer has pointed out the importance of a thorough *chromation* in order to obtain good results. He suggests treating the sections with Müller's liquid for eight to fourteen days prior to staining and then with 1 per 100 chromic acid for twenty-four hours. After this step, the sections must be briefly rinsed, first with water and then in alcohol before being stained with hematoxylin. The best results are obtained when using hematoxylin solutions ripened for at least six months. In the case of floating sections obtained from formalin-fixed material, they must be immersed for thirty minutes in 0.5 per 100 chromic acid, heating the well until vapors appear.

159. Kulschitzky-Pal's Procedure (Wolters). A combination of the preceding methods is recommended to avoid the yellowish background of the sections, thus allowing the most delicate myelin sheaths to be easily recognizable. This is achieved by staining the sections with acetic hematoxylin, immersing them for a few minutes in Müller's fluid, and then oxidizing and bleaching them as in Pal's method (**157**, Steps 4 and 5).

160. Spielmeyer's method.

1. Fix for thirty days in formalin, cut thick (25–35 μm) frozen sections and rinse them with water for one hour.
2. Leave the sections overnight in 2.5 per 100 *iron and ammonia alum*; use only violet crystals of alum to prepare the solution.
3. Rinse briefly with distilled water.
4. Immerse the sections for ten minutes in 70° alcohol. Gently shake the sections during this step.
5. Stain for two to twelve hours in a hematoxylin solution made by mixing 100 parts of water with 5 parts of stock hematoxylin solution; the latter reagent is a 10 per 100 hematoxylin solution in absolute alcohol ripened for at least six months. For this method to be successful the reagent must be matured. Spielmeyer even suggests using the same liquid several times.
6. Rinse with water.
7. Differentiate in the mordanting solution for half an hour or a little longer; the process must be monitored by removing a section from the differentiating solution from time to time, rinsing it with distilled water, and examining it under the microscope.
8. Rinse the sections thoroughly with water. If the results are not as good as expected, the whole procedure can be repeated with the same sections.
9. Dehydrate in graded alcohols, etc.

This method also can be run on gelatin- or celloidin-embedded material, although in the latter case it is advisable to increase the concentration of the mordant up to 4 per 100 and reducing its time of action to four hours; differentiation can be achieved using a mixture of iron alum (4 g), borax (2.5 g), potassium ferricyanide (2 g) and water (100 cc).

This procedure has become very popular because it renders very consistent results. Furthermore, it can be used on pieces preserved in formalin. It works nicely on tissue from humans and large mammals; in small ones the background can be somewhat dark, hampering the visualization of the most delicate sheaths.

161. Loyez's method. This method provides myelin staining in paraffin- or celloidin-embedded pieces without any chromation of the material, which can save a good amount of time. The modus operandi is as follows:

1. Fix in 10 per 100 formalin for at least eight days; the method will work nicely even in material that has been kept in formalin for several years.

2. Embed, preferably in celloidin or in paraffin if thin sections are needed. Cut sections, attach them to the slides, and transfer them to water.
3. Immerse the sections for twenty-four hours in a 4 per 100 solution of iron alum, using only those crystals of alum that have a violet color.
4. Rinse briefly with water and stain for twenty-four hours at room temperature (or, even better, at 37°C) in:

10 per 100 hematoxylin in alcohol	10 cc
Distilled water	90 cc
Saturated solution of lithium carbonate	2 cc

The alcohol solution of hematoxylin must be prepared at least six months in advance.

5. Rinse the sections carefully and then immerse them in 4 per 100 iron alum. This *first differentiation* must be stopped when the gray matter begins to fade.
6. Rinse with running tap water and end the differentiation using Weigert's reagent (**156**, Step 8) diluted 50/50 in water.
7. Dip the slides in distilled water to which a few drops of ammonia have been added and then rinse them thoroughly. Immersion in ammonia water is not essential, but it does intensify the coloration.
8. Dehydrate and mount.

Myelinated fibers are sharply stained in black against a pale-yellow background (in the brain cortex the background may be darker). The method works properly when sections are thinner than 10–15 μm; in thicker sections, the delicate myelinated fibers of the cortex may be lost.

The sections stained with Loyez's method can be counterstained with Unna's polychrome blue for the Nissl substance.

162. Schultze's method. This procedure is more sensitive for detecting thin myelin sheaths than those based on potassium dichromate; hence, it is especially useful for the study of the developing nervous system.

1. Fix small or thin nervous tissue fragments in 1 per 100 osmic acid (**8**).
2. Transfer the pieces to a 1 per 100 potassium dichromate solution for twenty-four hours. This reagent should be replaced several times.
3. Immerse the specimens for twenty-four hours in 50 per 100 alcohol; this step must be carried out in a dark flask.
4. Stain the blocks in a 0.5 per 100 solution of hematoxylin in 70° alcohol.
5. Rinse for one or two days in 70° alcohol; dehydrate, embed either in celloidin or paraffin, and cut thin sections (5 to 10 μm).

163. Marchi's method.

Fix small central nervous system samples in Müller's liquid (**5**) for eight to twenty days and then place them for one to two weeks in the following mixture, which must be changed daily:

Müller's liquid	2 parts
1 per 100 osmic acid	1 cc

Rinse for twenty-four hours in running tap water, dehydrate in alcohol, and embed in celloidin; cut thick sections and, without counterstaining, mount the sections in Canada balsam without coverslip (**68**).

This is an excellent method for visualizing the secondary degenerations that take place in the nervous system as a result of severing the neuronal nuclei or the myelinated tracts. With this staining procedure the normal myelin sheaths appear in a gray or pale-brown color, whereas the degenerating nerve fibers show trails or rows of small lipid droplets colored deep black.

The best results with Marchi's method are obtained when the animal is sacrificed fourteen to sixteen days after surgery. In the case of humans, this procedure can be used successfully if the patient dies eight to ten days after the lesion has occurred. Longer survival periods result in the resorption of degenerated myelin.

Some important observations. The tissue fragments to be treated with Marchi's method must not exceed 3–4 mm in thickness, because osmium solutions have a very low penetrating capacity as a result of their low diosmotic power. Nevertheless, the nervous centers must not be sliced before induration; the best procedure is to fix the brain in toto for five or six days in 10 per 100 formalin. Once the tissue is somewhat hardened, the degenerating areas are carefully dissected, avoiding any mechanical damage. The selected pieces are rinsed in running tap water in order to remove the excess of formalin and then transferred to Müller's liquid. Formalin fixation should not exceed the recommended period, because it may render artifacts in the preparations (the pseudogranules of Marchi). A prolonged immersion in Müller's fixative also must be avoided because the specimens can become so brittle that sectioning proves very difficult.

Coloration, even with Marchi's procedure, is obtained only if the chrome-osmium mixture acts on all the faces of the tissue slices; thus, a thin cotton sheet must be laid at the bottom of the flask and the pieces placed on it before pouring the mixture over them.

Finally, it is advisable that the embedding period in celloidin needs to be as short as possible, never exceeding four days. Sections can be obtained even without embedding; in this case, the specimens are indurated in alcohol, stuck to a wooden cube with collodion or gum Arabic, and sectioned with a sliding microtome.

164. Benda's method. This method is really a combination of two different techniques. It stains normal myelin sheaths with the Spielmeyer's procedure and degenerating ones with scarlet red.

1. Fix in formalin and cut frozen sections.
2. Run the method of Spielmeyer (**160**), skipping Step 4.
3. Stain with scarlet red (see Herxheimer's method, **222**).

Myelin is stained a blue to black color, and the lipids produced in myelin degeneration are stained in red.

14

Coloration of the Macroglia, Microglia, and Oligodendroglia

MACROGLIA

165. Weigert's method for macroglia. This method specifically demonstrates the fibrils of the fibrous astrocytes by staining them blue. In the cell expansions, these threads appear clearly separated whereas in the cell body their appearance is lumpy due to the crisscrossing of the fibrils. The epithelial cells and the protoplasmic astrocytes (also called spider-like cells and penniform cells) are not stained by this technique.

Here is the *modus faciendi*:

1. Fix brain slices not thicker than 5 mm, in 20 per 100 formalin for four days, changing the liquid daily. The method only works properly in fresh specimens of human brain; in animals, the results are very variable. For some specimens, 5 per 100 potassium dichromate can be used instead of formalin.
2. Immerse the pieces for eight days in Weigert's mordant (*Gliabeize*):

Water	100 cc
Chrome fluoride	2.5 g
Glacial acetic acid	5 cc
Neutral copper acetate (powder)	5 g
Formalin	10 cc

To prepare this mixture, chrome fluoride must be dissolved in boiling water; while boiling, add the acetic acid and the copper acetate and withdraw the flask immediately from the Bunsen burner. Add the formalin when the liquid has cooled down to room temperature.

3. Rinse briefly with water and embed in celloidin or, better still, in paraffin. Cut 15–20 μm thick sections.
4. Reduce the sections for about ten minutes in 0.33 per 100 potassium permanganate.

5. Rinse briefly with water and immerse the sections for one to two hours (until the brownish tone they acquired in the permanganate disappears) in the following liquid:

Chromogen (Höchster)	5 g
Formic acid (Sw 1.20)	5 cc
Distilled water	100 cc

Just before use, mix 90 parts of this reagent with 10 parts of 10 per 100 sodium sulfite.

6. Rinse briefly with distilled water (two changes) and stain for some minutes in: Saturated solution of methyl violet in 70° alcohol 100 cc

5 per 100 oxalic acid   5 cc

Methyl violet must be dissolved by gentle warming and once cooled to room temperature mixed with oxalic acid.

7. Blot the sections with blotting paper and immerse them for thirty seconds in a saturated iodine solution in 5 per 100 potassium iodide.
8. Bleach in a 50/50 mixture of xylene and aniline oil.
9. Rinse carefully with xylene in order to remove the aniline oil and mount either in Canada balsam or in d'Ammar resin, both dissolved in xylene.

Gliofibrils and nuclei are stained blue, whereas the protoplasm and connective fibers remain colorless. This method is rather unreliable; Spielmeyer recommends treating the sections for twenty-four hours with 2.5 per 100 iron alum immediately before Step 4.

166. Pötter's modification of Weigert's method.

1. Fix fresh brain fragments for four or more days in 10 per 100 formalin then embed in paraffin.
2. Immerse for four days at 40°C in Weigert's mordant for neuroglia (**165**).
3. Rinse for ten minutes with distilled water.
4. Immerse the sections for three days in a liquid containing 80 cc of distilled water and 20 cc of *Agfa's* methylhydroquinone developer. This must be carried out in the dark and at room temperature.
5. Rinse thoroughly with distilled water and stain for one to three days with Victoria blue (from Grübler). The staining solution is made dissolving the dye up to saturation in warm water, boiling gently for one hour, and leaving to cool and filter.
6. Blot the sections and treat them for some seconds with the iodine-iodide solution (**165**).
7. Differentiate in xylene plus aniline oil (three parts xylene; 1 part aniline oil); check the differentiation with the microscope.
8. Rinse several times with xylene to remove the aniline oil and mount in balsam. Glial fibers are stained deep blue against a colorless background.

167. Anglade's Procedure.

1. Fix for four days in the following liquid:

   7 per 100 sublimate   1 vol.
   Fol's liquid (**23**)   3 vols.

2. Rinse for two hours with running tap water.
3. Dehydrate in alcohol or acetone and embed in paraffin.
4. Immerse the sections in the Victoria blue solution (**166**, Step 5); during the staining period the liquid must be hot but not boiling.
5. Drain the slides and immerse them in Gram's solution:

   Iodine   1 g
   Potassium iodide   2 cc
   Distilled water   300 cc

6. Differentiate in:

   Xylene   1 part
   Aniline oil   2 parts

7. Clarify in xylene and mount in Canada balsam.

Neuroglial fibers and nuclei are stained deep violet. The method renders results similar to those of Weigert's procedure.

168. Benda's method.

1. Fix fresh material for at least two days in 90°–94° alcohol.
2. Treat the pieces for twenty-four hours with 10 per 100 nitric acid.
3. Immerse for another twenty-four hours in 2 per 100 potassium bichromate.
4. Transfer directly to a 1 per 100 solution of chromic acid; this reagent should also act for twenty-four hours.
5. Wash for one day in running tap water and embed in paraffin.
6. Immerse the sections for twenty-four hours in 4 per 100 iron alum.
7. Rinse briefly with running tap water.
8. Stain for two hours in a diluted solution of sodium sulpho-alizarinate (Kahlbaum).

This solution is prepared by dripping a concentrated alcoholic solution of this dye onto distilled water until an amber yellow color appears.

9. Rinse briefly with distilled water and wipe the sections with filter paper.
10. Drip 1 per 1000 toluidine blue over the slides until the sections are covered by the dye; heat with a flame until vapors begin to appear and then withdraw from the flame and allow an additional fifteen-minute staining period. If staining is carried out at room temperature, the sections must stay in the dye for one to twenty-four hours.

11. Rinse in 1 per 100 acetic acid or in a very weak solution of picric acid.
12. Blot the sections with filter paper, immerse in absolute alcohol, and differentiate with creosote under the microscope; differentiation usually takes about ten minutes.
13. Clarify thoroughly in xylene and mount in Canada balsam.

Gliofibrils are stained deep blue against a reddish background; nuclei and fibrin threads have a bluish tinge.

169. Holzer's procedure. This method is more constant than Weigert's for staining the fibrous neuroglia of the human brain.

1. Fix in either 10 per 100 formalin (five to eight days) or in a 50/50 mixture of formalin and 96° alcohol and leave for at least twelve days, after which time the tissues must be immersed in 10 per 100 formalin for three more days.
2. Embed in either paraffin or in celloidin. Frozen sections also may be used, but they must be immersed for several hours in 50° alcohol. Mount on clean glass slides.
3. Cover the sections with:

1 per 100 Phosphomolybdic acid	5 cc
96° Alcohol	15 cc

This step must be repeated two or three times.

4. Drain off excess liquid and gently blot the sections with filter paper, but be very careful not to dry the sections completely.
5. Press the sections with a strip of filter paper wetted with a 20/80 mixture of 96° alcohol and chloroform; this must be done quickly or the sections will dry out.
6. Cover the sections with some drops of:

Crystal violet (crystals, Meister Lucius, Hoechst)	0.5 g
Absolute alcohol	2 cc
Chloroform	8 cc

After not more than *two to five seconds*, the sections will be covered by a film of a metallic-green color.

7. Immediately pour some drops of 10 per 100 potassium bromide over the slide and let it act until the sections turn blue.
8. Blot the sections with blotting paper and differentiate with a freshly prepared mixture of aniline oil and chloroform (aniline oil, 6 cc; chloroform, 9 cc; ammonia, one drop); differentiation must be stopped when the milky clouds formed when adding the differentiating solution disappear.
9. Rinse several times with xylol and mount in balsam.

Gliofibrils are deeply stained in a blue-violet color. The perinuclear cytoplasm of the gliocytes also is shown. This method also stains the connective tissue.

170. Mallory's method.

1. Fix for four days in 20 per 100 formalin then place the samples for a further four days in a saturated solution of picric acid; end fixation by immersing the specimens for four additional days in 5 per 100 ammonium bichromate at 37°C.
2. Embed in celloidin.
3. Immerse for fifteen to thirty minutes in 0.5 per 100 potassium permanganate.
4. Rinse with distilled water and bleach the sections with 1 per 100 oxalic acid.
5. Rinse several times with distilled water and stain for twelve to twenty-four hours in:

Hematoxylin	0.1 g
Distilled water	80 cc
10 per 100 Phosphotungstic acid	20 cc
Hydrogen peroxide	0.2 cc

Hematoxylin must be dissolved in lukewarm water and then left to cool to room temperature before adding the other components.

6. Rinse briefly with water, dehydrate, clarify in origanum oil and xylol, and mount in Canada balsam.

Gliofibrils are stained in blue and connective tissue in pink.

171. Held's method for staining the *glia marginalis* (1909).

1. Fix thin tissue slices for one to six days (at 37°C) in:

Müller's liquid (5)	100 cc
Sublimate	3 g
Acetic acid	3 cc
Formalin	0.5 cc

The acetic acid and formalin must be added just before use.

2. Embed in celloidin.
3. Treat the sections for five minutes in a solution of caustic soda (80° alcohol, 100 cc; **sodium hydrate**, 1 g).
4. Rinse in distilled water.
5. Immerse for some minutes in 5 per 100 iron alum.
6. Rinse briefly with distilled water and stain for twelve to twenty-four hours (at 50°C) in molybdic hematoxylin.

This dye is prepared by dissolving 1 g of hematoxylin in 100 cc of 70° alcohol and adding molybdic acid in excess; the solution has a blue color that changes gradually to deep black if vigorously shaken. The liquid thus prepared must be allowed to ripen for at least one year. To prepare the staining solution, drip this stock solution on distilled water until it turns deep violet.

7. Differentiate in 5 per 100 iron alum in order to bleach the connective tissue.
8. Rinse with water and counterstain with Van Gieson's picrofuchsin (**59**) for fifteen seconds.
9. Rinse in 96° alcohol until no more color is drained off; dehydrate, clarify, and mount.

This method stains the *glia marginalis* black, as well as the pial and perivascular limiting membranes of Held; collagen fibers are stained bright red.

Note: Much better results are obtained by fixing in formalin-bromide and staining with the methods of Del Río-Hortega (silver carbonate) or Cajal (ammoniacal silver oxide).

172. Alzheimer's method for staining neuroglial cells and blood vessels.

1. Fix in alcohol and embed in celloidin. Fixation also can be performed in Weigert's mordant (**165**), but in this case the pieces need to be rinsed with water for several hours and then cut with the freezing microtome.
2. Place the sections for a short time in a well containing distilled water to which some drops of saturated molybdic acid solution have been added. Then immerse them in saturated molybdic acid for two to twelve hours. (One hour is enough for celloidin sections.)
3. Rinse briefly with distilled water (two changes).
4. Stain for one hour in Mann's liquid:

1 per 100 Methyl blue[1]	35 cc
1 per 100 Eosin (w.g.)	35 cc
Distilled water	100 cc

5. Rinse with distilled water until no color drains off.
6. Rinse briefly with 96° alcohol until the sections become pale brown (one to two minutes).
7. Absolute alcohol, xylol, and Canada balsam.

This splendid procedure stains the gliofibrils, cylinder-axes, neuroglial ameboid cells, and connective fibers in blue, whereas myelin and erythrocytes are red. Protoplasmic glia is poorly demonstrated, however, as is to be expected with aniline methods.

173. Cajal's gold-sublimate method (1913).

1. Fix fresh human brain slices for two to six days (one-month maximum) in:

Formalin	15 cc
Distilled water	85 cc
Ammonium bromide	2 g

2. Cut frozen sections, not thinner than 30–40 μm (*EN 39*).

Chapter 14: Macroglia, Microglia and Oligodendroglia

3. Rinse briefly with distilled water and impregnate in a freshly prepared mixture of:

1 per 100 Brown gold chloride (Merck)	10 cc
Sublimate (needle-like crystals, Merck)	0.4–0.6 g
Distilled water	50 cc^2

Pour this fluid into a Petri dish until the liquid level is about 0.5–1 cm; use 5 cc of gold solution for each section.

The reagent must act only on one face of the sections, which must be carefully laid out flat at the bottom of the dish.

Staining has to be carried out in complete darkness or at least under subdued light; the staining period is four to eight hours at 18°–22°C, although for especially difficult specimens, the temperature can be raised to 25°–30°C and the time shortened to two or three hours (de Castro). In either case, the best indicator is the color of the sections, which are deep purple when properly impregnated.

4. Rinse with distilled water and fix in:

5–10 per 100 Sodium hyposulfite	20 cc
Sodium bisulfite (Normal solution)	4–6 drops

5. Rinse the sections with 70° alcohol, mount them on clean slides, and blot them with blotting paper; alcohols, origanum oil, xylene, and Canada balsam.

When the reaction is successful, protoplasmic astrocytes are purple-red whereas the neurons are pink or pale violet; nerve fibers are not visible.

The best results with this procedure are achieved in adult human brains, although it renders acceptable images in cat and dog brains, but not so good in rabbit brains. Nevertheless, in the hands of skillful investigators, like Achúcarro and de Castro, splendid colorations can be obtained even in reptiles, birds, and amphibians.

Remarks: The temperature is critical to obtain selective staining. Temperatures below 12°C hamper the impregnation of protoplasmic glial cells. For the human brain the optimal temperature is 18°–20°C and the reaction is completed after three to six hours; temperatures over 22°C result in a loss of contrast. On the other hand, the human cerebellum, medulla, and spinal cord need higher temperatures and shorter impregnation times (two or three hours at 22°–26°C). For other mammals, a temperature of 24°–26°C is necessary. Vertebrates phylogenetically distant from humans (reptiles, amphibians, and fish) may require as much as 28°–32°C for only one or two hours (de Castro).

The prevailing color of properly stained sections is either purplish or reddish-violet. In order to assess the color of the sections properly, they should be immersed in distilled water. A pale violet (or pale pink) hue indicates underimpregnation, in which case, the section must be returned to the gold bath. During the last half hour, the staining needs to be very carefully controlled (preferably with observation under the microscope), because even a very short (ten to fifteen minutes) overimpregnation may render the preparation useless. This is due to the formation of a dusty gold precipitate over the sections.

It must be kept in mind that protoplasmic astrocytes are very prone to autolysis and, therefore, the tissue must be as fresh as possible. Our best preparations have been made from human brains obtained from autopsies performed only two to six hours after death; although in winter, when temperatures are very low, good results can be obtained up to twenty-four hours after death.

Finally, let us mention that formaldehyde eventually destroys the aurophilic substances in the tissue and thus the reaction must be carried out as soon as possible. It is pointless to extend the fixation to more than three days, when the induration ability of formalin is fully achieved, although nice protoplasmic astrocytes still can be obtained in pieces kept for up to two weeks in the fixative. In the case of fibrous astrocytes, the fixation time can be longer (two months or even more), especially when using pathological material. This neuroglial type is more finely demonstrated if ammonium bromide is replaced by urea nitrate, although with this formula protoplasmic astrocytes are not shown.

174. Del Río-Hortega has proposed a modification of Cajal's former method that is especially recommended for *gliomata*, although it also can be successful in normal material.

1. Fix for thirty days or more in Cajal's formalin-bromide (**2**); cut frozen sections.
2. Rinse in distilled water. In some cases, results are improved by rinsing the sections first in ammoniacal water and then with water with acetic acid.
3. Impregnate in:

1 per 500 Gold chloride	50 cc
Crystallized sublimate	0.5–1 g

   Warm gently to dissolve and add:

Glacial acetic acid	30 drops

   Place this mixture in a well, immerse the sections in it, and put it in the oven (30°–35°C) until the specimens show either a pale or deep purple color; in the latter case go directly to Step 5.

4. Reduce in 5 per 100 oxalic acid for fifteen to thirty minutes; the sections will become deep purple.
5. Rinse with distilled water and fix in 5 per 100 sodium hyposulfite. Rinse again, dehydrate, clarify, etc.

175. Cajal's method with formalin and uranyl nitrate. This method was originally developed to demonstrate the Golgi apparatus, but it also stains in a most reliable manner the protoplasmic glia, and especially two of its distinctive characteristics, namely, the *gliosomes* and the *lipoid inclusions*.

Chapter 14: Macroglia, Microglia and Oligodendroglia

1. Fix thin (2–3 mm) slices of fresh nervous tissue for twenty-four to forty-eight hours in Cajal's formalin-uranyl nitrate mixture (**136**).
2. Rinse briefly with distilled water and immerse the pieces in 1.5–2 per 100 silver nitrate for two or three days at room temperature.
3. Dip in distilled water and reduce in the formalin-hydroquinone mixture (**136**) without sulfite. Rinse and embed in paraffin.

In some cases, it is useful to gold-tone the sections (**175**). This procedure enhances the contrast of the stained structures; it also allows counterstaining with either toluidine blue or Unna's polychrome blue, resulting in beautiful preparations that facilitate perfect analysis of the nuclear morphology (de Castro).

This method can be used in all the vertebrates, though the best results are obtained in man and young mammals. Nevertheless, one should be forewarned that only the superficial sections can be used, due to the poor penetration of the reagents. However, in deeper sections, although the neuroglial protoplasm is not impregnated, gliosomes and lipoid inclusions can be identified.

176. Staining of glial cells with ammoniacal silver oxide (Cajal, 1920).[1] Ammoniacal silver oxide has been used successfully by several authors (Montesano, Perusini, Achúcarro, etc.) to stain the glial cells of the white matter. We have recently developed a modification of this procedure that is most reliable and impregnates the astrocytes of both white and gray matters; the *microglial cells* are also impregnated, especially in pathological material.

1. Fix for more than four days in formalin-bromide (**2**).
2. Cut 20–35 µm thick frozen sections.
3. Immerse the sections for four hours (use a 37°C oven in winter) in:

Distilled water	50 cc
Formalin	6 g
Ammonium bromide	3 cc

Alternatively, the blocks may be immersed in this liquid for some minutes at 50°–55°C prior to sectioning, as suggested by Del Río-Hortega.

4. Rinse briefly with distilled water (twice) to remove the fixative.
5. Impregnate the sections for five to ten minutes at room temperature in a well containing:

Ammoniacal silver oxide	5 cc
Distilled water	15 cc
Pyridine	4–8 drops

We prepare the ammoniacal silver oxide as follows: Pour twelve drops of 40 per 100 caustic soda on 10 cc of 10% silver nitrate, so that a dark brown precipitate is formed. Pour out the supernatant and wash the remaining precipitate five times with distilled water. Add 60 or 70 cc of distilled water and dissolve with ammonia.

Because special care must be taken to avoid an excess of ammonia, it is preferable to leave some precipitate undissolved.

6. Warm the well gently (40°–45°C) using an alcohol burner until the sections become a Turkish tobacco color.
7. Dip in distilled water.
8. Reduce in 15 per 100 plain formalin or in a 20 per 100 solution of chalk-neutralized formalin.
9. Rinse the sections two or three times in plenty of tap water.
10. Tone in 1 per 500 yellow gold chloride. This step can be carried out at room temperature or in the oven at 37°C, as suggested by Del Río-Hortega. In the first case, toning is achieved after several hours and in the second one in just ten to twenty-five minutes.
11. Fix in 6 per 100 sodium hyposulfite to which a small volume of alcohol (some milliliters) and some grains of sodium bisulfite have been added.
12. Rinse thoroughly with water and then in 33 per 100 alcohol. Mount the sections on glass slides, dehydrate in alcohol, and clarify with origanum essence, oil of cloves, or carbol-xylol, xylol, and Canada balsam or d'Ammar resin.

This procedure gives absolutely consistent results in the nervous centers of vertebrates. White and gray matter astrocytes are clearly shown, although the latter may fail to be stained if the fixation time exceeds fifteen days or if the silver solution is too diluted. Needless to say, extremely fresh material is required to demonstrate protoplasmic astrocytes.

To stain microglial cells, the sections need to be removed from the ammoniacal silver oxide when they become a yellowish color[3]; in this case, the heating of the well (Step 6) can be omitted, though it hastens the reaction.

This procedure also stains the Nissl substance (using a very diluted silver solution) and the connective tissue fibers of both neural and non-neural organs.

177. Achúcarro's method (1911–1912). This ill-fated scholar devised a procedure to stain the neuroglial cells and connective tissue that has proved to be a general-purpose method, as shown by the recent work of Tello, Del Río-Hortega, Ranke, Calandre, Havet, Sacristan, Fortun, Fañanas, and many other Spanish and foreign authors.

Here is the last formula proposed by Achúcarro:

Fixation. Fix tissue slices not exceeding 2–3 mm in thickness in 20 per 100 formalin with enough drops of ammonia added to give an alkaline reaction when tested with litmus paper.
Sections. Not thicker than 10 µm.
Mordant. Immerse the sections in 10 per 100 tannin, flatten them, and warm gently; avoid the formation of bubbles. The sections will stiffen.
Wash. Once the mordant has cooled to room temperature, the sections are transferred to water to which some ammonia drops have been added until the sections recover the flexibility.

Chapter 14: Macroglia, Microglia and Oligodendroglia

Impregnation. A very diluted ammoniacal silver oxide solution (two to three drops of silver oxide per 10 cc of distilled water) is used to complete this step. Impregnation must stop when the tissues begin to turn yellow to brown.

The silver oxide solution, which is similar to Bielschowsky's, is prepared as follows:

10 per 100 Silver nitrate   5 cc
40 per 100 Caustic soda   5 drops

Wash the precipitate several times, dissolve with ammonia, carefully avoiding any excess, and make up to 25 cc with distilled water (*EN 37*).

Reduction. Reduce for five minutes in ammoniacal formalin (see Fixation). This method renders exquisite impregnations of the macroglial cells and the reticular network of the extracellular matrix of all tissues, including the perivascular connective tissue of the brain. For this purpose, see also the *first variation* of Del Río-Hortega (**145**) of this procedure.

178. Del Río-Hortega has modified the original method of Achúcarro in order to improve the staining of the protoplasmic and fibrous neuroglia. This modification is usually known as the *fourth variation* of Achúcarro's method.

1. Fix for several days in 10 per 100 formalin or, even better, in Cajal's formalin-bromide (**2**).
2. Cut frozen sections and treat them at 50°–55°C with an aqueous solution of brominated tannin (tannin, 3 g; ammonium bromide, 1 g; water, 100 cc).
3. Immerse the sections in ammoniacal water (distilled water, 20 cc; ammonia, 4 drops) until they become transparent and flexible again.
4. Stain in 10 per 100 ammoniacal silver oxide. (See the preparation of this reagent in **145**.) The impregnation must be carried out in two wells and must be stopped when the sections acquire a pale-yellow color.
5. Flatten the sections in water until they become an even yellow color.
6. Reduce in 10 per 100 chalk-neutralized formalin.
7. Rinse, dehydrate, etc. Very dark sections can be gold-toned.

179. Del Río-Hortega's method for astrocytes (1918) (*EN 40*).

1. Fix blocks of brain tissue in 10 per 100 formalin or in formalin-bromide (**2**). The fixation must not exceed twenty days if protoplasmic astrocytes are to be stained.
2. Cut frozen sections.
3. Rinse in plenty of distilled water in order to remove completely any trace of formalin; at least three changes are required.
4. Impregnate the sections in ammoniacal silver carbonate, prepared as follows:

    10% Silver nitrate solution   5 cc
    Saturated lithium carbonate solution   15 cc

The resulting yellowish-white silver carbonate precipitate must be washed once or twice in distilled water, then up to 55 cc of distilled water is added, after which ammonia is slowly dripped onto the solution until the precipitate is dissolved.

Pour 10 cc of the solution into a glass well, add three drops of pyridine and then immerse the sections, heating the solution up to 50°C. Remove the sections when they turn brown (three to five minutes). Throughout this procedure, the well must be covered with a watch-glass.[4] Any remaining solution must be kept in a dark flask.

5. Carefully dip the sections in distilled water.
6. Reduce in 10–20 per 100 neutral formalin.
7. Tone at 50°–60°C in 1 per 500 gold chloride solution until the sections become deep purple.
8. Fix for thirty to sixty seconds in 5 per 100 sodium hyposulfite.
9. Rinse, dehydrate, etc.

When the results are not satisfactory, Del Río-Hortega suggests using one of the following variations: (a) impregnation for ten minutes at 40°C in 2 per 100 silver nitrate prior to Step 4; (b) addition of one or two drops of pyridine per each cc of silver carbonate solution for a finer rendering of the gliofibrils; or (c) substitute 80° alcohol for the distilled water in Step 5, to improve the impregnation of immature, poorly differentiated cytoplasms.

This procedure is useful in the study of some types of gliomata.

180. Lugaro's method for staining the protoplasmic neuroglia (1932).

1. Use 3–4 mm thick blocks of human nervous tissue, indurated in 18% formaldehyde for three to eight days in the ice box.
2. Transfer the specimens directly to the silver solution (see below) at room temperature. Each block should be placed in a tightly closed flask with 10 cc of this solution.
3. After three hours, add 7 cc of 25% formaldehyde to each flask.
4. After five to eight days, rinse the blocks with running tap water to remove the superficial black precipitate. Cut 35 μm thick frozen sections.
5. Dehydrate, clarify, and mount on balsam.

Preparation of the silver baths:
The following solutions must be made just before use:

Solution A: 9% sodium hyposulfite.
Solution B: 2% silver bromide solution in 9% sodium hyposulfite.
Solution C: 0.3% silver iodide solution in 9% sodium hyposulfite.

The author suggests making eight working mixtures, combining the *A*, *B*, and *C* solutions in different proportions in this order:

Parts

Solution A		4	5	6	7	8	9	10	11
Solution B		16	15	14	13	12	11	10	9
Solution C	1–2	2	4	5	6	7	8	12

When the formaldehyde is added to the mixture of silver solutions it produces the precipitation of colloidal silver sulfide inside the tissue. This compound impregnates the gray matter glial cells selectively, especially its gliosomes and a *paranuclear body* of possible lipid nature.

181. Bolsi's modification of Cajal's ammoniacal silver oxide method (1926).

1. Fix the tissue in formalin.
2. Cut frozen sections.
3. Immerse the sections for thirty minutes at 50°C in the following mixture:

Pyridine	5 cc
Acetone	5 cc
Distilled water	15 cc
Ammonium bromide	1 g

This mordant can be replaced by 3.6 per 100 oxygenated water or by a saturated solution of oxalic acid.

4. Rinse the sections and treat them with ammoniacal silver oxide as described in **176**; reduce in 5 per 100 formalin, rinse, tone with gold, and fix in hyposulfite. Mount in Canada balsam.

Bolsi has demonstrated that his mordanting mixture also can be combined with Cajal's silver nitrate-pyridine method, thus allowing astrocyte impregnation in floating sections of formalin-fixed material.

182. Some years ago one of us suggested the possibility of staining macroglia and microglia without using ammoniacal silver.[2] Here is the procedure we used:

1. Fix for twenty-four hours in formalin bromide and transfer the pieces to 12 per 100 formalin, where they can be stored indefinitely. Cut frozen sections.
2. Impregnate and reduce all the sections at the same time by immersing them in a well containing:

2 per 100 Silver nitrate	10 cc
Pyridine	6–10 drops
Formalin	10–15 drops

Heat the well gently using an alcohol burner until the sections turn deep brown (five to ten minutes).

3. Rinse, tone heavily in 1 per 500 gold chloride, and fix in 5 per 100 sodium hyposulfite. Because this formula is rather inconstant, we no longer use it.

183. Method for staining the glioblasts. Del Río-Hortega (1932) has proposed a variation of his silver carbonate method for impregnating both mature and immature glial cells. It is based on the ability of alcohol to enhance the impregnation of the cytoplasm, either when associated to the silver solution or prior to reduction.

1. Fix in 10 per 100 formalin or in formalin-bromide; cut 10–15 μm frozen sections. Embed the specimens in gelatin before sectioning.
2. Rinse with ammoniacal water.
3. Immerse the sections in a mixture containing equal parts of ammonia, pyridine, and water. This solution must act for at least ten minutes (or up to several days) at room temperature, or five minutes at 50°C.
4. Without rinsing, immerse the sections for ten to fifteen minutes at 50°C in the following solution:

2 per 100 Silver nitrate	10 cc
Pyridine	30 drops
95° alcohol	30 drops

5. Impregnate in the following mixture until the sections are deeply stained:

Ammoniacal silver carbonate	10 cc (**179**, Step 4)
Pyridine	30 drops
95° alcohol	30 drops

6. Rinse the sections, one by one, with 80° alcohol.
7. Rinse for some minutes with 96° alcohol. This step can be carried out at room temperature, although it is preferable to heat the reagent slightly with a flame.
8. Reduce in 1 per 100 formalin.
9. Tone in 1 per 500 gold chloride; this step must be performed first at room temperature (until the sections turn gray) and thereafter at 50°C until the sections become purple to violet.
10. Fix in 5 per 100 sodium hyposulfite, rinse, and mount.

This technique yields a light, but extremely delicate, impregnation of the astrocytic cytoplasm, both in adult and immature cells (spongioblasts, astroblasts) showing their relationship with the blood vessels. The nucleus is not stained.

The author recommends omitting Step 3 when trying to stain the cells of partially differentiated glioblastomas of the astroblastic or oligodendrocytic types.

DEMONSTRATION OF THE GLIOSOMES AND MITOCHONDRIA

184. These organelles, first reported by Held and Alzheimer, have been analyzed by Nageotte, Mawas, Fieandt, and especially by Achúcarro, who has stained them with his own method using tannin and ammoniacal silver oxide. These structures are clearly demonstrated by the uranyl-formalin method (see **175**) if the pieces are fixed for one or two days; the best images are obtained from sections cut at some depth from the block, given that in the more superficial ones the glial cytoplasm is completely blackened.

Excellent images also can be obtained using Achúcarro's procedure (**177**) or Del Río-Hortega's more recent one (**186**). The latter even allows, in some cases, a clear-cut differentiation between the two main constituents of the neuroglial protoplasm, that is to say, gliosomes and mitochondria, although their relationship is not understood.

Some old methods, such as Altmann's (58) and Fieandt's (185) must be mentioned, although the latter is rather complicated and does not show up the processes of the gray matter astrocytes; the images are thus rather confusing, causing even such illustrious neurologists as Held or Oppenheim to err.

185. Fieandt's method.

1. Fix extremely fresh tissue fragments, not thicker than 2 mm, in Heidenhain's mixture containing sublimate and trichloroacetic acid:

Sublimate	70 g
Sodium chloride	6 cc
Distilled water	1000 cc
Crystallized trichloroacetic acid	20 g
Glacial acetic acid	10 cc

2. Immerse the pieces in 96° alcohol for five to seven days. The reagent must be replaced, three times on the first day and then daily.
3. Dehydrate for two or three days in absolute alcohol and then pass the specimens successively through cedarwood oil (one day), *ligroin* (twelve hours) and ligroin-paraffin (twenty-four hours). Embed in paraffin (at 52°–54°C), cut 5 µm sections, mount them on glass slides (see **41**), and deparaffinize them.
4. Treat the sections first with 96° alcohol and afterward with:

Crystallized iodine	1 g
96° alcohol	10 cc

5. Remove iodine with 96° alcohol.
6. Bleach the sections with 0.25 per 100 sodium hyposulfite for one hour.
7. Rinse two or three times with distilled water and blot the sections with filter paper.
8. Stain for twelve or fourteen hours in:

Crystallized hematoxylin	0.5 g
Distilled water	400 cc
10 per 100 phosphotungstic acid	100 cc
Oxygenated water (Merck)	1 cc[5]

9. Blot the sections with blotting paper and differentiate them in a freshly prepared reagent containing:

Crystallized iron sesquichloride	5 g
Absolute alcohol	50 cc

The differentiation process takes at least one hour and needs to be monitored under the microscope.

10. Blot once more with bibulous paper.
11. Rinse briefly with distilled water (twice) until the sections become bluish.
12. Dehydrate for twenty-four hours in absolute alcohol and clarify in origanum oil, xylene, and Canada balsam.

Gliosomes and glial fibers of fibrous astrocytes are deep-blue, whereas the cytoplasm is lightly stained either in blue or gray; cylinder-axes and collagen fibers appear gray-yellow. As with all the methods performed on thin sections that stain the protoplasm faintly, it is impossible to trace the expansions up to their final destination.

186. Del Río-Hortega's method with iron alum and silver carbonate. Del Río-Hortega developed three variations of his silver carbonate method that render excellent results for the impregnation of the chondrioma and gliosomes of glial cells.

187. *(a) "Cold" staining method (EN 41).* This formula is used mainly to stain the chondrioma.

1. Fix 2–3 mm thick pieces in the following liquid:

Formalin	10 cc
Distilled water	90 cc
Pure iron alum	6–8 g

The specimens must remain in this reagent for two or three days at 25°–35°C or four to eight days at 10°–20°C; the solution must be filtered before use.

This fixative can be replaced by Cajal's formalin-uranyl nitrate (3); in which case, fixation takes two or three days.

2. Cut 10 μm frozen sections. Because the specimens turn very brittle in the fixative, excessive freezing must be avoided.
3. Rinse the sections first with ammonia water and afterward in plenty of distilled water.
4. Stain in ammoniacal silver carbonate for one to five minutes, depending on the room temperature.

Preparation of the silver solution: Mix 5 cc of 10 per 100 silver nitrate with 15 cc of 5 per 100 sodium carbonate; wash the precipitate and dissolve by dripping ammonia onto it. Add distilled water to make a final volume of 55 cc–75 cc. This reagent must be kept in a dark flask.

5. Place the sections in distilled water and leave them undisturbed for fifteen to thirty seconds. The selectivity of the method depends on this step; if it is omitted, only the gliosomes will be shown.
6. Reduce in 1 per 200 formalin, tone in 1 per 600 gold chloride, and fix in sodium hyposulfite. Rinse with water, dehydrate, clarify, and mount.

This technique stains the mitochondria of glial cells completely and occasionally those of neurons. When Cajal's formalin-uranyl nitrate fixative is used, only the gliosomes are stained, particularly those of ***interfascicular oligodendroglia***.

188. *(b) "Warm" staining method (EN 41).* This formula is especially suitable for staining gliosomes.

1. Carry out the first three steps of the above technique.
2. Impregnate in silver carbonate to which has been added three drops of pyridine for each 10 cc of solution, until the sections become a pale tobacco color. This step must be carried out at 45°–50°C.[6]
3. Remove the sections from the silver bath and place them in a Petri dish containing distilled water. Wait two or three minutes, then agitate the sections gently and transfer them one by one to the reducing solution.
4. Reduce in 10 per 100 formalin.
5. Tone and fix as in the preceding formula.

This technique stains the gliosomes of all glial cell types and also the neuronal chondrioma. Furthermore, any particular type of granulations can be enhanced by simply changing the concentration of the reducing solution. Thus, gliosomes are better stained using 5–10 per 100 formalin, whereas the chondrioma of neurons and **gliocytes** need lower concentrations (1 per 400 and 1 per 100, respectively). Impregnation of the oligodendroglial mitochondria is enhanced by the addition of twenty drops of 96° alcohol to the silver bath.

189. *(c) Double impregnation formula.* This alternative method should be used when the former two fail to stain the mitochondria; it can be used to stain the chondrioma and the cytoplasmic granules of the ependymal cells.

1. Fix as in either variation *(a)* or in the following liquid for three or four days:

Formalin	10 cc
Distilled water	90 cc
Ammonium bromide	2 g
Iron alum	6–8 cc

2. Cut thin frozen sections, rinse them twice with ammonia water and then in distilled water.
3. Immerse the sections for some minutes in 2 per 100 silver nitrate, heating the well gently with a flame.
4. Dip the sections in distilled water and impregnate for one minute in silver carbonate.
5. Rinse briefly with distilled water and reduce in 1 per 100 formalin.
6. Stain at room temperature and intensify the staining by gently heating the vessel.
7. Fix in sodium hyposulfite, rinse, dehydrate, clarify, and mount.

IMPREGNATION OF OLIGODENDROGLIA AND MICROGLIA

190. Del Río-Hortega's method for impregnating microglia (1921).[3] This important procedure, which is widely used nowadays, was developed as a result of two improvements to the original technique for staining macroglia (**179**): (1) warming the pieces in formalin-bromide and (2) reducing the sections before they become tanned by the silver solution.

Here is the modus operandi:

1. Fix thin slices of nervous tissue for one to three days in Cajal's formalin-bromide liquid (**2**). Once the fixation is complete, immerse the slices in a well containing fresh fixative and heat with the flame from an alcohol burner (at 50°–55°C) for ten minutes.
2. Cut 25–30 μm thick frozen sections.
3. Rinse the sections in ammoniacal distilled water (20–30 cc of water, several drops of ammonia).
4. Rinse briefly with distilled water.
5. Impregnate for five to ten minutes at 15°–20°C in a concentrated solution or for ten to twenty minutes in a weak solution of silver carbonate. The preparation of this liquid must follow the rules previously described (**178**); the composition is:

10 per 100 silver nitrate	5 cc
5 per 100 sodium-potassium carbonate	20 cc
Ammonia (sufficient drops to dissolve the precipitate)	
Distilled water	15–20 cc

6. Reduce for some minutes in a large Petri dish containing 1 per 100 formalin. While the reduction takes place, the formalin must be stirred vigorously. Care must be taken, however, not to damage the sections; in our experience, the best way to do this is by blowing air vigorously onto the surface of the liquid.
7. Before the reducing becomes turbid, transfer the sections to tap water.
8. Tone in 1 per 500 gold chloride (ten to fifteen minutes at room temperature or slightly fewer if warming gently).
9. Fix in 5 per 100 sodium hyposulfite.
10. Rinse, dehydrate in graded alcohol, clarify in carbol-xylol-creosote and xylol, and mount in Canada balsam.

This is the most reliable technique for demonstrating the regular microglia, the rod cells, and any class of mesodermal phagocytes of the nervous system.

Microglial cells are deep violet or almost black against an almost colorless background, where only the blood vessels and the neuronal nuclei can be faintly seen.

A prolonged impregnation period results in a loss of staining selectivity, because astrocytes are also revealed. On the other hand, this technique yields beautiful overviews of glial cells when performed on tissues fixed for ten minutes at 55°C in 10 per 100 formalin with 3 per 100 ammonium bromide (*EN 42*) added.

191. Impregnation of microglial cells with ammoniacal silver oxide (Cajal). As pointed out above (**176**), this reagent impregnates the microglia in formalin-bromide fixed material. It may be useful, however, to point out some requirements for the success of the method for this purpose.

1. The fixation period must not be longer than three days.
2. The sections need to be immersed in warm (50°C) formalin-bromide. Alternatively, hyperbromuration can be carried out on the block itself, as in Del Río-Hortega's method.
3. Impregnation in ammoniacal silver oxide must be stopped when the sections begin to color (e.g., when they turn a dull shade of yellow).

Results comparable to those using Del Río-Hortega's or Bolsi's methods can be obtained if these precautions are taken, especially in pathological human material (e.g., *general paralysis of the insane, senile dementia*). On the other hand, in laboratory animals (cat, dog, rabbit, etc.), microglia are not so strongly stained. Individual skill with this technique is of paramount importance. Our technician, Miss Serra (1921, Trabajos, vol. XIX), has obtained splendid preparations of *mesoglial* cells even in the frog's spinal cord; incidentally, ammoniacal silver oxide stains the gliofibrils of ependymal cells beautifully.

192. Bolsi's method for microglia (1927–1930).

1. Fix for twenty-four to forty-eight hours in Cajal's formalin-bromide.
2. Immerse the pieces for a long time (at least one or two months) in the following modification of the solution developed by Noguchi for staining spirochetae:

Pyridine	5 cc
Acetone	5 cc
Formalin	15 cc
Distilled water	75 cc
Ammonium bromide	3 g

3. Rinse briefly with distilled water, cut 15 μm thick frozen sections and place them in distilled water.
4. Immerse the sections in a porcelain crucible containing about 20 cc of the above mixture. Heat with an alcohol burner flame (45°–50°C) for ten minutes and then allow to cool to room temperature.

This step can be omitted if the pieces have been stored for several months in the mixture of pyridine, acetone, formalin, and bromide.

5. Place the sections for more than five minutes in the following solution:

Distilled water	160 cc
Glycerin	40 cc
Ammonia	100 drops

6. Without rinsing, impregnate for forty to sixty seconds in 2 per 100 silver nitrate.
7. Reduce the sections in a 2 per 100 formalin solution containing 0.05 per 100 gum arabic; this liquid must be replaced several times. During Steps 5, 6, and 7 the liquids must be stirred with a glass rod.

8. Rinse with distilled water and tone (if desired) in gold chloride; fix in sodium hyposulfite (hyposulfite, 5 g; 50° alcohol, 100 cc) to remove the unreduced silver.
9. Rinse again, dehydrate in graded alcohols, clarify in carbol-xylol (crystallized phenol, 1 part; xylene, 3 parts), and mount in Canada balsam.

Note that this technique uses neither Del Río-Hortega's ammoniacal silver carbonate, nor Cajal's silver oxide; the main staining agent is the ammoniacal silver nitrate, which is formed when the sections are transferred from the ammoniacal liquid of Step 5 to the silver nitrate. This method is not very consistent.

193. Silver oxalate procedure for microglia impregnation (Herrera, 1932). This author has succeeded in staining microglia with his silver oxalate method combined with Bolsi's liquid. Here is the *modus faciendi*:

1. Fix very fresh specimens for one to twenty days in:

Pyridine	2.5 cc
Acetone	2.5 cc
Formalin	15 cc
Distilled water	75 cc
Ammonium oxalate	3 g

2. Cut 25 μm thick frozen sections.
3. Rinse briefly with distilled water.
4. Stain the sections for one minute in silver oxalate. This solution is prepared by mixing:

5 per 100 Neutral potassium oxalate	20 cc
10 per 100 Silver nitrate	5 cc
Absolute alcohol	10 drops

Slowly drip 33 per 100 ethylamine (Schering) until the precipitate has just dissolved, then add distilled water to make up a final volume of 75 cc and store in a dark flask.

5. Reduce in 1 per 100 formalin, stirring the sections.
6. Dehydrate and mount as usual.

This method regularly renders good preparations of the microglial cells of normal and pathological brains.

194. A method capable of staining microglia in pieces that have been stored for a long time in formalin and using our formalin-bromide solution as a mordant would be very useful. However, our trials, as well as those of Del Río-Hortega, have failed, perhaps because these cells need the absorption of ammonium bromide *ab initio* to be impregnated. Gans has managed to obtain impregnations of the microglia in specimens stored in formalin for a year, even when embedded in celloidin. His method is as follows:

Chapter 14: Macroglia, Microglia and Oligodendroglia

1. Fix in formalin.
2. Cut 25 μm thick sections.
3. Immerse the sections for two hours in 2.5 per 100 ammonium bromide at 37°C.
4. Rinse briefly with ammoniacal water.
5. Impregnate for two hours in Del Río-Hortega's ammoniacal silver carbonate solution (**190**).
6. Reduce in formalin, rinse, tone, etc.

195. According to Metz and Spatz, lipid droplets can be stained in microglial cells impregnated with Del Río-Hortega's procedure if the sections are not heavily toned. The sections must be stained with scarlet red (see Herxheimer's method, **222**) after the sections are fixed in sodium hyposulfite. In this way, it is possible to show the fatty substances phagocytosed by the microglial cells.

These authors, as well as Del Río-Hortega, have combined silver impregnation with the reactions for iron demonstration, such as Turnbull's blue or Perls's blue. Both of these reactions must be carried out on sections fixed in sodium hyposulfite.

Turnbull's blue method must be performed as usual (see details in **229**), although some steps need to be shortened or silver impregnation will be lost. Hence, immersion in ammonium sulfide must not exceed ten to twenty minutes, and the treatment with potassium ferricyanide plus hydrochloric acid must not last longer than five minutes.

For Perls's reaction, the method recommended by Del Río-Hortega, the sections have to be immersed in freshly prepared 5 per 100 potassium ferrocyanide. The well is then gently heated until vapors appear (five to ten minutes), after which the sections are transferred directly to 5 per 100 hydrochloric acid and heated again for five to ten minutes. Rinse and mount.

Both techniques stain iron deposits deep blue, which stands out against the gray microglial cytoplasm stained with silver carbonate and gold chloride.

196. Demonstration of microglia in pathological specimens by the iron-staining method (Del Río-Hortega, 1927). This procedure is based on the affinity of pathological microglial cells for Prussian blue. In these conditions the iron fills the microglial cytoplasm almost completely, so that the cells are as well impregnated as with silver techniques, though with a bright blue color.

1. Fix fresh tissue slices for some days either in Cajal's formalin-bromide or in 10 per 100 formalin.
2. Cut 20–25 μm thick frozen sections.
3. Rinse for ten minutes in ammoniacal water (distilled water, 30 cc; ammonia, 20 drops) in order to remove the formaldehyde and bromide.
4. Rinse with abundant water.
5. Immerse for some minutes in 10 per 100 hydrochloric acid.
6. Place the sections in a well containing a freshly prepared mixture of:

5 per 100 Potassium ferrocyanide	45 cc
10 per 100 Hydrochloric acid	55 cc

Flatten the sections at the bottom of the well and then warm the solution to 55°C until it begins to turn bluish and turbid.

7. Rinse for some seconds with water made alkaline by the addition of 1 per 100 ammonia or soda carbonate. The sections will recover transparency and flexibility.
8. Rinse for some seconds in 1–10 per 100 hydrochloric acid.
9. Repeat Steps 6, 7, and 8.
10. Repeat these same steps yet again.
11. Rinse, counterstain with aluminous carmine and mount.

197. Del Río-Hortega's method for the impregnation of oligodendroglia (*EN 43*). This method can be used on brain material obtained from any kind of mammal, though it renders the best results in the white matter of adult cats or dogs; on the other hand, gray matter oligodendrocytes are not so consistently stained.[4]

1. Fix for twelve to forty-eight hours in Cajal's formalin-bromide liquid (**2**).
2. Once the fixation is complete, place the pieces in a well containing fresh fixative and heat with the alcohol burner for ten minutes at 50°–55°C.
3. Once the pieces return to room temperature, cut 20–25 μm thick frozen sections.
4. Rinse the sections in a Petri dish containing water to which ten to twenty drops of ammonia have been added; sometimes, better results are achieved if the sections are left overnight in ammoniacal water or in an equal parts of water, pyridine, and ammonia.
5. Rinse briefly with distilled water.
6. Impregnate for five to fifteen minutes in a freshly prepared and filtered concentrated solution of silver carbonate:

10 per 100 Silver nitrate	5 cc
5 per 100 Soda carbonate	20 cc
Ammonia	sufficient drops to dissolve the precipitate

7. Reduce in 1 per 100 formaldehyde or, after a brief rinse, in 10 per 100 formaldehyde. During this step, the sections must not be stirred.
8. Tone very carefully with gold and fix in sodium hyposulfite.

Some variations may sometimes improve the results, such as the immersion of the sections in 96° alcohol either before (two to twenty-four hours) or after impregnation (thirty seconds).

198. Del Río-Hortega's procedure with silver dichromate (1928). In some cases, the old Golgi method yields more valuable preparations than modern techniques. Del Río-Hortega has modified it for this purpose as follows:

1. Fix for two or three days, changing the fixative daily, in:

Potassium bichromate	3 g
Chloral hydrate	2–3 cc
10 per 100 Formalin	50 cc

2. Rinse briefly with distilled water.
3. Impregnate in 1.5 per 100 silver nitrate for two or three days.
4. Cut the sections and mount as in the regular Golgi method (see **73**, Steps 2–7); the preparations can be coverslipped following Poljak's procedure, although considerable skill is required to avoid damaging the sections.

Using this method in dogs, Del Río-Hortega has obtained splendid images of all the types of oligodendroglia in the white matter, although the results are not as good as results in the gray matter.

199. Oligodendroglia staining with the bichromate-formalin variations of the Golgi method (Cajal). Kenyon's old Golgi method (1897) for invertebrates and its modifications by Sánchez (1916) and Cajal and Sánchez (1915) (see **84**) can also be used for the demonstration of oligodendroglial cells, although the impregnation is not as complete as with the formula described above (**198**).

These methods can be carried out in two different ways. A first possibility is to immerse fresh blocks of tissue in a mixture of potassium bichromate and formalin (3–5 per 100 bichromate, 85 cc; formalin, 15 cc). An alternative procedure is to place the specimens consecutively in formalin and bichromate. We have had better results with the latter procedure, the modus operandi of which is as follows:

1. Brain slices not thicker than 3–4 mm, obtained from adult cats, dogs, or rabbits, are indurated for two to five days in 15 per 100 formalin.
2. Without rinsing, they are transferred to:

Potash bichromate	3–5 g
Water	100 cc
Formalin	15 cc

This liquid must be allowed to act on the pieces for three to five days.

3. Impregnate for two days in a solution containing 1 per 100 silver nitrate and 1 per 100 chloral hydrate.
4. Cut and mount in the usual way for the Golgi methods (**73**).

In some cases, it may be worthwhile trying double impregnation. The results depend largely on the length of the fixation period.

This procedure shows the white matter oligodendrocytes quite nicely, especially in the deeper regions of the blocks, where they become impregnated either individually or in small groups. In the gray matter, the method also stains the neurons, thus obscuring the oligodendroglial cells. It is noticeable that this procedure, like Río-Hortega's method with chloral and bichromate, impregnates the Purkinje and granule cells of the cerebellum and the pyramidal cells. Unmedullated axons are, nevertheless, resistant to the stain.

200. Penfield's modification of Del Río-Hortega's method for impregnation of the oligodendroglia (1921). Penfield has modified Del Río-Hortega's method following suggestions published by Globus (1927). Here are the details:

1. Fix either in 10 per 100 formalin or in Cajal's formalin-bromide. The fixation period can be prolonged indefinitely, but must never be shorter than one week.
2. Cut 20 μm thick frozen sections and place them in 1 per 100 formalin.
3. Rinse with distilled water and leave the sections overnight in ammoniacal water (fill a large well with water and add 25 ammonia drops).
4. Immerse the sections in Globus's liquid for one hour in the oven at 38°C:

Distilled water	95 cc
40 per 100 Hydrobromic acid	5 cc

5. Rinse briefly with distilled water (three changes).
6. Immerse for one to six hours in 5 per 100 soda carbonate.
7. Without rinsing, immerse the sections for three to five minutes in a diluted formula of ammoniacal silver carbonate (**187**). The sections should become a dull yellow color.
8. Reduce in 1 per 100 formalin. Rinse, tone, fix, etc., as in the regular Del Río-Hortega method.

According to Penfield, this procedure stains both microglia and oligodendroglia well, especially in pathological material. Furthermore, the author claims that it can be used on pieces that have been fixed and stored in formalin for a long time, although reliable results are obtained only in pieces fixed in formalin-bromide for fewer than five or eight days.

201. Impregnation of oligodendroglia with silver oxalate (Rodríguez). This technique is a minor modification of Herrera's procedure to stain microglia.

1. Fix for one to three days in:

Pyridine	2.5 cc
Acetone	2.5 cc
Formalin	15 cc
Distilled water	75 cc
Neutral potassium oxalate	3 g

2. Cut 25–30 μm thick frozen sections.
3. Immerse the sections for twenty-four hours in a 1:1 mixture of the fixative and 3 per 100 ammonium oxalate.
4. Rinse briefly with distilled water.
5. Stain for one minute in silver oxalate (see **193**, Step 4).
6. Reduce in 1 per 100 formalin, stirring the sections.

15

Methods to Demonstrate the Connective Tissue

In the nerves and nervous centers, as in the rest of the organism, a supporting connective tissue can be found. This tissue forms the **neurilemma** and the protective envelopes of the neuraxis (meninges) and supplies the delicate adventitial layers of the blood vessels in the nervous system and the connective skeleton of the peripheral nerves and autonomic and sensory ganglia (endoneurium). Because it plays a significant role in some neuropathological processes, especially inflammation and healing, we shall describe the most important methods for demonstrating the connective tissue.

METHODS FOR STAINING THE CONNECTIVE TISSUE

202. Almost all the techniques described elsewhere in this book (see Chapter 6 of Section One) can be used to stain the collagen fibers. The most suitable procedures are Cajal's trichromic method (**61**) and Calleja's (**62**) and Gallego's (**63**) variations on it. Other methods that produce good results are Mallory's techniques with phosphotungstic (**57**) or phosphomolybdic (**56**) hematoxylins, or with anilines (**65**), and, finally, Heidenhain's "Azan" (**66**) and van Gieson's (**59**)[1] procedures. Romanovsky's (**60**), Pappenheim's (**64, 254**), and Nissl's (**103**)[2] methods are very useful for the demonstration of all the cellular types of the exudates, especially Cajal's *cyanophilic cells.*

203. Orcein stain for elastic fibers (Unna-Taenzer).

1. Fix in formalin or in any liquid containing sublimate; cut either frozen or celloidin sections and rinse them with distilled water.
2. Immerse for thirty to sixty minutes in a 1 per 100 solution of orcein in 70° alcohol, containing 1 per 100 hydrochloric acid. This stain can be used immediately after preparation.
3. Rinse briefly with distilled water and with 96° alcohol.
4. Differentiate in absolute alcohol until the elastic fibers stand out against an almost colorless background.
5. Clarify in xylene and mount.

Results: The elastic fibers are stained a reddish-brown.

Nuclei can be counterstained with hematoxylin or with weak aqueous solutions of toluidine blue, methylene blue, or Unna's polychrome blue. Any of these complementary stains must be performed before differentiation.

204. Weigert's method for elastic fibers.

1. Fix in any of the liquids used in neurology, such as formalin, alcohol, sublimate, etc.
2. Cut frozen sections or embed the specimens in either paraffin or celloidin.
3. Stain for thirty to sixty seconds in Weigert's resorcin-fuchsin solution (see below).
4. Rinse in 96° alcohol and differentiate in absolute alcohol until the elastic fibers become a distinct deep-blue or black against a colorless background; differentiation can take several hours.
5. Clarify in xylol and mount in Canada balsam.

Nuclear counterstaining can be achieved with aluminous carmine; this step must be carried out before immersing the sections in Weigert's mixture.

Staining of the elastic fibers can be combined with the demonstration of tissue lipids; for this purpose, Fischer suggests mixing 74 cc of Weigert's reagent with 26 cc of distilled water and then dissolving Sudan III or scarlet red to saturation while warming gently. The sections must be immersed in this mixture for thirty to sixty minutes and then differentiated in a saturated solution of Sudan III or scarlet red in 70° alcohol. Rinse with water and mount in glycerin.

Preparation of the resorcin-fuchsin solution: Put 2 g of brilliant fuchsin, 4 g of resorcin, and 200 cc of distilled water in a porcelain well. Heat the mixture until boiling, stirring continuously. Add 25 cc of officinal solution (29%) of ferric chloride and keep the solution boiling for five more minutes. Allow the liquid to cool to room temperature and filter. Place the filter paper *containing the solid residues of the reagents* inside the porcelain well and pour 200 cc of 96° alcohol over it. Boil again while stirring to disintegrate the filter paper. (Be careful not to approximate the flame to the edge of the well, or the solution will ignite!). Allow the solution to cool, make up to 200 cc with 96° alcohol, and add 4 cc of hydrochloric acid. This stain maintains its selectivity for elastic fibers for up to six weeks.

IMPREGNATION METHODS FOR CONNECTIVE TISSUE

205. Some years ago we[1] used the reduced silver nitrate method combined with fixation in acrolein for the demonstration of the connective sheaths of the blood capillaries of the central nervous system. With this procedure, this delicate adventitial envelope appears as a meshwork of thin filaments that are stained black. The technique is as follows:

Chapter 15: Demonstrating Connective Tissue

1. Fix thin tissue slices for twenty-four hours in:

   33 per 100 Acrolein in alcohol   4 cc
   Distilled water   40 cc

2. Rinse for twenty-four hours in running tap water.
3. Immerse for one day in ammoniacal alcohol (96° alcohol, 50 cc; ammonia, 5 drops).
4. Rinse briefly with water and impregnate for five days in 1.5 per 100 silver nitrate, at 37°C.
5. Rinse and reduce as usual (**114**).

206. Cajal has proposed another fixative to demonstrate the adventitia of the blood vessels and the connective bands perforating the brain.

1. Fix the pieces for one day in a mixture of:

   Pyridine   20 cc
   Formalin   30 cc
   Distilled water   30 cc

2. Follow the method described in the preceding paragraph (**205**) from Step 2 onward.

207. Achúcarro's method with tannin and ammoniacal silver (**177**) renders excellent results for connective tissue impregnation; it is, however, somewhat inconsistent; thus, the following variations proposed by Del Río-Hortega should be preferred.

208. Reticulin impregnation with Del Río-Hortega's second variation of Achúcarro's method.

1. Fix in 10 per 100 formalin or in Bouin's liquid[3]; pieces fixed and stored in alcohol for long periods also yield excellent results.
2. Cut 10–15 μm thick frozen sections.
3. Immerse in a 1 per 100 alcoholic solution of tannin for five minutes at 50–55°C. At lower temperatures (40°–45°C), the sections must be treated for fifteen to thirty minutes.
4. Remove the sections from the tannin solution while they are still warm and dip them in distilled water.
5. Pass the sections through three wells, each containing 10 cc of distilled water and 1 cc of ammoniacal silver oxide (see the preparation of this liquid in **145**). When the solution in the first well begins to turn yellow, transfer the sections to the second one. In the same way, when the liquid in this well starts to color, move the pieces to the last well, where the solution must remain colorless and the sections are unevenly stained a pale-yellow color. Throughout the whole impregnation the sections must be gently stirred with a hooked glass rod.
6. Transfer the sections to distilled water and leave them flattened and undisturbed until they acquire a homogeneous and intense color.

7. Rinse for thirty seconds in a new bath of distilled water and reduce in 20 per 100 neutral formalin.[4] Rinse and mount as usual.

Results: Reticulin threads are impregnated in a deep-brown or black color, whereas collagen fibers turn a russet shade.

209. Collagen bundles are better shown by Del Río-Hortega's *third variation* of Achúcarro's method. This procedure is identical to the former one up to Step 5, but the sections become a brownish-yellow (instead of pale-yellow) color in the silver baths. Once impregnated and rinsed with plenty of water, the sections are not reduced, but directly toned in 1 per 500 gold chloride until they become deep violet. Toning must be held at 40°–45°C and usually takes about fifteen minutes. Fix in 5 per 100 hyposulfite, rinse, and mount.

Results: Collagen bundles are reddish-purple or deep violet, whereas reticulin fibers are barely visible. Elastic fibers also are impregnated, although they are more selectively demonstrated with the *first variation* (**145**).

210. The subpial and perivascular connective sheaths of nervous centers, as well as the interstitial tissue of nerve trunks (neurilemma, endoneurium), can be also beautifully shown by Cajal's modification of Bielschowsky's method (**176**). The pieces can be fixed in either in 10 per 100 formalin or in formalin-bromide, although the latter renders better results. The sections must be impregnated until they become a tobacco color; rinse, reduce, etc.

211. The classic Bielschowsky's method (**109**) yields worthwhile results for connective tissue impregnation providing that the fixation period is short.

When the material is brittle, Maresch's modification can be used, because it works on paraffin sections. The procedure is much the same as the original one, but the paraffin sections are allowed to float for one or two days in 2 per 100 silver nitrate at 30°C. The remaining steps need to be prolonged for up to thirty or forty minutes. Another possibility is to mount the paraffin sections on coverslips (*EN 44*) and then deparaffinize and stain them.

The best fixatives for connective tissue are formalin and alcohol, although Bielschowsky's method (but not Maresch's modification) also works on bichromate-fixed tissues.

212. Del Río-Hortega's silver carbonate method also yields good images of the perivascular connective tissue. This author has proposed two techniques: (a) single-impregnation formula and (b) double-impregnation formula. The first reveals the astrocytes and the connective meshwork, whereas the second only shows the latter.

First formula. The procedure is carried out as in the original silver carbonate method (**187**): (a) Fix in formalin or in formalin-bromide; (b) cut frozen sections and rinse them with water; (c) impregnate *strongly* at 45°–50°C in pyridinated silver carbonate (silver carbonate, 10 cc; pyridine, 30 drops); (d) rinse with water and reduce in 10 per 100 formalin; (e) tone in gold chloride and fix in hyposulfite.

Second formula. (a) Fix in formalin or in formalin-bromide, cut frozen sections, rinse with water, and immerse them for five minutes in 1 per 100 potassium permanganate; (b) bleach in 5 per 100 oxalic acid; (c) rinse first in ammoniacal water and then in distilled water; (d) immerse the sections for ten minutes in 2 per 100 silver nitrate, at 45°–50°C; (e) impregnate at 45°–50°C until the sections are *deeply* stained with pyridinated silver carbonate (one drop of pyridine for every milliliter of silver solution); (f) rinse with distilled water (occasionally with the addition of one to two pyridine drops), and reduce in 1 per 100 formalin; (g) tone in gold chloride, hyposulfite, etc.

SUPRAVITAL STAINING WITH ACIDIC DYES

213. This is presently very fashionable for studying the components of the reticuloendothelial system but also can prove useful in determining the histiocytic nature of various nervous system components, especially in some experimentally induced pathological conditions in which the blood vessels are no longer able to impede the diffusion of the dyes into the tissues. Thus, the dyes can now easily reach the phagocytes.

214. Staining with trypan blue (*Trypanblau*, Goldmann). Prepare a 0.5–1 per 100 solution of trypan blue in water or, preferably, in saline. Immediately before use, filter and sterilize it.[5] This reagent must be injected every two or three days until the skin and mucous membranes turn deep blue. The injections can be subcutaneous, intravenous, or intraperitoneal, but in no case must the dose of a single administration exceed 0.5–1 cc/20 g–body weight.

Once the animal is sacrificed, the tissues are fixed for one or two days in either 10–20 per 100 formalin or in 5 per 100 sublimate. The specimens can be cut with the freezing microtome or embedded in celloidin or paraffin; counterstain the nuclei with carmine.

215. Lithium carmine can be used instead of trypan blue. The preparation of this stain is as follows: Make a saturated solution of lithium carbonate at room temperature.

1. Dissolve 100 cc of this reagent in 2.5 g of high-quality carmine (G. Hollborn); this step must be carried out in a bain-marie.
2. Filter the stain and use while still warm. This colorant is used just as trypan blue. Nuclear counterstain can be provided by hematoxylin. The connective tissue is stained bright red. Mount on clean glass slides.
3. Cover the sections with:

1 per 100 Phosphomolybdic acid	5 cc
96° Alcohol	15 cc

   This step must be repeated two or three times.
4. Drain off excess liquid and gently blot the sections with filter paper, but be very careful not to dry the sections completely.
5. Press the sections with a strip of filter paper wetted with a 20/80 mixture of 96° alcohol and chloroform; this must be done quickly or the sections will dry out.

6. Cover the sections with some drops of:

Crystal violet (crystals, Meister Lucius, Hoechst)	0.5 g
Absolute alcohol	2 cc
Chloroform	8 cc

After not more than *two to five seconds*, the sections will be covered by a metallic-green film.

7. Immediately pour some drops of 10 per 100 potassium bromide over the slide and let it act until the sections turn blue.
8. Blot the sections with blotting paper and differentiate with a freshly prepared mixture of aniline oil and chloroform (aniline oil, 6 cc; chloroform, 9 cc; ammonia, 1 drop); differentiation must be stopped when the milky clouds that formed when the differentiating solution was added disappear.
9. Rinse several times in xylol and mount in balsam.

Gliofibrils are deeply stained in a blue-violet color. The perinuclear cytoplasm of the gliocytes is also shown. This method also stains the connective tissue.

16

Methods for the Demonstration of Substances Produced by Alterations of the Cell Metabolism

Now is an appropriate moment to describe the methods for demonstrating some of the substances produced by the components of the nervous tissue (neurons and nerve fibers, glial cells, and mesodermal elements), under both normal and pathological conditions. In the former, these substances result from the metabolism and turnover of cells, whereas in the latter they are products of degenerative or regressive processes affecting the nervous centers or peripheral nerves.

216. The visualization of fatty substances originating from the breakdown of myelin sheaths was previously mentioned when Marchi's and Benda's methods were described (**163, 164**). In previous chapters, we also have reported Cajal's uranyl-formalin method (**148**), which stains lipid granules, as well as discussed Spatz's, Metz's, and Del Río-Hortega's (**195, 196**) procedures for the demonstration of iron and fatty inclusions of pathological microglial cells.

The next paragraphs will describe Alzheimer's methods for staining the granules that appear in pathological glial cells. This first group of techniques is followed by another, describing procedures useful in identifying the various substances that appear as a result of degenerative or necrobiotic processes. Finally, we will mention some microchemical reactions capable of showing iron, glycogen, lipids, lime, etc.

It should be borne in mind that general staining methods, such as Nissl's, Weigert's, Spielmeyer's, and Pappenheim's, are very helpful for obtaining an overview of the pathological process before deciding which specific method should be used.

DEMONSTRATION OF SOME CELL GRANULES

217. Alzheimer's method for the fuchsinophilic granules. This method renders images that are complementary to those obtained with the fuchsin-light green technique (**141**).

1. Fix for twenty-four hours in 10 per 100 formalin.
2. Immerse in Flemming's concentrated mixture (**10**) for eight days.
3. Rinse for twelve to twenty-four hours with running tap water, embed in paraffin and cut 2–4 µm thick sections.
4. Dewax, transfer the sections into water, and subject them to the mordant action of a saturated solution of copper acetate (one hour at 37°C).
5. Rinse twice with distilled water and stain for thirty minutes in:

10 per 100 Hematoxylin in alcohol	10 cc
Distilled water	87 cc
Saturated solution of lithium carbonate	3 cc

6. Rinse briefly with distilled water, dehydrate, clarify, and mount.

Result: The various types of granules are deep-blue against a pale background; the protoplasm is stained in a yellowish-gray or blue shade. Neurosomes are also shown.

218. Alzheimer's method for the fibrinoid granules. This method is similar to Weigert's for fibrous glia staining. The fresh specimens are fixed directly in the mordant (**165**, Step 2), rapidly embedded in celloidin (the embedding must take fewer than three days), and sectioned. The sections are then stained according to Weigert's procedure (**165**), although the volume of soda sulfite added to the formic acid-chromogen mixture should be smaller (2 cc of sulfite per 90 cc of mixture).

Result: The fibrinoid granules located in the soma and processes of neuroglial cells, as well as those in perivascular spaces are intensely stained in blue; nuclei are also the same color. In some cases, gliofibrils are also visible.

219. Alzheimer's method for the demonstration of basophilic-metachromatic substances (protagonoid substances).

1. Cut frozen sections of formalin-fixed material; the fixation period should be short. Specimens briefly fixed in alcohol also can be used.
2. Stain for one hour in 1 per 100 toluidine blue.
3. Rinse with distilled water.
4. Bleach with alcohol. This step should be stopped when the myelin sheaths are almost colorless but still clearly visible.
5. Xylol and balsam.

Results: The basophilic-metachromatic substances are stained in red. According to Alzheimer these substances are presumably identical to those described by Reich as π-granules (**256**), which appear inside glial cells and in the perivascular spaces. In the dorsal roots, Reich's π-granules are present inside Schwann cells.

220. Alzheimer's procedure using the May-Grünwald stain.

1. Cut frozen sections of specimens briefly fixed in formalin.
2. Briefly treat the sections with a heavily diluted solution of osmic acid (add two drops of osmic acid to the volume of water contained in a watch glass).
3. Rinse with water and stain for one minute in the May-Grünwald liquid.[1]
4. Rinse with water, dehydrate in acetone, clarify in xylol, and mount in balsam.

This staining method is selective for the degeneration products of neurons and glial cells in amaurotic idiocy (Spielmeyer-Vogt variety).

DEMONSTRATION OF FATS AND LIPOID SUBSTANCES

221. Staining methods using osmic acid. This reagent is reduced by neutral fats, especially by triolein and oleic acid, which are stained black; other fatty substances turn a brownish shade. Due to a secondary reduction process, fats sometimes may be shown in black after treating the tissue for a long time with a mixture of water and 70°–80° alcohol. The correct way of using osmic acid already has been described (**8**); other fixatives, such as Flemming's (**10**), Laguesse's (**12**), Altmann's (**11**), and Cajal's (**13**) mixtures also can be used.

When the pieces previously have been fixed in formalin, osmic acid still can be used after sectioning with the freezing microtome. The sections are rinsed with water and 70° alcohol to remove excess osmium and mounted in glycerin. The choice of this mounting medium is due to the fact that the osmium-impregnated fat is rather soluble in xylene, benzene, toluene, ether, etc. On the other hand, neither chloroform nor cedarwood oil dissolve the fat previously treated with osmium so readily. Hence, these substances may be used as intermediate agents between alcohol and paraffin whenever lipids are to be demonstrated in osmium-fixed material embedded in paraffin.

222. Staining with scarlet red (Herxheimer). The procedure is as follows:

1. Fix the specimens in formalin and cut frozen sections.
2. Rinse the sections for some minutes in 50° alcohol and immerse them for two to five minutes in a covered well containing:

70° Alcohol	50 cc
Acetone	50 cc
Scarlet red	0.2–0.3 g

The staining solution must be stored in a tightly stoppered flask and filtered just before use.

3. Rinse briefly with 70° alcohol and afterwards in distilled water.
4. Counterstain the nuclei for ten minutes in diluted Ehrlich's hematoxylin (hematoxylin solution, 10 drops; water, 20 cc).

5. Rinse with running tap water and mount in glycerin.

The fatty substances are stained orange-red and the nuclei blue. The scarlet red mixture can be replaced with a saturated solution of Sudan III in 70° alcohol.

223. Lorrain and Smith's Nile blue sulfate method. This method is based on the unique property of Nile blue to stain the neutral fats brilliant red and the fatty acids and other fatty substances bluish-violet. Kleeberg's modification (1923) of the original method is the following:

  1. Fix in formalin and cut frozen sections.
  2. Rinse with water and stain for twenty minutes in an aqueous saturated solution of Nile blue sulfate.
  3. Rinse briefly with water and differentiate in 1 per 100 acetic acid, monitoring with the microscope.
  4. Rinse with water for one to two hours.
  5. Mount in glycerin.

Cell nuclei are also stained deep blue.

224. Ciaccio's method. This method was proposed for the demonstration of lipids.

  1. Fix small pieces for one or two days in:

5 per 100 Potassium bichromate	80 cc
Formalin	20 cc
Acetic acid	5 cc

  2. Immerse the specimens directly in 3 per 100 potassium bichromate (five to eight days).
  3. Rinse for twenty-four hours with running tap water; then dehydrate, clarify in either benzene or carbon sulfide, and embed in paraffin.
  4. Cut sections, mount them on glass slides, dewax, and immerse them for some minutes in 70° alcohol.
  5. Stain for thirty to sixty minutes at 35°C in a Sudan III solution; coloration must be carried out in a tightly stoppered flask in order to avoid evaporation. The staining reagent is made as follows:

Acetone	5 cc
80° Alcohol	95 cc

Place this mixture in a bain-marie at 50°C, add Sudan III up to saturation, allow to cool, and filter. Sudan III can be replaced by Nile blue (see **223**).

  6. Dip in 50° alcohol and rinse thoroughly with distilled water.
  7. Counterstain with either hematein or diluted Ehrlich's hematoxylin (**222**); rinse again with running tap water and coverslip the sections using glycerin or Apathy's liquid (**71**).

Lipids are stained yellowish-orange.

225. Kawamura's modification[1] of Ciaccio's method is highly recommended, especially when only formalin-fixed material is available.

1. Cut frozen sections and immerse them for twenty-four hours in Ciaccio's fixative (**224**) and then in 3 per 100 potassium bichromate for an additional day.
2. Rinse successively with water, 70° alcohol, and 90° alcohol. Immerse for one hour in a 1:1 mixture of absolute alcohol and xylene.
3. Pass the sections through alcohols of decreasing strength to 70° alcohol.
4. Stain with Sudan III (**224**) or Nile blue (**223**).

The remaining steps must be carried out as described in previous methods.

226. Schaffer's method for staining lipids and prelipids. This interesting procedure was conceived for the demonstration of the degenerative products that are stored by the neurons in the Tay-Sachs variety of amaurotic idiocy.[2]

1. Fix thin tissue slices (0.5–1 cm) for two or three months at 37°C in 5 per 100 potassium bichromate.
2. Rinse with running tap water for one day and embed the pieces first in celloidin and then in paraffin (*EN 45*).
3. Cut thin sections (about 6 μm thick) and mount them on albumin-glycerin coated glass slides.
4. Dewax and immerse for three to seven days in 5 per 100 potassium bichromate, at 37°C.
5. Rinse thoroughly with water and stain for one to two days in Weigert's hematoxylin, at 37°C (**156**, Step 6).
6. Rinse thoroughly with water and differentiate in Pal's liquid (**157**, Step 5) monitoring with the microscope.
7. Immerse the sections in a warm, saturated lithium carbonate solution until they become a deep blue color.
8. Rinse with water and counterstain with picrofuchsin (**59**).
9. Rinse briefly with water, dehydrate, clarify, and mount in balsam.

Results: The degenerative *lecithinoid granules* are stained deep blue, the *semilecithinoid granules* ash-gray, and fuchsinophilic granulations are bright red whereas the perikaryon acquires a rosy hue.

DEMONSTRATION OF FERRIC PIGMENTS

227. In this section, we shall point out the more useful techniques for iron demonstration, particularly because the absorption and transport of iron in some lesions and the localization of ferric pigments in normal structures (*substantia nigra, globus pallidus, nucleus ruber, putamen,* etc.) have recently become interesting topics for the neurologist.

228. The demonstration of ferric pigments can be achieved in unfixed material (Spatz), but microscopic analysis should always be carried out after a short induration in alcohol or neutral formalin.[2] Sections can be obtained with the freezing microtome, although celloidin- or paraffin embedding also may be used. Care must be taken to avoid any contamination of the pieces or the sections by liquids or instruments containing iron. Thus, extremely clean glassware[3] and iron-free reagents must be used; furthermore, the sections must be handled with glass hooks.

229. Turnbull blue (ferrous ferricyanide) method (Tirmann-Schmelzer-Hueck). This is the most reliable and precise method for the demonstration of iron.

1. Rinse the sections carefully with distilled water and immerse them for twelve to twenty-four hours in a concentrated solution of ammonium sulfide. This solution should be clear-yellow and it should never be kept for more than two to three weeks.
2. Rinse thoroughly with distilled water and place the sections for about fifteen minutes in a freshly prepared mixture of 20 per 100 potassium ferrocyanide and 1 per 100 hydrochloric acid (1:1). In this step the iron sulfide is transformed into ferrous ferrocyanide (Turnbull blue).
3. Rinse several times with distilled water and counterstain with Grenacher's carmine (**42**). Rinse, dehydrate, clarify, and mount in balsam. Iron is bright-blue, whereas the nuclei are red.

230. Prussian blue reaction (Wicklein-Falkenberg). The sections, once rinsed with distilled water, are immersed for thirty to sixty minutes in a freshly prepared mixture containing hydrochloric acid and potassium ferrocyanide:

1 per 100 Hydrochloric acid	25 cc
2 per 100 Potassium ferrocyanide	8–10 drops

Rinse thoroughly with distilled water, counterstain with carmine (**42**), etc. Iron becomes deep blue. The 2 per 100 potassium ferrocyanide solution must be prepared immediately before use.

DEMONSTRATION OF NON-FERRIC PIGMENTS

231. The non-ferric pigments are important constituents of the neuron protoplasm because they are constantly present and increase with aging and with several pathological conditions. The methods for pigment demonstration already have been discussed in Chapter 3 (**147–149**), so we shall now just comment on the types of pigments and their differential staining.

232. There are two types of non-ferric pigments in the nervous system; one of them is dark or brownish and is related to melanin, while the other, known as lipopigment or lipofucsin, is fatty and has a yellow color.

The melanin pigment, most abundant in the neurons of the *locus niger* and *locus coeruleus*, is very resistant to chemicals, although it is bleached by chlorine water

Chapter 16: Alterations of the Cell Metabolism

and destroyed by strong acids or alkalis; this pigment is stained with the silver methods.

The lipopigment can be extracted with mixtures of alcohol and xylene and is stained with Sudan III, scarlet red, Nile blue, Weigert's hematoxylin, and osmic acid.

Both types of pigmentary substances are thus well defined on morphological grounds and also on the basis of their chemical constitution and genesis; they represent different, but independent, stages of cell metabolism.

GLYCOGEN DEMONSTRATION

233. Whenever glycogen needs to be demonstrated, for instance in some developmental and pathological processes, the method of choice will be Best's carmine.

234. Best's procedure for glycogen demonstration.

1. Fix very fresh specimens in absolute alcohol and embed in celloidin; cut 15–20 μm thick sections.
2. Stain the nuclei deeply with either hematein or hematoxylin (Böhmer, Ehrlich, Delafield, etc.).
3. Rinse thoroughly with running tap water and stain for five minutes in a freshly prepared mixture of:

Best's carmine stock solution	2 cc
Ammonia	3 cc
Methanol	3 cc

The stock solution is prepared by mixing the following components in a small flask:

Carmine	2 g
Powdered potassium carbonate	1 cc
Potassium chloride	5 cc
Distilled water	60 cc

Boil this mixture gently for a few minutes. Allow it to cool to room temperature and add 20 cc of ammonia. This reagent is kept in a tightly stoppered bottle in a cool place, but even with these precautions it must not be used any later than one or two months after preparation.

4. Differentiate for one to five minutes in:

Methanol	40 cc
Absolute alcohol	80 cc
Distilled water	100 cc

5. Absolute alcohol, xylene, and balsam. Glycogen is stained a vivid red and nuclei blue.

DEMONSTRATION OF AMYLOID SUBSTANCE AND CORPORA AMYLACEA

235. The main histochemical property of amyloid substance is its metachromatic staining with iodine (**238**) or with some basic aniline dyes.

236. Amyloid matter staining with methyl-violet or gentian-violet (Schmorl). This procedure can be carried out in specimens fixed in formalin, alcohol, or sublimate. The sections, once rinsed with distilled water, are stained for twelve to twenty-four hours in a diluted solution of either methyl-violet or gentian violet (one to two drops of a 2 per 100 solution of any of these dyes in 20 cc of distilled water). The sections are then rinsed and mounted in glycerin or in Apathy's syrup gum.

Following this simple procedure, which avoids the usual differentiation in acetic acid, the amyloid is very selectively stained in a red or violet-red color, whereas the nuclei are shown in deep blue and the background is pale blue. In any case, if differentiation in acetic acid is desired, the staining solution must be more concentrated (1 per 100). The stain must act for some minutes, followed by differentiation carried out for two or three minutes in 2 per 100 acetic acid. The amyloid substance is red or violet-red and the nuclei blue; the background is pale blue.

237. Amyloid staining with iodine green. Immerse the sections for twenty-four hours in 1 per 300 iodine green, then rinse with water and mount them on glass slides; blot the sections and coverslip with glycerin, levulose, or Apathy's syrup gum.

The areas containing amyloid substance are violet-red; other parts are stained green.

238. Corpora amylacea. The corpora amylacea are promptly stained by almost any dye after formalin fixation, though they show a high affinity for hematoxylin, especially when used as in Weigert's method (**165**). With this procedure, they are stained either deep brown or yellow.

The histochemical properties of these bodies resemble those of amyloid, because they also are stained metachromatically by iodine and the aforementioned basic aniline dyes.

According to Lafora, corpora amylacea can be distinguished from the amyloid substance using the following reactions:

1. Weak Lugol's solutions stain the corpora amylacea in violet and the amyloid substance in brown.
2. Concentrated Lugol's solutions or iodine solutions turn the *corpora* a reddish brown color that changes to deep red after sulfuric acid treatment; the *amyloid substance*, on the other hand, is blue-violet or greenish.
3. Thionine or cresyl-violet stain the corpora amylacea blue-violet and the amyloid substance pale blue.
4. Russel's method (**240**) stains the hyaline substance bright red and the corpora amylacea green.

Stümer has proposed other criteria to identify corpora amylacea:

1. The previously mentioned iodine affinity.
2. Best's carmine method (**234**) stains them pale red and glycogen deep red; staining of corpora amylacea is unaffected by digestion with saliva or by prolonged immersion in water.
3. Corpora amylacea are stained by Nile blue sulfate and neutral red (similar to soaps and fatty acids).
4. Corpora amylacea are not stained by Sudan III.

DEMONSTRATION OF HYALINE DEGENERATION

239. The transparent hyaline substance, a degenerative product, is usually located in the connective tissue and in the wall of the blood vessels, especially in the precapillaries. It will be properly fixed by any liquid (except those containing osmic acid); Van Gieson's method stains it orange-red.

240. Russel's method. Stain the sections (previously rinsed with water) for ten to thirty minutes in carbol-fuchsin[4]; rinse successively with water (three to five minutes) and absolute alcohol (one and a half minutes). Differentiate in carbol-iodine green (iodine green, 1 g; 5 per 100 phenol, 100 cc), dehydrate briefly in absolute alcohol, clarify, and mount.

The hyaline substance is stained deep red and the nuclei pale green.

CALCAREOUS SUBSTANCES

241. The calcareous substances are beautifully stained with hematoxylin; however, the coloration is not specific, because the pseudocalcareous bodies that are so frequently found in the dentate nucleus, pallidum, Ammon's horn, etc. are also stained. Therefore, it is preferable to use selective methods, such as Roehl's, Kossa's, and Cajal's.

Fixation must be carried out in alcohol, because aqueous solutions (including formaldehyde), dissolve lime to some extent even when used for only short periods.

242. Roehl's method. (A) Paraffin-embedded or frozen sections are placed for five minutes in an ammoniacal solution of copper sulfate (excess ammonia should be minimal). (B) Rinse with water and stain for fifteen minutes in Weigert's iron hematoxylin (**156**, Step 6). (C) Differentiate in 50 per 100 diluted Weigert's borax-ferrocyanide solution (**156**, Step 8). (D) Rinse, dehydrate, clarify, and mount.

Lime is stained black.

243. Kossa's method. Immerse the sections for thirty to sixty minutes in 1–5 per 100 silver nitrate, rinse with abundant distilled water, and counterstain the nuclei with safranin. Calcareous substances are stained deep black.

244. Cajal's reduced silver nitrate method. Cajal's studies on experimentally induced degeneration and regeneration processes of the nervous system have proved that this method distinctly stains the calcified cells black. This procedure has the additional advantage of revealing the cells and fibers of the region.

Any variation of this method is suitable for the present purpose, although the best results are obtained after fixation either in plain alcohol or in ammoniacal alcohol (**115, 116**). Pyridine fixation (**119**) is even capable of staining the lime granulations of blood thrombocytes.

17

Methods for the Demonstration of the Peripheral Nerves under both Normal and Pathological Conditions

245. The histological study of the nerve trunks is a most delicate task due to the extreme fragility of peripheral nerve fibers. Thus, it requires some skill, both in the handling and excision of the nerve and in the choice of the most suitable fixative for the demonstration of a given structure. Careless maneuvers, such as an excessive pressure exerted with tweezers or the fingers, torsion or stretching of the nerve, desiccation, and poor fixation can all produce profound alterations in the morphology of myelinated fibers, resulting in the formation of "-pseudostructures" or artifacts.

Therefore, bearing in mind the complexity and delicacy of the myelinated fiber, we shall mention those fixation and staining procedures especially apt for the demonstration of each of the components of these structures.

246. Fresh examination of the medullated nerve tube. The observation of unfixed specimens provides useful information about the structure of the nerves. The procedure, according to Nageotte, is the following: A thin nerve is preferable, such as frog's sciatic nerve, and should be carefully peeled. Then, the straight arms of a "U"-shaped sheet of tin are slipped under the nerve and the tips of the "U" are folded around the specimen, thus immobilizing it in a stretched position. The nerve is sectioned at the sides of the "U" and transferred to a glass slide. The nerve must be moistened right away with aqueous humour of the same animal and then coverslipped. The resulting preparation is sufficiently diaphanous to allow a good illumination for observing the superficial myelinated fibers. Providing that the procedure has been performed carefully, the nerve fibers will be intact, and Ranvier nodes, myelin sheaths, and Lantermann's incisures will be identifiable.

DEMONSTRATION OF RANVIER NODES

247. Silvering method for the demonstration of Ranvier crosses. The procedure for demonstrating these structures is similar to the silvering method for endothelia. The first step is to use threads to tie both ends of a freshly excised nerve trunk to a piece of wood so that the nerve is firmly stretched throughout the whole procedure. The specimen is then immersed for twelve to twenty-four hours in 0.5–1 per 100 silver nitrate, after which it is rinsed with distilled water and indurated in alcohol. The nerve can now be released from the holder and either teased with needles or embedded in paraffin or celloidin.

The Latin-shaped crosses of Ranvier and their cementing discs are black; the so-called Fromann's striae of the cylinder-axis and the profiles of the perineural endothelial cells also are impregnated.

248. Ranvier nodes also are visible after teasing nerve trunks fixed with osmic acid. (See more details about the use of this reagent for peripheral myelin staining in **261**.) In order to obtain preparations showing isolated nerves, mechanical dissociation can be performed on osmium-fixed nerve trunks.

METHODS TO STAIN THE SCHWANN CELLS

249. The Schwann cell nuclei are distinctly stained using the usual procedures with basic anilines and hematoxylin, already described in the first part of this book. However, if the protoplasm of these elements is to be stained, specific methods are required. We describe those techniques that have rendered good results for this purpose below:

250. Nageotte's method for the demonstration of Schwann cells.

1. Fix the nerve trunks for several hours in Dominici's liquid (**16**).
2. Rinse with water and dissociate the nerve fibers on a glass slide.
3. Stain briefly in Heidenhain's iron hematoxylin.
4. Dehydrate, clarify, and mount in balsam.

This technique stains the Schwann cell protoplasm deeply; nuclei are dark gray.

251. Cajal's procedure using formalin-uranyl and ammoniacal silver.

1. Fix fresh nerve trunk fragments for (at least) twenty-four hours in:

Formalin	15 cc
Uranyl nitrate	1 g
Water	100 cc

2. Rinse the blocks with distilled water.
3. Dissociate the main nerve fascicles (it is not necessary to isolate single fibers) and immerse for four to ten hours (or even more) in ammoniacal

silver. This reagent is prepared by dripping ammonia onto a 1 per 100 silver nitrate solution until the precipitate initially formed by ammonia is dissolved and the solution becomes transparent again.
4. Rinse briefly with distilled water and reduce for six to twelve hours in:

Formalin	5–8 cc
Water	100 cc
Hydroquinone	1.5 g
Anhydrous sodium sulfite	0.25 cc

5. Rinse briefly, first with water and then with 70° alcohol.
6. Embed in celloidin or delicately dissociate on a glass slide.

The cytoplasm of Schwann's cells is a translucent brown color. Inside the cytoplasm, a network of thick longitudinal fibers originating in the perinuclear region can be seen. Arising from these fibers, thinner, transverse trabeculae are shown and are conspicuously anastomosed.

252. Doinikow's method.

1. Immerse fresh nerve trunks for twenty-four hours in Orth's fixative (**6**) and indure them afterward in Muller's liquid (**5**) for several days.
2. Immerse the blocks for eight to ten days in Marchi's osmium-bichromate mixture (**163**).
3. Cut celloidin sections or dissociate the nerve trunk.
4. Immerse for one hour in a saturated solution of phosphomolybdic acid.
5. Rinse with water and stain for twenty-four hours in Mann's liquid:

1 per 100 *Methyl blue*[1]	35 cc
1 per 100 Eosin (w.g.)	45 cc
Distilled water	100 cc

6. Rinse briefly with distilled water and dehydrate in 96° and absolute alcohol consecutively.
7. Tone the sections in alkaline alcohol until the blue color changes to bright red. Alkaline alcohol is made by adding 10 drops of 1 per 100 sodium hydroxide (NaOH) to 60 cc of absolute alcohol.
8. Rinse with absolute alcohol and immerse the sections in acetic alcohol (absolute alcohol to which a few drops of acetic acid have been added) until the blue color returns.
9. Rinse again with absolute alcohol, clarify briefly in carbol-xylol and xylene, and mount in paraffin oil. The coverslip can be sealed with d'Ammar resin or any other cementing substance.

The Schwann cell protoplasm is deeply stained. The myelin appears pale-red and the myelin framework russet red; the products of myelin degeneration appear black, gray, or brown. Connective fibers are stained blue. This procedure also renders good results when the postfixation step in Marchi's liquid is omitted.

253. Nemiloff's procedure with methylene blue. This technique is almost identical to Dogiel's post vital staining method with weak solutions of Ehrlich's methylene blue.

The nerve trunks are moistened with a 1/8 per 100 solution of methylene blue for one or two hours in a 37°C oven. (See **88, 91** for further details on the method and how to prepare the staining solution.) The pieces are then either teased or fixed in ammonium molybdate for two to six hours; in the latter case, the specimens can be dehydrated briefly, embedded in paraffin (the embedding period must not exceed forty minutes) and sectioned as thinly as possible.

The cell body and the processes of Schwann cells are stained blue. This technique also demonstrates the mitochondria and neurofibrils of the axon, the Schmidt-Lantermann clefts, the spinous double bracelet, and, occasionally, the spiral apparatus of Rezzonico.

254. Some general purpose methods can be used to complement the results from specific techniques for the axon, the myelin sheath, or Schwann cells. Allow us to mention Cajal's trichromic method, Mallory's methods with hematoxylin or with basic anilines, and Unna's polychrome methylene blue and Unna-Pappenheim methyl green-pyronin.

Unna's method is used on paraffin sections of material fixed in alcohol, formalin, or Orth's liquid. The sections, once dewaxed, are stained for ten minutes in polychrome methylene blue (Grübler), then rinsed with water for two or three minutes, and differentiated in a 25 per 100 solution of Unna's glycerin-ether mixture (*Glizerinäthermischung*, Grübler).

Differentiation will never exceed thirty to sixty seconds and must be monitored under the microscope. When differentiation is complete, rinse with plenty of water, dehydrate briefly, clarify, and mount.

The Unna-Pappenheim method must be carried out in material fixed in Orth's, Zenker's, or Helly's liquids. The sections are immersed for fifteen minutes in the Pappenheim methyl green-pyronin stain (*Pyronin-Methylgrün*, Grübler) at 37°C, then dipped in distilled water and differentiated in 70° alcohol. Dehydrate directly in absolute alcohol, clarify in xylene, and mount as usual.

255. Supporting network of the Schwann cell. Some time ago De Cattani and other Italian histologists reported the existence of a fibrillary network surrounding the myelin sheath. This structure frequently has been ignored because the techniques needed for its demonstration were rather unreliable. It is possible, however, that some of these filaments were observed by Nemiloff, Cajal (1912), and Sánchez y Sánchez, who were able to confirm their existence using the formalin-uranyl nitrate method (**136**).

Sánchez (1916) obtained brilliant results with this method in the fish *Cyprinus auratus*. The pieces must be indurated for eight to twenty-four hours and then sectioned in the freezing microtome; gold-toning is advisable. Sánchez's results are similar to those obtained by Cajal in mammals, though in fish the network is more intricate.

256. Reich's method for staining the protagonoid granules (called π-granules by Reich).

1. Fix for several days in Müller's liquid. This is the recommended fixative for staining these granules specifically.

2. Rinse with water and cut 20 μm thick frozen sections.
3. Stain for five minutes in 1 per 100 toluidine blue or thionine.[2]
4. Rinse briefly with distilled water.
5. Differentiate first in 80° and then in 96° alcohol until the sections turn pale blue.
6. Immerse in absolute alcohol until no stain is drained off.
7. Clarify in xylene and mount in balsam.

When the differentiation has been properly done, the protagon granules π-granules) are stained carmine-red, whereas the nuclei are a very pale blue color; the myelin sheaths are pale-blue, if stained at all. Sometimes Unna's plasma cells are also colored.

257. Reich's method for staining the π and μ granules, Reich's granules.

1. Induration in Orth's fixative.
2. Rinse and cut 15 μm thick frozen sections.
3. Stain for twenty-four hours at 37°C in carbol-fuchsin (acid fuchsin, 1 g; 5 per 100 phenol, 100 cc).
4. Differentiate for half a minute in 1 per 100 potassium permanganate.
5. Immerse in Pal's mixture (**157**, Step 5).
6. Repeat Steps 4 and 5 until the sections become pale pink.
7. Rinse with water and stain for half a minute in 2 per 100 toluidine blue.
8. Dehydrate in 80°, 90°, and 100° alcohol.
9. Clarify in xylene and mount in balsam.

Nuclei and connective tissue are stained blue, the π-granules are a pale purple-red, and the μ granules an intense fuchsin-red. The latter structures are possibly formed by a lecithin-like substance, but this group probably includes structures of a heterogeneous nature. According to Doinikow, some of them may be identical to the *Ezholz granules* and are stained by Sudan III and scarlet red.

258. Nageotte's procedure to reveal the Schwann cell syncytium (*EN 46*) of the unmyelinated fibers.
The nerve trunks are fixed for twenty-four hours in Ranvier's "one-third" alcohol (absolute alcohol, 28 parts; water, 72 parts). The pieces are then immersed in a weak nitric acid solution (1 per 1000) until the collagen fibers swell (this takes from several hours to one day). Finally, the specimen is teased on a glass slide, stained with hematein, and differentiated with Cajal's picro-indigo carmine mixture (**61**). Mount either in glycerin or in balsam.

259. Nageotte has proposed another technique for revealing the relationship between the axon and Schwann cells in Remak's fibers.

1. Fix thin sympathetic nerves obtained from cat, dog, or rabbit in 1 per 100 osmic acid for twenty-four to thirty-six hours.
2. Rinse for some hours with distilled water.
3. Embed in paraffin and cut sections as thinly as possible, never thicker than 3–5 μm.

4. Mount the sections on glass slides, dewax and stain them with methylene blue.
5. Rinse briefly with water and mount in glycerin or in balsam.

260. For more methods to stain Remak's fibers, see **275–280**.

METHODS FOR MYELIN STAINING

261. The classic procedure of Schultze with osmic acid should be preferred to more modern methods when trying to study the fatty covering of nerves. This method works very well in normal material and even better in degenerating nerves. In order to obtain good fixation, small animals must be chosen (frog, guinea pig or newborn cat, rabbit or dog), so that the nerve trunks are thin. In addition, this material provides a small connective scar in regenerating nerves.

The procedure is as follows:

1. Pin the nerve to a sheet of cork and immerse it in a large volume of 1 per 100 osmic acid.
2. Rinse for twenty-four hours with water; renew the water several times.
3. Embed either in celloidin or in paraffin; in the last case, terpineol or cedarwood oil must be used as intermediate agents. Cut thin sections.
4. Counterstain with hematoxylin, carmine, or safranin.
5. Rinse and mount in either Apathy's liquid or balsam.

The osmic acid method is especially valuable for the study of both stages of degeneration–regeneration. The first stage consists of the early changes undergone by myelin sheaths (eight to ten days after nerve transection), whereas in the second stage the myelination of the fibers that penetrate the scar in the distal stump (thirty to thirty-five days after the nerve injury) can be seen. Needless to say, the regenerating nerve fibers are not stained by this method until they acquire the myelin sheath on the tenth day after surgery; the demonstration of the fibers in these early stages requires the use of axon-staining methods.

262. As osmium fixation is not suitable for very thick pieces. The best fixatives for such specimens are 10–15 per 100 formalin, 3 per 100 potassium bichromate, or Müller's liquid; the latter reagent should be allowed to act for at least two to four weeks. Material fixed by any of these procedures can be stained by all the myelin methods, such as Weigert-Pal's (**157**), Kulschitzky's (**158**), Spielmeyer's (**160**), and Loyez's (**161**).

263. The extent of myelin degeneration in the distal stump of the transected nerve trunks can be examined using Benda's (**164**) or Marchi's (**163**) methods. If the latter method is to be carried out on frozen sections, they must be placed in water and then immersed for two to three days either in 1 per 100 potassium bichromate or in Müller's liquid. The sections are then placed for three days in Marchi's liquid, in the dark, after which they are dehydrated, clarified, and mounted in balsam. Staining of the lipid droplets can be enhanced by immersing the sections in 1 per

Chapter 17: Demonstrating Peripheral Nerves

100 osmic acid once they have been treated with Marchi's liquid. Osmic acid must act for several hours at 37°C.

264. Lipid droplets and other products of degeneration that appear at the distal stump also can be stained with Sudan III and scarlet red (see Herxheimer method, **222**). Formalin fixation is advisable.

265. Nageotte's procedure to show myelin mitochondria. According to Nageotte, the myelin sheath is nothing but a colossal compound mitochondrion. This idea is based upon the results provided by some techniques that are more or less specific for mitochondria. Here is the method he proposed:

1. Fix rabbit peripheral nerve trunks or spinal cord roots at 37°C for twenty-four hours in:

Potassium bichromate	5 g
Distilled water	100 cc
Acetic acid	1.5–2.5 cc

Special care must be taken to avoid softening of the specimens during the extraction procedure.

2. Rinse with plenty of water, dehydrate, embed in paraffin, and cut thin sections (2–5 μm).
3. Mount the sections on glass slides, dewax, and transfer them to water.
4. Carry out Altmann's method (**58**) from Step 5 onward.

The myelin sheaths of those nerve fibers that are not swollen show radially arranged rod-shaped structures. Axon mitochondria are barely stained.

The best fixative for this method, according to Tupa, is Helly's liquid (Zenker's liquid, 50 cc; formalin, 2.5 cc); this reagent must act for several hours, after which the pieces are immersed for a short time in 5 per 100 potassium bichromate. Counterstaining can be achieved with Heidenhain's iron hematoxylin.

LANTERMANN INCISURES; SPIRAL APPARATUS; SPINOUS DOUBLE BRACELET; NEUROKERATIN NETWORK (EN 47)

266. In osmium-stained preparations, the myelin sheath appears occasionally interrupted by slanting, funnel-shaped channels that are known as Schmidt-Lantermann incisures.

267. The Schmidt-Lantermann clefts also can be demonstrated in formalin-fixed nerves after staining with hematoxylin and acid fuchsin (Nageotte). The procedure is as follows:

1. Fix nerve trunks in formalin and tease them on a glass slide with histological needles.
2. Immerse the specimens in alcohol in order to remove the fatty components of the myelin and stain them immediately with hematoxylin or with hematein.

3. Rinse with water and mount either in glycerin or, after dehydration and clearing, in balsam.

The Lantermann incisures and their limiting membranes appear to be disrupting the neurokeratin network, which is stained violet.

268. Cajal's method with formalin-pyridine-manganese. This technique is a variation of the reduced silver nitrate method.

1. Fix nerve trunk fragments for twenty-four hours in the following liquid:

Formalin	6 cc
Pyridine	10 cc
Manganese nitrate	0.5 g
Water	40 cc

2. Rinse for twenty-four hours in order to remove pyridine from the tissue.
3. Immerse for twenty-four to forty-eight hours in 1.5 per 100 silver nitrate.
4. Rinse briefly with water and reduce for some hours in a liquid containing 1 g of hydroquinone, 5 cc of formalin, 80 cc of water, and 0.25 g of anhydrous soda sulfite. Rinse with water and either tease or embed in celloidin.

This technique vigorously stains the funnel-shaped membranes of the Schmidt-Lantermann incisures in dark-brown; the **Segall rings** and the **Rezzonico-Golgi apparatus** also are shown.

269. Nageotte's procedure to demonstrate the spiral apparatus. Nageotte used Altmann's method to visualize the Rezzonico apparatus. For this purpose, thin nerve trunks obtained from adult rabbits or guinea pigs must be used. The pieces must be fixed for one day in Laguesse's liquid (**12**), and then rinsed and embedded in paraffin. The sections, which must be very thin, have to be mounted on glass slides, dewaxed, and stained following Altmann's method (**58**). The author recommends removing the chrome from the tissue prior to staining. For this purpose, we use the same technique proposed by Cowdry for the plastosomes, namely, oxidation in 0.25 per 100 potassium permanganate for twenty or thirty minutes and then bleaching of the sections with 5 per 100 oxalic acid for thirty to sixty seconds.

Nageotte's method stains the filaments of the Rezzonico apparatus bright red, whereas myelin appears rosy; neurofibrils are more strongly stained than myelin.

270. Finally, allow us to point out that the spiral apparatus can be occasionally shown by the formalin-uranyl nitrate method, as proved by Cajal in mammals and by Sanchez y Sanchez in fish. The procedure is the same as for staining the Golgi apparatus (**136**).

271. Nageotte's technique for staining the spinous double bracelet. According to Nageotte, this is the most suitable technique to show these organelles in their most typical form.

1. Fix nerve trunks for two weeks in 5 per 100 potassium bichromate at 37°C.

2. Rinse the pieces with water for one day and embed them in paraffin.
3. Cut thin sections longitudinally, mount on a glass slide, dewax, and immerse in water.
4. Stain the sections as in the original Benda's method for mitochondria, or, preferably, as in Altmann's method (**58**).

The spinous double bracelet, which is regularly located before or after Ranvier's nodes, is stained deep-red; the granules of the Schmidt-Lantermann incisures also are shown.

272. Ehrlich's method for staining the spinous double bracelet and neurofibrils. Although Nageotte was the first to describe this structure precisely, other authors had previously observed it impregnated with methylene blue. It is interesting that Cajal actually drew it in some of his works, although he never mentioned it in the text.[1]

To demonstrate the spinous double bracelet using the Ehrlich-Dogiel method, both the intravascular injection and the lubrication methods (**87–89**) can be used. To stabilize the stain, fixation with ammonium molybdate (**95**) is the method of choice.

After lubricating the pieces with methylene blue, the axonal and myelin mitochondria are frequently stained, as well as the cylinder-axis fibrils, as mentioned in Nemiloff's procedure (**253**). Needless to say, to stain any of these structures consistently, the nerves must be undamaged. Nageotte distinguishes two phases in the methylene blue staining of neurofibrils: a first stage of incomplete staining, in which the neurofibrils are stained in patches, resembling mitochondria, and a second stage, when complete impregnation is achieved.

273. Artifactual distortions of myelin. Lantermann's reticulum and neurokeratin network. According to Nageotte, the neurokeratin framework is nothing but the Lantermann's reticulum, once the fatty substances have been extracted. Both reticula are actually artifacts produced by the same process, not real structures of the nervous tissue. In fact, if we follow Nageotte's advice and stain the myelinated fibers by means of a weak (0.25%) solution of osmic acid, followed by bleaching with hydrogen peroxide and staining with acid fuchsin, a thick reticulum is demonstrated. This network, the *Lantermann's reticulum*, is formed by crisscrossing trabeculae that are coarser when the fixation is poor. This image is homologous to the *neurokeratin network* that appears in nerve fibers fixed with formalin, dehydrated with alcohol-ether, and stained with hematoxylin. The only difference between both reticula is that the neurokeratin fibers appear thinner due to the improved lipid extraction attained by the alcohol. Lantermann's reticulum also is demonstrated in osmium-fixed fibers exposed to the action of turpentine essence, which removes the unsaturated lipids.

DEMONSTRATION OF THE CYLINDER-AXIS AND NEUROFIBRILS

274. Bethe and Mönckeberg's method to demonstrate the neurofibrils of the myelinated fibers.

1. Fix thin nerve trunks for twenty-four hours in 0.25 per 100 osmic acid.
2. Rinse with water for six hours.

3. Treat the nerves with 96° alcohol for twelve to twenty-four hours.
4. Rinse again with water for four hours.
5. Immerse the pieces for six to twelve hours in 2 per 100 sodium bisulfite containing one to three drops of hydrochloric acid for every 10 cc.
6. Rinse with water for two to four hours.
7. Dehydrate with alcohol, clarify in xylene, and embed in paraffin.
8. Cut 2–3 µm thick sections and mount them on uncoated glass slides.
9. Transfer the sections to water and immerse them in a warm (20°–30°C) 1–4 per 100 ammonium molybdate solution.
10. Rinse several times with water and stain for five minutes in 0.1 per 100 toluidine blue; this step must be carried out at 50°–60°C.
11. Rinse briefly with water, dehydrate in alcohol, clarify either in toluene or xylene, and mount in balsam.

Neurofibrils are stained reddish-violet and the myelin a pale shade of gray. If myelin staining is so strong as to mask the neurofibrils, the sections must be thoroughly clarified in toluene (Step 11). This method will only work properly if the sections are very thin.

275. Bulk impregnation formulae of Cajal's reduced silver nitrate method that are particularly suitable for the study of degeneration and regeneration processes of nerve trunks. Several formulae of Cajal's method are very selective for the impregnation of the cylinder-axes of myelinated nerve fibers. Furthermore, this technique is the method of choice for showing the changes that take place in the axon and axonal sprouts during the degeneration and regeneration processes, as proven by Perroncito, Cajal, Nageotte, Lugaro, Tello, Rossi, Deineka, Sala, Rojas, de Castro, etc.

When dealing with the demonstration of regeneration phenomena, such as the course of sprouting fibers through the scar of distal stump, etc., the following advice must be kept in mind:

1. The sections of the impregnated blocks must not be thinner than 30 to 40 µm, so that newly formed fibers can be followed for a long distance.
2. To avoid shrinkage and curling of the regenerating nerves, regardless of the induration method, the nerves must be loosely pinned to a clean, smooth cork.[3] The pins must be removed when the pieces are to be immersed in the silver bath. Overlooking this simple precaution has caused experienced authors to miss the invasion of the distal stumps by the nerve sprouts due to the poor alignment of both ends. This problem is especially prominent in thin paraffin sections that only should be used to assess the fine structure of the growing axons and ***Bügner's band***.

276. Formula with ammoniacal alcohol (see **116**). This formula is suitable for the demonstration of axons, providing that the volume of alkali added to the alcohol is not excessive: Three ammonia drops for every 50 cc of alcohol are sufficient. This rule also should be observed when the aim is to study the central or peripheral stumps of a transected nerve one or more months after surgery, that is to say, once the initial swelling has disappeared. On the other hand, the early stages of the process require larger volumes of ammonia, about six to eight drops for every 50 cc of alcohol.[4]

Results: Axons are the only nerve constituents that are stained. Adult axons are stained orange to brown, whereas young ones are deep-red or dark brown. Nuclei, although visible, are only faintly stained; the background is pale yellow.

277. Formula with pyridine (119). This is the technique of choice for the following purposes: (a) to study the development and maturation of nerve trunks; (b) to stain the myelinated and unmyelinated axons of the nerve trunks; and (c) to analyze the first stages of the regeneration process.

Results: This procedure sharply stains the neurofibrils of the developing and regenerating axons. In the latter case, splendid images of the so-called metamorphic region (*EN 48*) of the growing axon can be obtained. Nuclei remain almost unstained. Remak's fibers are impregnated in a brownish-red or orange color. Toning of the sections is not recommended.

278. Formula with chloral hydrate (117). This method yields very consistent results, besides producing almost no shrinkage or swelling of the tissue. Furthermore, it stains both the adult and the regenerating axons, though it fails to impregnate the nerve fibers during normal neurogenesis. Nuclei can be identified without any further staining with anilines. Finally, allow us to say that this is perhaps the best formula of Cajal's method to demonstrate Remak's fibers, under both normal and pathological conditions.

The results are similar to those reported for the ammoniacal alcohol formula, though the fine unmyelinated fibers and the newly formed ones are more deeply stained.

279. The formulae that contain hypnotics and nitric acid (**118**) are especially useful in the study of the normal and pathological sympathetic axons. One of us (de Castro) has obtained excellent results using these procedures to analyze the degeneration and regeneration of the pre and postganglionic autonomic nerves. This technique does not stain the connective tissue, and thus renders highly limpid impregnations of the neural elements. If the sections are thin enough, gold-toning can be combined with subsequent nuclear counterstaining with anilines or hematoxylin.

Result: The unmedullated nerve fibers are a brown or reddish color against a limpid yellowish (or pale-orange) background. As in the previous formula, medullated axons also are stained.

280. Bielschowsky's method. In order to reduce the staining of the connective tissue of nerves, this author suggests rinsing the sections with acetic acid prior to reduction. The procedure is as follows:

1. Carry out steps 1 to 5 of the regular Bielschowsky method (**109**).
2. Immerse the sections in a weak solution of acetic acid (one to two drops per 20 cc of distilled water) until the color of the sections turns from brown to yellowish.
3. Reduce, tone, etc., as usual; no acetic acid should be added to the toning solution.

Result: The connective tissue fibers are stained violet, whereas the cylinder-axes are dark brown; sometimes myelin appears reddish. Schwann cells can be colored either with hematoxylin-eosin or with the van Gieson method.

Despite this modification, Bielschowsky prefers the bulk impregnation (**111**) for the study of peripheral nerve trunks.

281. Doinikow's modification of Bielschowsky's procedure.

1. Stretch the nerve trunks and attach to a cardboard strip; then fix them in 20 per 100 formalin for at least one month.
2. Rinse briefly with water and immerse for one or two days in pyridine; thick nerve trunks must be sectioned longitudinally with a straight razor blade prior to immersion in pyridine.
3. Rinse with tap water for twelve to twenty-four hours and then rinse the specimens several times with distilled water.
4. Impregnate for four to five days in 2 per 100 silver nitrate at 35°C.
5. Rinse briefly with distilled water and immerse the pieces for four to eight hours in Bielschowsky's ammoniacal silver.
6. Dip several times in distilled water and reduce for twelve to twenty-four hours in 20 per 100 formalin.
7. Rinse, dehydrate, embed in celloidin, and section.

282. Miskolczy's Variation of Bielschowsky's method. This technique is recommended by its author for the impregnation of thick human nerve trunks, either normal or regenerating.

1. Fix in formalin; then remove the fixative by rinsing the blocks with distilled water.
2. Degrease the specimens by passing them through graded alcohols and xylene; the pieces must remain for at least two hours in the latter reagent.
3. Transfer the pieces to water through graded alcohols.
4. Impregnate for two to seven days in 10 per 100 silver nitrate.
5. Rinse the specimens with distilled water and immerse them for two to five hours in Cajal's ammoniacal silver oxide (**176**).
6. Rinse briefly with distilled water and immerse the blocks in a weak solution of acetic acid (one to two drops per 20 cc of distilled water) in order to reduce the staining of the connective tissue.
7. Reduce for twenty-four hours in 20 per 100 formalin. The reducing solution must be replaced when milky clouds appear.
8. Embed in paraffin, section, mount on glass slides, tone, and fix.

DEMONSTRATION OF THE CONNECTIVE TISSUE OF NERVE TRUNKS (ENDONEURIUM, PERINEURIUM, AND EPINEURIUM)

283. The connective tissue fibers and cells that form the skeleton of the peripheral nerve trunks can be readily demonstrated by the procedures described in Chapter 15, **202–212**.

Cajal's reduced silver nitrate method also yields excellent staining of the connective tissue if the specimens are fixed in formalin-acetone (**134**). The endothelium lining the vaginal cavities of the perineurium as well as *Henle's sheath* can be visualized by the silvering method developed by Ranvier for the demonstration of the *Latin crosses* (see **247**).

284. Cajal's procedure for staining the peritubular connective sheath (*EN 49*). This technique is a minor modification of the reduced silver nitrate method.

1. Fix the nerve trunks for twenty-four hours in the following mixture:

Formalin	8 cc
Pyridine	15 cc
Water	40 cc

2. Rinse with running tap water in order to remove the pyridine and formalin from the blocks.
3. Dissociate the nerve trunks grossly and immerse them for several hours in 1 per 100 Bielschowsky's ammoniacal silver oxide (**109**).
4. Reduce in a hydroquinone-formalin-sulfite mixture (**268**, Step 4).
5. Dissociate the nerve delicately and mount.

This method reveals that each medullated nerve tube is surrounded by a connective sheath impregnated with a brown color and with a granular appearance.

18

Methods for the Demonstration of Peripheral Nerve Endings

285. Three types of histological methods t reveal the morphology of the peripheral nerve endings: (1) the old procedures using gold chloride; (2) supravital staining methods, such as Ehrlich's; and (3) silver impregnations carried out either en bloc or on sections. The latter, with the exception of the Golgi techniques, show the neurofibrillary skeleton of the nerve endings, staining the neuroplasm only faintly, if at all. On the other hand, Golgi's and Ehrlich's methods, as well as those using gold chloride, color the entire protoplasm of the nerve fiber without distinguishing any particular organelle.

These three groups of techniques act differently on each type of nerve ending—a fact that possibly is related to the varying structure of the terminals. Thus, when trying to demonstrate the autonomic *excito-secretory* endings, which have little fibrillary substance, Golgi's and Ehrlich-Dogiel's are recommended, because Cajal's, Gros's, or Bielschowsky's techniques are not suitable for this purpose. On the other hand, the latter methods (but also the Golgi and methylene blue procedures) render superb results for the visualization of *visceral endings*, either of a *sensory* or of an *effector* nature. Finally, if our aim is to study the *somatomotor* or *somatosensory* endings, which contain plenty of neuroplasm and neurofibrils, any of the previously mentioned methods will be useful. (An exception to this rule is Golgi's black reaction, which is only satisfactory in embryos or very young animals.)

GOLD CHLORIDE METHODS

286. These methods are the oldest ones used for the demonstration of nerve endings in the striated muscle and in the skin (somatosensory). They have evolved from Cohnheim's classic procedure and are based on the same principle: the simultaneous action of an acid and gold chloride on fresh tissues, with further reduction of gold either by light or other means. In these methods, metal instruments cannot be used for section handling; indeed, only extremely clean glassware must be used.

287. Loewit-Fischer's procedure. Immerse fresh muscle fragments in a one-third solution of formic acid until the tissue becomes transparent (about one minute), and then place the pieces for one or two minutes in 0.5–1 per 100 yellow gold chloride, where they will become straw-colored. The specimens are then returned to the formic acid solution, where they should remain for twenty-four hours in the dark. It is sometimes useful to treat the specimens for a further twenty-four hours with a concentrated solution of formic acid, so that a more complete gold reduction is achieved. The method is completed by dissociating the specimens and mounting them in glycerin.

The terminal arborizations are violet; deep and superficial zones show too much background and thus must be discarded.

288. Ranvier's method for the demonstration of motor end-plates and corneal nerves.

Treat small tissue fragments with filtered lemon juice until they become transparent (five to fifteen minutes). The juice should be freshly prepared and must be squeezed from a ripe lemon. The pieces are then transferred to a 1 per 100 gold chloride for twenty or more minutes and reduced as in the previous method.

289. Ranvier's second formula for staining motor end-plates. This technique is more reliable than the previous one. Immediately before use, prepare a mixture of 1 per 100 gold chloride (eight parts) and formic acid (two parts). Boil this liquid three times and once it has cooled to room temperature, immerse the pieces in it for ten to sixty minutes. Rinse briefly with water, reduce for twenty-four hours in 25 per 100 formic acid, and immerse the pieces in glycerin for one or more days. Formic acid and glycerin must act under a diffuse light.

According to Ranvier, boiling the gold-formic mixture is of great importance, because it enhances the affinity of gold for muscle tissue.

290. Ruffini's procedure. Similar to the previous techniques, this is a variation of the original Loewit-Fischer method. This is its modus operandi:

1. Immerse fresh tissue fragments in 20 per 100 formic acid until they become transparent. This step takes from ten to thirty minutes, depending on the thickness of the specimen; the success of the method depends on the extent of the formic acid treatment.
2. Dry the specimens with a clean cloth and immerse them for twenty to thirty minutes in 1 per 100 gold chloride; the reaction must be carried out inside a red bell jar.
3. Dry the pieces again with a very clean cloth and treat them for twenty-four hours with 20–25 per 100 formic acid, keeping them in the dark. Use as little formic acid as possible (the pieces should barely be covered by the solution). The concentration of the formic acid must be lowered to 10–15 per 100 for embryos or invertebrates.
4. Dry the pieces and immerse them for eight days in glycerin, under a diffuse light.
5. Dissociate the specimens or embed them in celloidin or paraffin; in the latter case, cut thick sections.
6. If the sections are overstained, they can be decolorized in a mixture of glycerin and 1 per 100 potassium ferrocyanide. Rinse thoroughly with water and mount in glycerin.

Chapter 18: Demonstrating Peripheral Nerve Endings

This is the best gold-based method to date. It renders magnificent images of the nerve endings in hairs, muscles, mucous membranes, periosteum, etc., and it is the only method capable of showing the ultraterminal fibrils in the muscle fascicles, described by Ruffini (*EN 50*). Needless to say, this technique allows carmine counterstaining.

291. Golgi's gold chloride method. This author has proposed immersing small, fresh pieces in 0.5 per 100 arsenious acid until they become transparent (ten to twenty minutes). The blocks are then placed for twenty to thirty minutes in a 0.5 per 100 solution of potassium and gold chloride where they will turn a straw-yellow. Rinse with water and reduce for twenty-four hours in 1 per 100 arsenious acid (in sunlight). Dissociate and mount in glycerin.

DEMONSTRATION OF NERVE ENDINGS WITH THE GOLGI METHOD

292. The nerve endings of parenchymatous organs, which are almost impossible to stain with neurofibrillary methods, are beautifully shown by the original rapid Golgi method (**73**) and even better by Cajal's double impregnation technique (**74**). In fact, we owe most of our knowledge of the autonomic fiber endings to the Golgi method or its variations by Cajal (**74**), Juschtschenko (**78**), Timofejew (**79**), etc. The Golgi indirect procedure (**77**) also renders nice results.

As usual for Golgi-type methods, numerous trials are necessary to demonstrate the richness and morphology of the innervation of a given gland. It must be borne in mind, however, that the Golgi method is not suitable for all tissues or animal species. In organs containing a lot of muscle, or in connective or adipose tissues, the Golgi method usually fails to impregnate the endings properly. Our best results have been obtained in mice, guinea pigs, rabbits, and bats, whereas results were not as good in cats and dogs.

Finally, it should be pointed out that, when using young animals, these techniques are very consistent for revealing the intraepithelial sensory endings (larynx, esophagus, urethra), the terminal arborizations of medium and small blood vessels, and the *interstitial sympathetic neurons* of Cajal.

DEMONSTRATION OF PERIPHERAL NERVE ENDINGS WITH EHRLICH'S METHYLENE BLUE PROCEDURE

293. Ehrlich-Dogiel's supravital staining method (**87–100**) is one of the most selective for the demonstration of motor and sensory endings, either somatic or autonomic. It can be used in almost all organs and tissues, although in exocrine glands, hypophysis, and thyroid its results are poorer than those of the Golgi method.

The best preparations are obtained using the techniques of intravascular injection (**89**) or the method of repeatedly lubing the blocks with the dye (**91**). The following requisites must be fulfilled:

1. The animal must be thoroughly bled, so that even the smallest blood vessels are emptied.

2. The blood vessels of the chosen organ must be completely filled with a warm (37–38°C) methylene blue solution. If the lubing technique is used, the dye must be allowed to penetrate deeply inside the block.
3. Carefully cut slices from the specimens and expose them to air in order to allow the reduction of the stain.
4. Fix whenever the nerve terminals are selectively stained (see also, the rongalite procedure, **101**).

NEUROFIBRILLARY METHODS CAPABLE OF DEMONSTRATING THE NERVE ENDINGS

294. Almost all the silver methods previously described for the impregnation of central axons and neurofibrils (Cajal, Bielschowsky, Schultze-Gros) can be used successfully for staining nerve endings. Here, we shall mention only those which are specific for the various types of endings.

There are three possible situations when trying to study nerve endings: (A) When only formalin-fixed material is available: In this case, we must use either the original Bielschowsky's method or some of its variations (Boeke, Gros, Agduhr), or use the reduced silver nitrate method in sections (Cajal, Schultze). (B) When fresh material is available: Cajal's method should be attempted, using the most adequate formula (see **295**). (C) When the material is stored in alcohol: We must use the formulae of the Cajal's method, which include alcohol fixation (**115–116**).

295. Fixation formulae for Cajal's reduced silver nitrate method. Almost all of the formulae of Cajal's method are suitable for impregnating nerve endings. The best results are obtained using techniques without fixation (**114**), or fixed with ammoniacal alcohol (**116**), hypnotics (**111–118**), or pyridine (**119**). For all of them it is advisable to use newly sacrificed animals or, in the case of human material, only a few hours postmortem. Impregnations in young animals produce more regular and complete results than in adults. In the following paragraphs we shall comment on the results of each formula individually.

296. The formula without fixative (**114**) can be used to impregnate the large somatic terminal arborizations, either motor or sensory (corpuscles of Pacini, Meissner, Herbst, Grandry, tendon end-organs, and nerve endings in the striated muscles). As in the case of the central nervous system, the addition of alcohol or methyl alcohol to the silver bath may improve the delicacy of the impregnation.

This variation is most reliable, staining the terminal arborizations a brown or reddish color against a pale-yellow background. However, its main shortcoming is the poor penetration of the reagents so that only the sections obtained from the superficial areas of the block are properly impregnated.

297. The ammoniacal alcohol formula (**116**) is the best technique for nerve endings, although it has been criticized for inconstancy. This is largely due to either the use of impure alcohol or an excess of ammonia in the fixative (two to three drops of 36° (*EN 51*) ammonia for each 50 cc of alcohol are sufficient). When the method is successful, the neurofibrils are neatly stained a solid-brown or black-coffee color, standing out against a yellowish background in which the nuclei are delicately outlined. This formula admits gold-toning and complementary counterstaining. It can be successfully

Chapter 18: Demonstrating Peripheral Nerve Endings

used to reveal the sensory end-organs and the motor endings of both smooth and striated muscles. Furthermore, it is also useful for the study of the degeneration and regeneration processes of nerve endings (Cajal, Tello, Perroncito, Nageotte, Marinesco, etc.), although in this case the ammonia content must be increased to four to six drops in 50 cc of alcohol.

298. Pyridine (**119**) is one of the most constant fixatives of Cajal's method for the peripheral nerve endings in young animals (Tello). In this material, it renders superb impregnations of the sensory end-organs of skin and mucous membranes and also of motor end-plates. Cajal and Tello have proven the excellence of this procedure for the study of the histogenesis of the nerve endings. Gold-toning is not recommended in this formula because it brings up the background.

299. Fixation in chloral hydrate (**117**) is especially suitable for the demonstration of almost all types of peripheral endings, including autonomic ones. This method is better than the preceding one when working with adult material. We usually dissolve the chloral hydrate in a mixture of water and alcohol (**21**), because in this way, gold-toning and aniline counterstaining are easier to perform (de Castro).

300. When attempting to study the nerve endings of organs that have abundant connective tissue, the formulae with hypnotics and nitric acid (**118**) must be used. These procedures render a homogeneous and very faintly stained background (de Castro) thus allowing gold-toning and counterstaining. This advantage may be of critical importance if a topographical analysis of the endings is needed.

301. The mixtures of fixatives, such as chloral-alcohol-pyridine (**120, 329**) can also provide valuable results for the study of the peripheral nerve endings. The fixative recently proposed by Martínez Pérez (1932) for skin endings also yields nice impregnations. The *modus faciendi* is as follows:

1. Prepare a saturated solution of chloral hydrate in pyridine and then drip distilled water onto it until milky clouds begin to appear. Stir until the liquid clears. If the solution does not become completely transparent, add one or two drops of pure pyridine.

Immerse the pieces for twenty-four hours in this reagent.

2. Rinse for twenty-four hours with running tap water and treat for the same time in ammoniacal alcohol (ammonia, 4 drops; alcohol, 50 cc). The remaining steps are carried out as in the original Cajal's method (**119**, Steps 5 and 6).

302. Dogiel's formula with alcohol and formic acid. This author has used the following fixative to study the innervation of the Herbst-Grandry corpuscles:

90° Alcohol	100 cc
Formic acid	1–2 cc

The pieces are fixed in this liquid for one to two days, then are rinsed with 2–2.5 per 100 silver nitrate and impregnated in this reagent for five to six days at 37°C. Rinse carefully with distilled water and reduce as usual (**114**, Step 3).

Regrettably, the results obtained by us with this technique are far from satisfactory.

303. Golgi's modification of Cajal's method (135). Golgi's suggested changes to the original reduced-silver procedure allow not only the staining of the reticular apparatus, but also of some peripheral endings (corpuscles of Pacini and Herbst-Grandry, intraepithelial endings, preganglionic endings). This has been proven by Dogiel, Lawrentjew, Kolossow, Katmanow, etc. The procedure of Dogiel, Deineka, and Lawrentjew is as follows:

1. Fix the pieces for eight to ten (or even more) hours in a mixture of formalin, arsenious acid, and 96° alcohol (see **135**, Step 1).
2. Rinse briefly with 2 per 100 silver nitrate and impregnate the pieces in this reagent for five to seven days.
3. Rinse with distilled water and follow the original method (**135**, from Step 3 onward).

Results: In gold-toned sections, the neurofibrils are deep-violet or black against a pale, though somewhat grainy, background. The nuclei are clearly shown but should be counterstained with carmine.

304. Bielschowsky's procedure. This method renders excellent results in large nerve endings but fails to demonstrate the finest endings in the sympathetic system. Furthermore, it may generate confusing images because the fine reticulin fibers, which also are impregnated, can be taken for axons. Bulk impregnation (**111**) is more reliable than section impregnation (**109**).

305. Boeke's modification of Bielschowsky's method. The modification proposed by
Boeke yields better results than the original method:

1. Fix for two weeks (or, preferably, for two months or more) in 12 per 100 neutral formalin; formalin must be neutralized with $MgCO_3$.
2. Rinse briefly with distilled water and immerse for three days in pyridine.
3. Rinse for eight hours with distilled water, changing the water several times.
4. Impregnate for five to six days in 3 per 100 silver nitrate at 37°C.
5. Rinse briefly with distilled water and immerse the pieces for twenty-four hours in Bielschowsky's ammoniacal silver oxide (**111**, Step 4).
6. Rinse for two or three hours with distilled water changing the water several times.
7. Reduce for one day in 20 per 100 neutral formalin.
8. Rinse, embed in paraffin, cut sections, and tone them with gold chloride. Mount in balsam.

This method renders beautiful impregnations of the sensory and motor endings, and, occasionally, of the sympathetic terminals. Boeke's periterminal network (*EN 52*) is also sometimes shown.

306. Bielschowsky-Gros method. This technique yields nice results for the demonstration of nerve endings and autonomic ganglia in material stored in 12–20 per 100 neutral formalin for long periods (although never exceeding one year). Stöhr Jr. (1932) suggests fixing the pieces in 50 per 100 neutral formalin for a few days. For further details of this method, see **112**.

307. Lawrentjew has proposed a simple and most reliable modification of the Gros method, the *modus faciendi* of which is as follows[1]:

1. Fix fresh pieces for one hour in Lawrentjew's AFA mixture:

96° Alcohol	1 part
Formalin neutralized with magnesium carbonate	1 cc
Saturated aqueous solution of arsenious acid	1 cc

Before fixation, the pieces (intestines, esophagus, vagina, skin, etc.) should be spread out and pinned to a paraffin sheet.

2. Transfer the pieces, without rinsing, to 20% neutral formalin. In this step, the specimens can be detached from the paraffin. The pieces remain in this liquid for a period ranging from four to seven days to four to six months. However, if fixation proceeds for more than two months, the impregnation becomes slow and unspecific.
3. Rinse with water for three to five minutes and section with the freezing microtome. The sections, which must be thick, are placed in water with a few drops of formalin.
4. Immerse the sections in 20% silver nitrate for one to five minutes.
5. Transfer the sections to a 20% formalin solution. The formalin should be diluted with tap water, not distilled water. The formalin solution is poured into four wells, so that the sections can be transferred consecutively from one well to the next one after milky clouds appear in the solution. The whole step must not exceed one or two minutes.
6. Immerse the section in a small amount of ammoniacal silver placed in a watch glass. In this way, the impregnation can be monitored under the microscope and thus be stopped at the right time. The ammoniacal silver bath is prepared as follows:

Six to eight milliliters of 20% silver nitrate are poured into a measuring cylinder, after which ammonia is dripped onto it until the brown precipitate that appears with the first drops of ammonia finally disappears. A small volume of the final mixture is transferred to a watch glass and a few more drops of ammonia added. The longer the period in which the sections are immersed in the silver nitrate solution, the more ammonia is required. As a rule, five to six drops of ammonia are enough to demonstrate the nerve elements, but in some cases up to twelve to fifteen drops are necessary.

The impregnation of the nervous structures is completed after a few minutes. It starts with a lemon-yellow coloration and then darkens to brown and finally to black. When the aim is to demonstrate only the neurofibrils, the impregnation must be stopped before the somata turn black. Heavy impregnations must only be used when the primary objective is the visualization of the nerve endings.

7. Rinse the sections with ammoniacal water (distilled water, 5 cc; ammonia, 4 cc) for one minute. Rinse thoroughly with distilled water. Tone and mount as in the original procedure (**112**).

308. Cajal's method for frozen sections. We already have described this procedure (**129**), which was originally developed for staining central neural endings in formalin-fixed tissues. However, it also renders excellent results for the demonstration of the sensory and motor peripheral nerve endings, as one of us has proved.[1] The neurofibrils of the terminal arborizations are most delicately outlined in violet after gold-toning, standing out against a background in which the tissue structure is clearly defined. The periterminal reticulum of the motor end-plates (*EN 52*) is shown in a similar manner as when stained by Boeke's technique.

309. The following modification (Cajal, 1925) of the hydroquinone method (**129**) yields superb results for the impregnation of both peripheral and central nerve endings:

1. Frozen sections of formalin-fixed material are immersed for one or two hours in:

Distilled water	10 cc
96° Alcohol	10 cc
Ammonia	10 drops

2. Dip the sections in water in order to remove the excess of alkali and impregnate for one to twenty-four hours in 2 per 100 silver nitrate. This step will take only a few minutes if the bath is heated with an alcohol burner to 45°–50°C.
3. Rinse briefly with alcohol and reduce in the hydroquinone solution (**129**, Step 3).

This technique is most reliable: the best animals for this purpose are the adult cat and rabbit.

310. Schultze's method. This method is recommended by Stöhr Jr. who has made good impregnations of the nerve endings of the meninges, choroid plexuses, and blood vessels. It is similar to a previously described technique (**131**), but the concentration of the soda *lye* must be 10 parts of stock solution in 50 parts of water and the concentration of the silver nitrate must be increased to 10 per 100. According to Stöhr, the impregnation quality is even better if a very weak reducing solution is used (dilute the regular hydroquinone solution 80–120 times).

METHODS TO DEMONSTRATE THE NERVE TRUNKS AND NERVE ENDINGS IN ORGANS PROTECTED BY BONE TISSUE

311. The study of the nerve endings of the teeth, the labyrinth (organ of Corti and vestibular apparatus), and the bone marrow requires the use of certain special decalcification formulae for Cajal's and Bielschowsky's methods so that the specimens can be sectioned without losing their affinity for colloidal silver. The techniques explained below are equally useful for the study of the central nervous system, nerve roots, and spinal and sympathetic ganglia in small animals where it is difficult to dissect these structures from the surrounding bone. There are two types of procedure: short ones, in which fixation and decalcification take place at the same time (de Castro) and long ones, in which they are carried out separately (Bielschowsky, Agduhr, Hubert, Guild, Cajal, Lorente de Nó, Tello).

Decalcification times for the methods below have been explained elsewhere (**25, 28, 30, 119**). For the impregnation and reduction steps, see **119**.

312. Bielschowsky's decalcification procedure (1908). The main steps of this method are the following:

1. Fix for several days in 20 per 100 formalin.
2. Immerse the pieces in 5 per 100 nitric acid until the lime is completely removed, frequently replacing the liquid.[2]
3. Rinse thoroughly with water to remove the excess of acid.
4. Immerse the pieces for some days in 20 per 100 formalin.
5. Rinse for one hour with water, cut frozen sections, and place them in distilled water.
6. Immerse the sections for twenty-four hours in 4 per 100 silver nitrate in the dark.

The remaining steps are identical to Bielschowsky's method for nerve trunks (**280**).

To achieve good results in specimens that have been stored for a long time, Bielschowsky and Bruhl recommend carrying out the procedure twice and stress that it is absolutely necessary to rinse the sections thoroughly prior to transferring them to the ammoniacal silver hydroxide bath.

313. Agduhr's modification of Bielschowsky's en bloc staining method.

1. Fix for a week in 20 per 100 neutral formalin.
2. Decalcify in 5 per 100 nitric acid and return the pieces to formalin.
3. Rinse with running tap water and immerse the specimens for a week in pyridine.
4. Rinse with distilled water for ten days, changing the water daily.
5. Impregnate for ten days in 3 per 100 silver nitrate at 18°C. This step must be carried out in the dark.
6. Rinse with distilled water and immerse for twenty-four hours in ammoniacal silver oxide (in the dark). This reagent must be prepared in the same way as the original Bielschowsky's silver solution (see **109**, Step 5), although the proportions of silver, soda, and water are slightly different: 10 per 100 silver nitrate, 10 cc; 40 per 100 sodium hydroxide, 20 drops; distilled water, 300 cc.
7. Bleach the connective tissue by immersing the pieces for twenty-four hours in 1 per 200 acetic acid.
8. Reduce as in the original Bielschowsky's method (**111**). In some cases, Steps 2 and 3 can be omitted.

314. Decalcification procedures for Cajal's method (de Castro, 1925). We have previously mentioned the advantages of using nitric acid in fixation with hypnotics in order to stain the central or peripheral endings with Cajal's method (**118**). The main use of these formulae, however, is to demonstrate the nerve endings in organs inside bone structures, as proved by one of us (de Castro) and confirmed by several authors (Lorente de Nó, Miskolczy, F. Rossi, Terni, Calderon). The *modus faciendi* is as follows:

1. Fix pieces less than 1 cm thick in one of these liquids:

    (A)

Chloral hydrate	0.5 g
96° Alcohol	50 cc
Distilled water	0.50 cc
Nitric acid	3–4 cc

    (B)

Ethyl urethane	2–3 g
96° Alcohol	60 cc
Distilled water	40 cc
Nitric acid	3–4 cc

    (C)

20 per 100 Somnifene (H. La Roche)	2–4 cc
96° Alcohol	60 cc
Distilled water	40 cc
Nitric acid	3–4 cc

    The pieces must be left in one of these liquids until completely decalcified. Usually, this takes two or three days,[3] and it is advisable to use large volumes of fixative and replace it daily. If the pieces are very thick, they must be sectioned into 3–4 mm slices once they are soft enough to be cut with a scalpel.

2. Rinse with running tap water for twenty-four to thirty-six hours.
3. Immerse the pieces for twenty-four hours in ammoniacal alcohol (96° alcohol, 50 cc; ammonia, 4–6 drops).
4. Rinse for some minutes with distilled water and impregnate for five to seven days in 1.5–2 per 100 silver nitrate at 38–40°C. In this step, the pieces should turn brown (Cajal's ripening stage).
5. Rinse and reduce as usual (**114**). Gold-toning and nuclear counterstaining with hematoxylin, carmine, or anilines is possible with both A and B fixatives.

These techniques stain all types of peripheral nerve endings well, including those of the teeth and bone marrow. The best results, however, are obtained from the inner ear, where magnificent preparations can be made of the nerve endings in both the organ of Corti and the *maculae* and *cristae* of the vestibular organs.

Chapter 18: Demonstrating Peripheral Nerve Endings

315. The following method, proposed by Lorente de Nó (1926), can also be used, although it is more tedious and less reliable than the preceding ones.

1. Fix for one day either in 50 per 100 pyridine or in ammoniacal alcohol (ammonia, 5 drops; alcohol, 50 cc).
2. Rinse with water for one day and decalcify with 3 per 100 nitric acid for twenty-four hours.
3. Rinse with ammoniacal water for several hours.
4. Immerse the pieces in ammoniacal alcohol or in a mixture of alcohol (50 cc) and pyridine (15 cc).
5. Impregnate for six to seven days at 38–40°C in 2 per 100 silver nitrate. Reduce in pyrogallol, etc.

316. Tello has recently (1932) developed a variation of Cajal's method that stains the nerve endings in the inner ear excellently as well as the protoplasmic reticulum of the hair cells. This formula combines fixation in pyridine with decalcification in a chloral-nitric acid bath similar to de Castro's (**314**). The procedure is as follows:

1. Fix for twenty-four hours in 50 per 100 pyridine.
2. Rinse with water for twelve to twenty-four hours.
3. Decalcify with:

Chloral hydrate	10–20 g
Water	100 cc
Nitric acid	5 cc

4. Rinse for one day with a large volume of water.
5. Ammoniacal alcohol, one day.
6. 1.5 per 100 Silver nitrate, five to seven days at 37°C.
7. Reduce, embed in celloidin, etc.

PROCEDURES FOR STAINING THE SYMPATHETIC AND DORSAL ROOT GANGLIA

317. No special methods are required to reveal the perikarya, cylinder-axis, or endings of the neurons of the sensory and sympathetic ganglia. Golgi's and Ehrlich-Dogiel's methods (**74, 78, 79**) and (**89, 91, 293**) render excellent results. In the latter, however, the quality is variable depending on the organ studied. For instance, in the sympathetic ganglia the fibers and nerve endings are shown, but the neurons are only poorly impregnated, whereas in the intestinal plexuses of Auerbach and Meissner and the spinal and heart nerve ganglia, the neurons are preferentially stained.

318. When studying the peripheral ganglia, neurofibrilar methods are better than morphologic methods (*EN 53*) in terms of both quality and consistency. We recommend the following techniques for this purpose:

En Bloc Staining

1. For the demonstration of neurons and cylinder-axes in the ganglia of humans and adult animals: Follow Bielschowsky's (**111**) or, preferably, Cajal's method, fixing the specimens in weak ammoniacal alcohol (**116**). Cajal's method also produces good results on unfixed specimens (**114**), after fixation with pyridine (**119**), somnifene (**118**), or the double fixation proposed by Ranson. The double fixation includes immersion of the pieces in ammoniacal alcohol for twenty-four hours, followed by a brief rinse and an additional twenty-four hours in pyridine. The remaining steps are the same as for Cajal's procedure (**119**).
2. For histogenetic and developmental studies, Cajal's methods with pyridine (**119**) or plain alcohol (**115**) are preferable. These methods are especially valuable when dealing with vertebral and prevertebral sympathetic ganglia from newborn humans or human fetuses, when strong silver baths (3% or 5%) are recommended (de Castro). Chloral hydrate fixation (**117**) is the method of choice for intestinal ganglia from late embryonic stages and the newborn.
3. The delicate axons of preganglionic fibers take the silver selectively when using Cajal's method after fixation in ammoniacal alcohol (**116**), pyridine (**119**), chloral hydrate (**117**), and somnifene (**118**).
4. For the study of pathological ganglia, we use Cajal's methods with ammoniacal alcohol or pyridine fixation in addition to Bielschowsky's.

Section Staining of Formalin-fixed Specimens

1. Bielschowsky's method (**109**) renders good impregnations of the neurons. The best results, however, are achieved using the modifications made by Gros (**112**) or Gros-Lawrentjew (**307**), and with the Schultze-Stöhr technique (**131**). Cajal's method carried out on sections (**318**) yields more complete impregnations of the somata and dendrites of the sympathetic ganglia neurons as demonstrated by one of us (de Castro).
2. The nerve endings in the sympathetic ganglia are hard to demonstrate by means of the impregnation procedures on sections. The most selective techniques are those of Gros (**112**) and Gros-Lawrentjew (**307**).
3. In pathological tissue, the aforementioned procedures of Bielschowsky, Gros (Herzog), Schultze, and Cajal render good results.

319. Cajal's method for floating sections. This method originally was developed to study the cerebellum,[2] but one of us (de Castro) has used it successfully to demonstrate the morphology of the somata and cylinder-axes of the human sympathetic ganglia neurons.

It does have, however, a disadvantage: The neurofibrillary network of the perikarya and dendrites is not clearly shown. The main steps of the method are:

1. Fix in 14 per 100 formalin for two weeks.
2. Cut 20–25 μm thick frozen sections and place them in the fixative.
3. Rinse briefly with distilled water (twice) and immerse in 2 per 100 silver nitrate to which a few pyridine drops have been added (one drop per milliliter). The sections must be maintained in this bath until they turn the color of tobacco (one to two days at room temperature or some minutes if heated to 45°C with the alcohol burner).
4. Dip in alcohol or, preferably, in alcohol with a few drops of the silver solution.
5. Reduce in a freshly prepared mixture of:

    | Hydroquinone | 0.2 g |
    | Formalin (Merck) | 30 cc |
    | Distilled water | 70–80 cc |

6. Rinse, dehydrate, clarify, and mount.

If the sections are not strongly impregnated, they can be gold-toned, as in Bielschowsky's method.

19

Techniques for the Demonstration of the Nervous Tissue of Invertebrates

320. In the present chapter we shall report the specific techniques for the study of the morphology and neurofibrillar network of the neurons of invertebrates. We will not repeat any previously described procedures that are suitable for invertebrate tissue if they need no modifications.

METHODS CAPABLE OF REVEALING THE MORPHOLOGY OF NEURONS

321. As for vertebrates, Ehrlich's and Golgi's methods are suitable for this purpose (see Chapters 1 and 2).

Induration for the Golgi method in the osmium-bichromate mixture is recommended when trying to stain thin axons or their delicate terminal arborizations. Cajal's double impregnation (**74**) renders particularly good results because of the fineness and sharpness of the silver precipitate. If neuronal perikarya are to be shown, it is advisable to use the formulae with formalin and bichromate (**80–83**). These methods sometimes yield impregnations as excellent as those obtained using the osmium-bichromate fixation. Sectioning requires celloidin-embedding, especially in the case of insects.

322. Ehrlich's method has been successfully used by Retzius and Sánchez in crustaceans and hirudineans. These authors use a 1 per 100 methylene blue stock solution diluted five to twenty times; the stain is injected in the body cavity of the living animal. After ten to twenty minutes, the animal is opened along the dorsal midline, and the ganglia exposed to air, so that the blue color is "regenerated." (See the basis of Ehrlich's method in **87**.) The staining of neurons and nerve fibers will be completed in one and a half or two hours; during this period the animal must be placed in a humid chamber and the ganglia sprinkled from time to time with the methylene blue solution. The specimens can be studied directly either by placing them on a glass slide (Retzius) or fixed with picrate or molybdate (**94, 96, 97**). Using the latter, permanent preparations can be obtained by squashing them between the glass slide and the coverslip (Sánchez y Sánchez), providing the ganglia are not too thick.

METHODS FOR STAINING NEUROFIBRILS

323. Apathy's procedure to color neurofibrils. This method has the following steps:

1. *Fixation.* Fix very small tissue fragments either in a saturated solution of sublimate containing 0.5 per 100 sodium chloride or in alcohol-sublimate (1:1 mixture of absolute alcohol and saturated solution of sublimate). For hirudineans, the best results are obtained with a 1:1 mixture of sublimate solution and 1 per 100 osmic acid (which must be freshly prepared). The fixation time ranges from four to twenty-four hours, depending on the thickness of the specimen.
2. *Removal of the sublimate.* The pieces are rinsed several times with distilled water and then immersed for twelve hours in an iodine-iodide solution (potassium iodide, 1 g; metallic iodine, 0.5; water, 100 cc). Afterward, they are placed for some hours in 95° alcohol and then transferred to iodinated alcohol (potassium iodide, 1 g; metallic iodine, 0.5; alcohol, 100 cc); this must act for eight to twelve hours in order to remove the sublimate crystals completely. Finally, the iodine is washed out with 96° alcohol.
3. *Paraffin embedding and sectioning.* Dehydrate the blocks in absolute alcohol and embed in paraffin, using chloroform as intermediate solvent. Cut 10 μm thick sections and stick them to the slide by capillarity or with albumin-glycerin. Dewax with chloroform, immerse in absolute alcohol, and place the sections in water for two to six hours.
4. *Impregnation.* Treat the sections for one day with 1 per 100 yellow gold chloride (Merck), in the dark.
5. *Reduction.* Dip the sections in distilled water or blot them dry with filter paper and immerse for twenty-four hours in 1 per 100 formic acid. This should be done by pouring the formic acid onto a glass well, where the glass slides are immersed obliquely, with the sections facing down in order to avoid the precipitation of gold on the surface of the sections. The well with the slides is exposed to indirect sunlight, for a whole day, to speed up the reduction. Two sheets of white paper (one under the well and another on the side opposite the incoming sunlight) are used to reflect the sunlight and accelerate this step. The optimal temperature for this step is 23°C. In winter, or in northern countries, the well must be exposed to direct sunlight.
6. *Section mounting.* Finally, the sections are rinsed with water and mounted either in Apathy's medium or as usual in balsam.

Results: This technique is very inconstant. The best results are obtained in hirudineans. The critical step is the photo-reduction of gold in acidulated water. According to Levi, the concurrence of the luminous, thermal, and chemical energies (of the acidulated water) is crucial to produce an energy state, without which the reaction does not take place. The neurofibrils are beautifully impregnated deep-violet or black.

324. Cajal's reduced silver nitrate method. As proved by one of us (Cajal) and also by Sánchez y Sánchez, Rina Monti, Azoulay, etc., this procedure renders excellent impregnations of the neurofibrillary lattice of the neurons of invertebrates. Especially good results are obtained in the ganglion chain of crustaceans and hirudineans and in the large neurons of insects and cephalopods. The steps of the different formulae of the method are those described previously, although the silver concentration needs to be somewhat raised. In the following paragraphs we will comment on the results of some specific formulae:

325. The technique without fixation (**114**) works nicely for hirudineans (*Hirudo medicinalis, Alaustomum*, etc.) when the silver nitrate is used at a 5–6 per 100 concentration and the impregnation is held for three to five days at 37°C. As Cajal pointed out some time ago, however, the reaction is consistently good in some of the batches of leeches delivered to our laboratory, whereas in others the method always fails.

326. Fixation in plain alcohol (**115**) renders superb impregnations of the neurofibrillary network in hirudineans (*Pontobdella, Glossiphonia algira*). This structure does not stain as well in insects or in cephalopods, although in these cases this technique demonstrates the axons and nerve endings beautifully. The silver nitrate concentration must be 3–5 per 100.

327. Fixation in ammoniacal alcohol (**116**) followed by impregnation for two or three days in 3–4 per 100 silver nitrate at 37°C results in excellent impregnations in several hirudineans (*Pontobdella, Glossiphonia, Hirudo*). Special care must be given to the proportion of alkali: Two or three drops of ammonia per 50 cc of alcohol results in a distinct staining of the neurofibrils, but when four to five drops are added, only the glial fibers are colored.

328. Fixation in 70–80 per 100 pyridine is useful for revealing neurons and especially nerve endings in the cephalopods (Cajal). Impregnate in 3–5 per 100 silver nitrate for three to five days in the oven.

329. Finally, we should not finish without mentioning Cajal's chloral-pyridine mixture (**120**), which renders good results when used to demonstrate the nerve endings in the muscles of crustaceans (D'Ancona). The proportions are: chloral hydrate, 5 g; pyridine, 20 cc; absolute alcohol, 40 cc; water, 40 cc. The fixation time is one day.

Methods for Demonstrating Some Pathogenic Microorganisms

Frequently the histopathologist needs to demonstrate the presence of the causative germ in pathological lesions of the nervous system. Thus, it is relevant to mention the methods used in neuropathology for the demonstration of pathogenic germs, such as the procedures capable of staining *Treponema pallidum, trypanosomes, tuberculosis bacillus* and, in the case of rabies, the so-called *Negri bodies*. Further knowledge about topics on bacteriology can be found in the Morbid Anatomy and Bacteriology treatises.

DEMONSTRATION OF THE SYPHILIS TREPONEMA

330. The following paragraphs are concerned with the silver impregnation methods for the demonstration of this germ in sections of either formalin- or alcohol-fixed brain or spinal cord (Levaditi's, Noguchi's, and Jahnel's procedures). Thus, we shall omit the so-called rapid methods, such as the darkfield examination of fresh brain tissue, the techniques of Burris and Fontana-Tribondeau, and the staining of smears with the Giemsa liquid.

331. Levaditi's method. This method is simply a variation of Cajal's reduced silver nitrate method.

1. Fix thin tissue slices in 10 per 100 formalin.
2. Immerse the specimens for twenty-four hours in 96° alcohol.
3. Immerse in distilled water until the pieces sink.
4. Impregnate for three days in 1.5 per 100 silver nitrate at 37°C.
5. Rinse briefly with distilled water.
6. Reduce for twenty-four hours in:

Pyrogallol	4 g
Distilled water	100 cc
Formalin	5 cc

7. Rinse with water, embed in paraffin, cut 5 μm thick sections, dewax, mount, and cover as usual.

When the method works properly, the spirochetae are stained deep-black against a pale-yellow background. The cells and fibers are weakly stained, but in some cases it may be extremely difficult to distinguish the germs from the thinner axons, which may become twisted by the action of the fixatives. Finally, we should point out that the first sections must be discarded because they are usually overimpregnated and contain silver precipitates.

332. Noguchi's method. This procedure is a modification of the Levaditi-Cajal method.

1. Fix in formalin, cut 5–7 mm thick slices and immerse them for five days in the following mixture:

Formalin	10 cc
Pyridine	10 cc
Acetone	25 cc
Alcohol	25 cc
Distilled water	30 cc

2. Rinse for twenty-four hours with distilled water.
3. Immerse the blocks for three days in 96° alcohol.
4. Rinse for an additional day with water.
5. Impregnate for three days at 37°C in 1.5 per 100 silver nitrate.
6. Rinse for two hours with distilled water.
7. Reduce as in the Levaditi's method.
8. Rinse, embed in paraffin, and cut sections as thin as possible (3–5 μm thick).

The treponemes stand out in a deep-black color against a pale-yellow background; gliofibrils are usually brownish.

333. Jahnel has proposed the following modification of Levaditi's method:

1. Steps 1, 2, 3, and 4 are the same as in the original method (**331**).
2. Rinse for two hours.
3. Reduce in a solution made of:

Pyrogallol	4 g
Distilled water	100 cc
Acetone	10 cc
Pyridine	10 cc

4. Rinse thoroughly with water and embed in paraffin. Cut very thin sections.

334. Jahnel has suggested another variation that consists in substituting Step 5 of Levaditi's method (**331**) with a sixty-minute rinse in pyridine. This technique is not

Chapter 20: Pathogenic Microorganisms

as selective as the previous ones, although it sometimes renders excellent results in mice with recurrent syphilis.

335. Jahnel's procedure with uranyl-nitrate and pyridine. This is the most reliable technique, to date, of impregnating the syphilis treponema in the central nervous system. Here is the modus operandi:

1. Small tissue blocks, not thicker than 2–4 mm, are indurated for a long time in either formalin or alcohol. (Excellent results are obtained after a fixation period of fifteen to twenty days.)
2. Immerse for one to three days in pure pyridine.
3. Rinse thoroughly with distilled water in order to remove pyridine.
4. Immerse the blocks again in 5–10 per 100 formalin for some days.
5. Rinse for twenty-four hours with distilled water and then immerse the specimens for one hour in 1 per 100 uranyl nitrate at 37°C.
6. Rinse for twenty-four hours in distilled water.
7. Place the blocks for three to eight days in 96° alcohol.
8. Hydrate the pieces by placing them in water until they sink.
9. Impregnate (five to eight days at 37°C in the dark) in 1.5 per 100 silver nitrate. Use a large volume of solution.
10. The remaining steps as in the Levaditi's method (**331**, from Step 6 onward).

This is an outstanding method for the demonstration of the syphilis treponema in the central nervous system, where it is stained deep black against a pale-yellow background. It does not work so well, however, in non-neural tissues; in these cases, Jahnel suggests lowering the uranyl nitrate concentration to 0.1–0.2 per 100.

336. Jahnel's method for section staining. If spirochetae can be regularly stained in sections, this should be the method of choice for studying tertiary neurosyphilis, because it would thus be possible to observe the cytoarchitecture of the nervous centers and the localization of the germs in adjacent sections.

1. Fix in formalin, cut frozen or celloidin sections, and immerse them for one to twelve hours in pyridine.
2. Rinse with several changes of distilled water.
3. Immerse for one hour in 96° alcohol.
4. Rinse briefly with distilled water.
5. Treat the sections for two hours with 5 per 100 soda-free uranyl sulfate or with Merck's uranyl nitrate at the same concentration and at 37°C.
6. Rinse briefly with distilled water (twice).
7. Impregnate for three to six hours in 1 per 100 silver nitrate at 37°C.
8. Reduce as in Liesegang's procedure for neurofibrils (**127**). The correct way to carry out this reaction is as follows: Place the sections in a well containing 5 cc of 0.25 per 100 silver nitrate and then add 20 cc of a 70 per 100 solution of gum arabic. Shake the well gently until both liquids are mixed and then add 25 cc of a freshly prepared 5 per 100 hydroquinone

solution. From this moment onward, while the reduction takes place, the bath must be gently stirred, while being careful not to disturb the sections, which should be spread out perfectly.

This step lasts about ten minutes, although it is better to stop it when the sections turn reddish-brown.

9. Rinse thoroughly with distilled water, dehydrate, clarify in xylene, and mount in balsam.

This method yields better results in frozen sections as compared with celloidin sections, which frequently show irregular precipitates. Furthermore, celloidin sections require an increase in the concentration of silver nitrate in the developer to 0.5 per 100.

DEMONSTRATION OF THE TRYPANOSOMES IN SLEEPING SICKNESS

337. Giemsa-Romanowsky's method.

1. Fix small pieces of brain tissue in 96° alcohol. Dominici's fluid (**250**, Step 1) or sublimate-acetic acid (**18**) also can be used, provided that the sublimate crystals are later removed with Lugol or diluted iodine tincture. Subsequently, the iodine must be removed with 0.5–1 per 100 sodium hyposulfite.
2. Embed in paraffin and cut 3–5 µm thick sections.
3. Dewax in xylol.
4. Dip the sections in absolute alcohol and blot with filter paper.
5. Immediately immerse the sections in:

Giemsa solution (Grübler)	10 drops
Distilled water	10 cc

The staining time ranges from thirty minutes to several hours; the solution must be changed after the first thirty minutes.

6. Differentiate in distilled water.
7. Dehydrate briefly with either alcohol or acetone, clarify in xylene, and mount in balsam.

The trypanosomes are strongly stained; their cytoplasm has a peculiar color, whereas the nucleus appears violet.

COLORATION OF NEGRI BODIES IN RABIES

338. Lentz's staining method.
It is well known that Negri bodies are most abundant in the Ammon's horn of humans and animals suffering from rabies. The way to demonstrate them is as follows:

1. Fix pieces of nervous tissue in alcohol. Zenker's liquid and sublimate also can be used, although, if they are, the excess of reagent must be removed from the pieces by rinsing them with water.
2. Embed in paraffin and attach the sections to uncoated glass slides (**38**).
3. Transfer the sections to water and color them for *one minute* in:

Eosin extra *B* (Höchst)	0.5 g
60° alcohol	100 cc

4. Rinse with water.
5. Stain for *one minute* in Loeffler's blue:

Saturated alcoholic solution of methylene blue *B* (Höchst)	30 cc
0.01 per 100 Potash lye	100 cc

6. Rinse with water and blot the sections with filter paper.
7. Differentiate in alkaline alcohol:

Absolute alcohol	30 cc
1 per 100 sodium hydroxide in absolute alcohol	5 drops

   Differentiation must proceed until the sections turn pale-red.

8. Differentiate again, until the neurons become bluish, in:

Absolute alcohol	30 cc
50 per 100 Acetic acid	1 drop

9. Rinse with absolute alcohol, clarify in xylene, and mount in balsam. Negri bodies are carmine-red, with the typical granules inside them stained in blue.

339. Negri bodies also are magnificently impregnated by Del Río-Hortega's *first variation* of (**145**) Achúcarro's method, as demonstrated by Fañanás and Del Río-Hortega. This procedure has the advantage of being easier and faster than those of Lentz and Heidenhain. Furthermore, it reveals more Negri bodies than any other technique and thus is a valuable diagnostic method.

DEMONSTRATION OF THE TUBERCULOSIS BACILLUS

340. Ziehl-Neelsen's Method. The best fixatives for this method are alcohol and sublimate-based liquids. Embed the pieces in paraffin and mount the sections on uncoated glass slides. The staining procedure is as follows:

1. Stain the sections for one or two hours in carbol-fuchsin (acid fuchsin, 1 g; alcohol, 10 cc; 5 per 100 aqueous solution of phenol, 100 cc) at 37°C.
2. Bleach the sections in alcohol-hydrochloric acid (70° alcohol, 100 cc; hydrochloric acid, 1 cc) and then rinse them with alcohol.
3. Counterstain with methylene blue for one to two minutes.
4. Rinse with water.
5. Dehydrate in alcohol, clarify in xylene, and mount in balsam.

341. Very good results also can be obtained using Schmorl's technique:

1. Stain the sections for thirty minutes with Böhmer's hematoxylin.
2. Rinse with water for half an hour.
3. Stain for one hour in Ziehl's carbol-fuchsin (**340**) at 37°C.
4. Differentiate in alcohol-hydrochloric acid and then rinse.
5. Rinse thoroughly with water and then immerse in alkaline water until the sections turn blue (alkaline water is made of ten parts of water and one part of saturated solution of lithium carbonate).
6. Rinse again with water (for ten minutes), dehydrate, etc.

Koch's bacilli are deep-red; neuroglial cells, neurons, and connective tissue fibers are stained in shades of blue.

EDITORS' NOTES

(1) The best lenses available in Cajal's time were apochromatic. Planapochromatic lenses were not widely used until much later.
(2) In Cajal's day, Köhler illumination was not commonly used. The advice about using a frosted glass bulb was due to the fact that the only way to use an artificial light source for a microscope was to follow Nelson's method.
(3) At that time, several scientists (Altmann, Benda, Nageotte, Regaud, Meves, etc.), coined different terms to name the same cytoplasmic granules ("mitochondria," "chondriomites," "plastosomes," "bioblasts," etc; see Vocabulary). They suggested a number of functions for them, from being elemental living particles (bioblastic granules), to cell respiration (mitochondrial granules).
(4) Lugol's solution.
(5) An officinal solution has different proportions, depending on the substance (see Vocabulary). For iodine, the officinal solution is 10% iodine in 96° alcohol.
(6) Held's misconceptions cited here by the authors are commented on in the Introduction of this book.
(7) *Astacus* is a species of crayfish.
(8) Cochineal is a dyestuff consisting of the dried bodies of the insect *Coccus cacti*, found on several species of cacti in Mexico and elsewhere. It is used for making carmine and, in the past, also as a general-purpose scarlet dye.
(9) *Haematoxylon Campechianum*.
(10) Hematoxylin ($C_6H_{14}O_6$) is not a stain by itself, but it acquires this property after it is oxidized to hematein ($C_6H_{12}O_6$). The loss of the two hydrogen atoms occurs without the addition of oxygen to the molecule, and it results in the appearance of a quinonoid chromophore on the ring that carries the oxygen (carbon 9). This complex oxidation process was called "ripening" in the time of Cajal and de Castro.
(11) Coplin jars.
(12) G. Grübler Gmbh. was a small factory at Leipzig where the dyes developed by the powerful German chemical industry were purified for micrographical purposes by Dr. Karl Hollborn. For more than half a century, and until it was destroyed during World War II, Grübler was the only supplier of reagents specifically tested for Histology. Its address, 71 Kronprinzenstrasse, can be found written in capitals in the laboratory notebooks of Cajal and his students.
(13) Cedarwood oil is no longer used as immersion oil.
(14) In Cajal's days, most ovens were preset to a fixed temperature. As a matter of fact, ovens that included a thermostat to change the temperature (that are so common today) were back then a luxury for most scientific laboratories.

(15) The purpose of mounting Golgi-impregnated sections on this kind of slide is to be able to observe the sections from both sides. This is necessary because these sections are often so thick as to prevent the examination of their deepest portions when using objectives of a great numerical aperture and, consequently, of a short focal length.

(16) As a matter of fact, time has proven unsuccessful in deteriorating most of the preparations made by Cajal, some of which are over one hundred years old! Thus, there are now in the Cajal Institute in Madrid preparations of Golgi-impregnated sections that retain the fine details of the structure of the nerve cells, as well preserved as they were described and drawn by the Master (the actual address of the Cajal Institute is Avenida Doctor Arce, 37; Madrid). These preparations have been used to illustrate neuronal morphology in general treatises on the structure of the cerebral cortex (A. Peters and E.G Jones (Eds.): "Cerebral Cortex. I. Cellular components of the cerebral cortex." Chapter 6 on "Nonpyramidal Neurons. General Account," by Alfonso Fairén, Javier DeFelipe and José Regidor. New York: Plenum Press, 1984. Also, J. DeFelipe and E.G. Jones (Eds.): *Cajal on the Cerebral Cortex*, Chapter VI. New York: Oxford University Press, 1988), and in confocal laser microscopy analysis (Boyde, A. "Three-dimensional images of Ramón y Cajal's original preparations, as viewed by confocal microscopy." TINS 15, 246–248, 1992).

(17) Here, the term "spongioblasts" refers to the amacrine cells of the retina.

(18) Sandarac is a resin that exudes from the tree Callitris quadrivalvis, native of northwest Africa; it was used in the preparation of spirit varnish and the pounce employed in rendering parchment fit to write upon.

(19) The methods described in the present chapter are no longer in use. In Cajal's day, however, they were of utmost importance, because they were routinely used to check whether the findings reported in analyses of Golgi-impregnated material were real, or were mere artifacts.

The aforementioned procedures reduce the histological artifacts to a minimum, but the preparations fade quickly. To obtain permanent preparations, the dye must be made insoluble both in water and in alcohol, an operation that was termed "fixation of the dye," or just "fixation," by Cajal (**94 to 99**). Specimens prepared in this way can be mounted after dehydration and clearing, and even embedded in paraffin or celloidin.

The chief limitation of these methods is their inconstancy. Although the ability of methylene blue to detect redox processes is unquestioned, this property alone cannot explain the selectivity of the dye for just a few neurons and nerve endings. Dr. de Castro, who used these methods with great frequency, wondered in the 1960s whether the selectivity of the reaction was due to some unidentified impurity present in certain batches of the dye. As a matter of fact, he complained that, despite his dexterity using these techniques, he only got good results with reagent that had been purchased before World War II.

(20) It must be kept in mind that, when dilutions of methylene blue are expressed as quotients, they are dilutions of the stock 1% solution.

At the time when the methylene blue procedure was developed, the regular scales used in the laboratories were not sensitive enough to weigh amounts of reagents smaller than 1 gram. This problem was thus overcome by preparing a stock solution to be later diluted to obtain very small concentrations.

(21) Nowadays, the flasks used in the laboratory for preparing solutions are made of Jena-type glass, which is neutral and stable under high temperatures. Cajal and

de Castro's specification about the type of glass to be used was due to the fact that most of the glassware used in the laboratories at the beginning of the century was made of general-purpose, acidic glass, while the neutral ones were extremely expensive.

(22) Epigraph number 90 is a transcription of the Methods section of Cajal's paper «Las células de cilindro-eje corto de la capa molecular del cerebro» ("Short axon cells in brain's molecular layer.") in Revista Trimestral Micrográfica, Vol. 2, pp. 104–127, 1897. In the present book, this text is located in such a place that it seems just a comment to the intravascular injection method. Yet, it actually refers to a combination of this technique and the lubing method, described in epigraph number 91, and, as such, it should be located after it. Its importance for staining the cerebral cortex layer I cells made the authors include it here as a variant of the injection method, to be used for this specific purpose.

(23) In 1891, Cajal described the existence of large cells with several long, axon-like protoplasmic expansions in layer I of the cerebral cortex of several animal species (Ramón y Cajal, S.: "Sur la structure de l'écorce cerebrale de quelques mammifères." La Cellule, 7:125–176, 1891). Because of their uncommon morphology, he named these neurons "special cells." Later, Retzius confirmed their existence in the brain of human fetuses, and proposed for them the term "Cajal cells" (Retzius, G.: "Die Cajal'sche zellen der grosshirnrinde beim menschen und bei saügetieren." Biol. Untersuchungen Neue Folge 4:1–9, 1894).

Yet, the descriptions of Cajal and Retzius were not absolutely identical.

Trying to fix this disparity, Kölliker used his authority to impose on the histologists of that time that the adult cells would be called "Cajal cells," and the fetal ones, "Retzius cells" (Kölliker, A.: "Handbuch der gewebelehre des menschen. Vol. II: Nervensystems des Menschen und der Tiere." Engelmann, Leipzig, 1896). It is widely accepted nowadays that both types are just one kind of neuron, eclectically called "Cajal-Retzius cells." (For a discussion, see: Marin-Padilla, M.: "Layer I cells," in A. Peters and E.G. Jones [Eds.] "Cerebral Cortex. I. Cellular components of the cerebral cortex." New York: Plenum Press, pp. 447–478, 1984).

(24) In 1850, Charles Gabriel Pravaz created a hollow silver needle, which adapted to the syringe, allowing injections of a small amount: the syringe with injection, or "syringes Pravaz."

(25) When the book was written, methylene blue staining was the only method that yielded images comparable to those obtained with the silver impregnation, and, because the chemistry involved in both types of processes was completely different, methylene blue happened to be an ideal method to ascertain the findings obtained with the Golgi method. Yet, the results of methylene blue staining varied, depending on which of the several variants was used. Thus, some authors reported findings that were in perfect accord with those from Golgi material, whereas others did not. This problem augmented several controversies that were the stuff of stormy arguments at that time.

One of the most notable of these discrepancies concerned the existence of the dendritic spines discovered by Cajal in 1888 using the Golgi method (Ramón y Cajal, S.: «Estructura de los centros nerviosos de las aves». Rev. Trim. Histol. Norm. Patol. 1:1–10, 1888). Several authors criticized this finding, which they considered to be just an occasional artifact produced by the precipitation of silver chromate. Besides, some authors reported that the spines were also absent in methylene blue-stained cortical pyramidal cells (Meyer, S.: "Die

Subcutane Methylenblauinjection ein Mittel zur Darstellung der Elemente des Zentralnervensystems." Arch. f. Mikrosk. Anat. 46, 1895), a fact that seemed to contradict Cajal's observations even more strongly. Kölliker's opposition to the existence of dendritic spines (Kölliker, A.: *Handbuch der gewebelehre des menschen. Vol. II: Nervensystems des Menschen und der Tiere.* Engelmann, Leipzig, p. 647, 1896) was especially significant to Cajal, because of the outstanding scientific prestige of the Würzburg's professor. Thus, determined to provide indisputable proof of the existence of dendritic spines, Cajal used a methylene blue staining protocol that was different from Meyer's. The procedure that solved the argument was the dye diffusion method (92), in which the dye was not injected subcutaneously, but directly deposited (either as a powder or in aqueous solution) on the surface of nervous system slices. The results of this and other variants of the methylene blue method regarding the dendritic spines were explained and discussed in an article that appeared in 1896 (Ramón y Cajal, S.: «Las espinas colaterales de las células del cerebro teñidas por el azul de metileno.» Revista Trimestral Micrográfica, 1:123–136, 1896). Paragraphs one to five of epigraph 100 are a word-by-word transcription of parts of the text in the latter article.

While this paper was in press, Dogiel published an article, using the methylene blue staining, in which he reported some findings that were opposed to Cajal's and even seemed to challenge the neuron doctrine itself (Dogiel, A. S.: "Die Nervenelemente in Kleinhirne der Vögel und Säugetiere." Arch. Mikrosk. Anat. EntwMech., 47:707–719, 1896). In the cited paper by Cajal, he only got the chance to include an addendum criticizing Dogiel's results and announced that he would deal with this problem in the near future. Subsequently, he rapidly wrote a comprehensive paper on the use of methylene blue in the central nervous system (Ramón y Cajal, S.: «El azul de metileno en los centros nerviosos.» Revista Trimestral Micrográfica 1:151–203, 1896). In this paper, he criticized in depth the methods used by Meyer and Dogiel, which produced confounding artifacts. Parts of the text of this paper were transcribed literally into the last paragraphs of epigraph number 100, beginning with the sixth paragraph.

Hence, epigraph number 100 is a combination of pieces of text from two independent articles, and this is the reason why its reading may seem challenging today.

(26) "Equivalent neurocytological images" was a term coined by Franz Nissl that meant that the morphology of the fixed and stained neurons was analogous to that of living cells.

(27) It may seem striking that this treatise explains numerous techniques that were already obsolete when the book was written. Furthermore, the purpose of many of them was actually to demonstrate that the neurons were not independent, but continuous structures. This sounds especially queer, considering that Cajal was the "father" of the neuron theory. Yet, it is easy to understand, considering that, at that time, the only way to ascertain the validity of a morphological observation was for it to be demonstrated independently by another scientist. Hence, it was advisable to communicate one's methods so they could be confirmed, and those used by other authors, so their findings could not. To better understand the reasons for including this vast array of neurofibrillary methods in the book, consult the Preface of this book on the historical environment of neuroanatomy at that time.

(28) Classic silver impregnation techniques, with the exception of the Golgi method, comprise the same three main steps, namely, (1) soaking the tissue in a silver

solution (impregnation), (2) reduction of the silver deposits in the tissue, and (3) gold-toning the reduced silver. There are many protocols for these basic reactions, but all of them are based on a small number of chemical processes. Impregnation can be achieved using either plain silver nitrate (as in Cajal's reduced silver nitrate method, 113) or different ammoniacal silver solutions. The latter are obtained by oxidation of silver nitrate in a strongly alkaline medium, achieved with sodium hydroxide (176), potassium hydroxide (109), or sodium carbonate (190, 197). Silver oxide is insoluble in water, so ammonia should be added to form soluble silver diamine ($Ag[NH_3]^{2+}$).

Reduction is achieved by using either formol in the case of ammoniacal silver impregnation or pyrogallol (or hydroquinone) for silver nitrate-impregnated tissues. In both cases, the result is the transformation of silver ions (Ag^+) in metallic silver (Ag^0), which forms visible aggregates inside the cells, and which cannot be extracted except by powerful oxidants.

Toning consists in replacing metallic silver with metallic gold. This reaction comprises the transformation of ionic gold (Au^{3+}) in metallic gold (Au^0), together with the ionization of the metallic silver atoms; ionic silver is further removed by sodium thiosulfate, which forms with it the water-soluble compound $[Ag(S_2O_3)^{2+}]$. The metal substitution needs to be carried out at an acidic pH, which is afforded by the own gold-chloride solution. Properly speaking, the chemical compound colloquially known as gold chloride is really tetrachloroauric acid ($AuCl_4^-$), which, once dissolved at the usual concentration (0.1–0.2%) has a low pH (2–4). Nevertheless, in some cases (for instance, in Bielschowsky's methods, 109) acetic acid was added to the gold solution in order to enhance the oxidative capability of the reagent. Gold toning is used in silver methods to enhance the contrast of the preparation. This effect can be obtained because metallic gold particles are smaller than metallic silver aggregates, and also because of the kinetics of silver substitution. In fact, the time needed to achieve the complete ionization of metallic silver aggregates is shorter than that used to generate a gold deposit of an equivalent size. Thus, a brief immersion of the sections in gold chloride will result in a noticeable removal of Ag^0, and in its replacement by small Au^0 particles. If toning is stopped at this stage, any area with small, but visible, Ag^0 deposits (as is the case of the background) will now be occupied by such small Au^0 aggregates as to render it colorless. On the other hand, this property works also in the opposite direction, so that any structure containing small Ag^0 deposits (i.e., weakly stained) may disappear after gold-toning because the size of the Au^0 particles may be unsuitable for their detection at the microscope.

All of the gold-toning techniques used either 1/300 or 1/600 yellow-gold chloride solutions. It may seem awkward nowadays that the concentration of the solution was expressed in such peculiar way. This was due to the fact that the gold chloride was sold in small glass vials containing 1 g of the substance. The usual practice at Cajal's lab was to heat the ampoule at the flame until the gold chloride began to melt; the vial was then dropped in a flask containing a given volume of cool distilled water, so that it exploded inside the water and even the last traces of the (then) extremely expensive chemical were dissolved. The fragments of the ampoule were left inside the flask, because they served as "markers" that the solution was "new" (i.e., not used). To tone the sections, a small volume of the "new" gold solution was poured in a well or in a Petri dish, and, once the procedure was finished, it was filtered and placed in a different flask. This used gold chloride was the one to be regularly employed, and only when the liquid was nearly colorless, were some drops of the precious "new" solution added to the well. The stinginess of this procedure illustrates the scant research funds available at that time in Spain.

The protocol for gold toning was somewhat different for paraffin-embedded and floating sections. In the latter case, the sections are transported with a glass rod from the water to a well containing the gold solution (regarding the handling of floating sections in Cajal's laboratory, see Translator's Note 41); 2 cc of 0.2% gold chloride are needed for each 10–20 μm thick section. Once immersed in the toning bath, the sections were unrolled with the aid of the glass rod. The aim of this maneuver was not only to avoid the appearance of wrinkles in the sections, but also to hasten mechanically the solubilization of the silver deposits. Once the sections were extended, the well was gently agitated. Toning was finished when the color of the sections changed from brown to gray or gray-violet, although in some methods toning had to be prolonged until the sections showed a deep violet tint. This gold reinforcement needs either twenty-four hours at room temperature, or just fifteen to twenty minutes, if the well is gently warmed at the flame (*EN 42*).

Once toning was over, the sections were immersed in sodium thiosulfate ("hyposulfite") to remove the unreduced silver. This operation is termed "fixation" throughout the whole of the book, though it has nothing to do with today's meaning of this term. In any case, it was held in a Petri dish of 8–10 cm in diameter filled with 5% sodium thiosulfate; the dish was placed onto a white background, to enhance light reflection. This trick was used in order to shorten as much as possible the action of thiosulfate, because the presence of this chemical during dehydration seemed to shrink the tissue, especially the gray matter. To shorten the thiosulfate action, the sections, which become fairly opaque to the naked eye after toning, were maintained in the "fixative" just until the glass hook could be seen through them, a maneuver that required some transillumination of the sections. After "fixation" was finished, the "hyposulfite" was completely removed by rinsing the section several times in large volumes of water (usually, 3×15 minutes).

Toning of paraffin sections only is used for Bielschowsky's method and for some variants of Cajal's reduced silver nitrate. The procedure is basically the same as the one just described for floating sections, though the gold solution should be placed in a sufficiently large Petri dish so as to allow the slides to be placed in a horizontal position. For the Cajal method, the procedure that rendered more delicate results was the one described in *EN 32*(e), which was colloquially known as warm-tone toning.

(29) Tap water is recommended instead of distilled water because silver chloride must be generated in the tissue for the method to work properly. Results are generally more constant and reproducible if, as recommended by de Castro, formaldehyde is dissolved in distilled water containing 0.1% calcium chloride.

(30) Gelatin-levulose (Heringa's medium) and plain levulose were water-soluble mounting media used in the past to avoid the dehydration and clearing of the sections.

(31) World War I.

(32) After the present book was published, following Cajal's death, the reduced silver method was thoroughly refined by Fernando de Castro; yet, these technical

improvements were known only to his direct students. The following paragraphs are a brief summary of de Castro's advice for success in obtaining superb results with the method.

a) *Fixation.* The best all-purpose fixatives are barbiturates and chloral hydrate. The barbiturate fixative most frequently used by de Castro was an equal-parts mixture of absolute ethanol (Merck), pyridine, and water, added to 1.8% somnifène. The latter component, which was a hypnotic originally developed by the Swiss firm Hoffman-LaRoche, is off the market since the early 1960s. It was a 1:1 mixture of 6.6% dietilaminic-diethylbarbiturate and 6.4% dietilaminic-allyl-isopropyl-barbiturate; the stock solutions of both barbiturates were prepared in ethylene-glycol. Chloral hydrate can be used as indicated in epigraph 117, but the results generally improve if it is used at 8% concentration in 50% ethanol. Just before use, the pH of the solution had to be raised to 8.5 with ammonia. The fixation time for either somnifène or chloral hydrate was sixteen to twenty-four hours at room temperature.

b) *Post-fixation treatment.* For most of the variations on Cajal's method, the fixative needed to be completely removed from the tissue once the fixation was over. The best way to do this was to rinse the pieces for at least sixteen hours in running tap water. This step was followed by a thorough rinse in deionized water (4×60 minutes), in order to remove some ions (chlorine, calcium, etc.) in the specimens, which react on their own with silver nitrate. Rinsing had to be avoided in those variants that comprise ethanol fixation (**115, 116**). When fixing in chloral hydrate mixtures, the pieces were briefly rinsed in deionized water (3×15 minutes), because tissues soaked in chloral hydrate are prone to swell when immersed in water. Once the specimens were fixed and the fixative removed (if necessary), they could be directly immersed in silver nitrate (120–122), though most formulae comprised a twenty-four-hour immersion in either plain ethanol or in ethanol with some ammonia drops added. In all cases, high-quality, absolute ethanol (Merck or equivalent) was used. The concentration of ammonia was critical for the final result. As a guideline, ammonia concentrations that rendered a pH of 10.5 to the ethanol resulted in excellent impregnation of axons, dendrites, and somata. Lower pH values, between 10 and 10.5, enhanced the axon impregnation (including axon terminals), but somata or dendrites were barely stained. If the pH value was over 11, the background was higher and obscured the finest details.

c) *Impregnation.* The standard procedure was to impregnate the pieces over seven days at 37°C in 2% silver nitrate. This step had to be performed in a wide-neck, glass-stopped dark flask, which was generally cleaned and rinsed in deionized water before the silver solution was poured in it. The volume of silver nitrate solution was around 25 cc for every 3-mm thick piece. The solution was replaced after the first day and whenever it looked turbid. The flask containing the pieces and the silver solution had to be gently shaken at least once a day, so that the specimens did not lie on the bottom always on the same face.

d) *Reduction and embedding.* When the impregnation had finished, the pieces were rinsed in deionized water (5×5 minutes') and placed in a dark flask containing a freshly prepared solution of 1.5% pyrogallic acid in 10% formol. It was of paramount importance to check that the pyrogallic acid was "white as snow," because it may have happened that even in just-opened flasks of this product, the reagent showed a grayish tonality. After twenty-four hours (at room temperature), the reductor was replaced by 5% formol for an extra hour. The pieces were then immersed in 70% ethanol; after a couple of hours, the liquid showed a greenish tint, due to the oxidized pyrogallic acid extracted from the tissue. The ethanol was then replaced until it remained colorless for at least twelve hours. Complete removal of pyrogallol from the tissue was important to prevent excessive shrinking during embedding. Tissue embedding could be done either in celloidin or in paraffin; the final quality of the slides was almost the same for both procedures, provided that the specimens were not overheated in the paraffin baths; as a rule, the oven temperature did not exceed 58°C.

e) *Gold-toning.* Sections obtained from specimens fixed either in somnifène or in chloral hydrate could be subjected to gold-toning. Toning could be achieved by immersing the dewaxed sections directly in 0.2% yellow gold chloride (125), though de Castro preferred to use the method of Veratti (135, Steps 5 to 7). In any case, toning was stopped when the sections took on a grayish color, because a longer gold treatment could mask the most delicate details.

(33) Neutral formalin (see 109) should not be confused with today's buffered formalin.

(34) As opposed to the staining of the axons in blocks of nervous tissue with Cajal's method.

(35) Cajal frequently used this title when referring to Camillo Golgi.

(36) While working at Alzheimer's laboratory, Nicolás de Achúcarro, one of Cajal's favorite disciples, developed a method for staining glial cells that was based on the combination of tannin as a mordant and of Bielschowsky's ammoniacal silver oxide as impregnating solution. The protocol of this method, which was the first one that rendered a complete visualization of the astrocytes, is included in epigraph 177. The original method was modified up to four times by one of Achúcarro's students, Pío Del Río-Hortega, in order to obtain more selective results. These modifications were known as first, second, third, and fourth variants of Del Río-Hortega to Achúcarro's method. The first variant (145) reveals centrosomes, mitochondria, elastic fibers, and glial cells cytoskeleton. The second variant (208) was developed for reticulin staining, while the third one (209) was more suitable to show collagen fibers. The fourth variant (178) was the one that stained protoplasmic and fibrous astrocytes.

(37) The original Biondi's liquid is a mixture of saturated solutions of Orange G (100 cc), acid fuchsin (10 cc), and methyl green (30 cc).

(38) For a review on the real nature of Golgi's reticular membrane, see Celio, M. R., Spreafico, R., De Biasi, S., Vitellaro-Zuccarello, L.: "Perineuronal nets: past and present." Trends Neurosci. 1998;21(12):510–515.

(39) Some of the methods developed by the Histology School of Madrid, and especially those described in this chapter, frequently have been faulted for their inconstancy. This inconstancy is due, in part, to the inaccuracy of the protocols and, in part, to the absence of some specific recommendations that were never included in the reports of the methods, because they were routine procedures in the labs of Cajal and of his students. These tricks have been included here as Translators' Notes for each method, but there are some recommendations that are common to all of these methods.

The first of these common rules is to use thoroughly cleaned glassware. The usual practice was to wash the glassware with plenty of soap, and then immerse it for twenty-four hours in nitric acid. The acid was washed out with running tap water and the tap water ions and salts washed out with distilled water.

Many of these procedures were carried out on floating sections, which could not be handled with metallic needles because the latter react with the silver and gold solutions used. The suitable way for carrying the floating sections through the various steps of the methods was to use a 2–3 mm diameter glass rod bent at a right angle at one of its ends. The bent segment, which was the one used to handle the sections, had to be 1.5–2 cm long, and its tip was thinned at the flame. The bent glass rod was kept in a large well filled with distilled water during the whole impregnation procedure, and it was rinsed before introducing it into any of the baths.

The chemicals used in these methods were of high quality. This advice was especially critical for water, which needed to be free of both organic matter and ions, because some of these, such as chlorine and bromine, could form photosensitive silver compounds that were reduced on their own. Needless to say, in Cajal's day, freshly deionized water was not available.

(40) The ammonical silver carbonate method was introduced by Del Río-Hortega (Del Río-Hortega, P.: «Noticia de un nuevo y fácil método para la coloración de la neuroglía y del tejido conjuntivo». Trab. Lab. Inv. Biol. Univ. Madrid, 15: 365–378, 1918) as an alternative to stain astrocytes, which by that time could only be properly visualized by the very inconstant method of Achúcarro (177). Nevertheless, it soon became evident that the new procedure was highly flexible, being capable, with minor modifications, of staining the mitochondria (187–189), the connective tissue fibers (212), and the neoplastic glial cells (179, 183). Micro- and oligodendroglia were, in fact, discovered by Del Río-Hortega using specific variants of his method (190, 197). The various protocols included here by Cajal and de Castro correspond only to those available when the present book was written. Yet, Del Río-Hortega developed more than forty variants during the 1940s, which were published in the journal that the Spanish histologist founded in Buenos Aires in his last days (see Del Río-Hortega, P.: «El método del carbonato argéntico. Revisión general de sus técnicas y aplicaciones en histología». I. Arch. Hist. Norm. Pat. (Buenos Aires), 1: 165–205, 1942; II. Arch. Hist. Norm. Pat. (Buenos Aires), 1: 329–361, 1943; III. Arch. Hist. Norm. Pat. (Buenos Aires), 2: 231–244, 1943). A thorough citation of all these techniques would go beyond the purpose of the present note, but it seems nonetheless convenient to include here some general comments that will allow a better understanding of the method, especially regarding the specifics of carrying out the impregnations.

The only way to succeed with this method is to keep in mind that the standard protocols are just starting points, rather than rigid procedures. For impregnating a given structure, one should chose the more convenient variant, then run it, look at the results and then modify the technique until the desired structures are revealed. These modifications can be done as the method is being performed, given that it does not take more than twenty to forty minutes.

In the first variant of the method, prior to silver carbonate impregnation the sections were immersed for thirty minutes in 0.1–1 M ammonia, pyridine, or an equal-parts mixture of ammonia, pyridine, and water. The former was used when the standard technique did not show properly the delicate glial expansions, such as those of oligodendroglia, microglia, or peripheral ganglia satellite cells. On the other hand, pyridine was used to enhance the "intracytoplasmic fibrils." Finally, the latter variant (equal parts of ammonia, pyridine, and water) was used for overfixed material. After this preliminary treatment, the method was run on one or two sections, which were mounted on glycerin and controlled under the microscope. If the outcome was not good enough, the ammonia concentration was raised, and the procedure tried again.

If the impregnation was in any way substandard, the silver carbonate concentration could be changed. Del Río-Hortega used three standard concentrations, which he called weak, medium, and strong. For the three cases, the starting point was mixing 3 parts of 5% sodium carbonate with 1 part of 10% silver nitrate. The precipitate, which had to have a milky or yellowish color (otherwise it was discarded), was dissolved with ammonia and added to twice the volume of water for the weak concentration, the same volume for medium concentration, or just 25% for the strong concentration.

The usual practice was to begin with the medium concentration procedure, unless otherwise stated. If the background was impregnated almost at the same time as the cells, strong carbonate had to be used. When the cells were not impregnated and the background was very pale, weak solutions were preferred. In any case, three to six drops of either 96% ethanol or pyridine could be added to the mixture, for every 10 cc of silver carbonate solution. Ethanol enhanced the impregnation of the hialoplasm, while pyridine did so with the cytoskeleton.

When, despite of all the aforementioned tricks, the results were not good enough, the formol concentration used in the reduction step had to be changed, simultaneously adjusting its best dilution, together with the impregnation time and the concentration of silver carbonate. A final resource was to reduce the sections in formol, while either remaining still or subjected to agitation. This trick was used to suppress the unspecific staining of cells, which begin to get impregnated nearly at the same time as the desired ones, and which can thus mask the result.

All the aforementioned variants could be combined in a vast variety of ways, for which the only guidelines were the experience, patience, and dexterity of the investigator. It was not uncommon at all that, after a long day of trials on difficult material, only two or three sections would turn out usable, although these were very valuable unquestionable for qualitative analysis.

(41) The terms, "cold" and "warm," were used by Cajal and his disciples to define a particular way of performing silver impregnation methods on floating sections. A warm impregnation began by introducing the sections into a well containing the impregnation solution, at room temperature. Then, the well was placed on an asbestos sheet supported by a tripod. Next, an alcohol burner was placed under the tripod, and regulated so that the flame was three centimeters long, and its tip was separated by two centimeters from the asbestos sheet. As impregnation proceeded, the well had to be gently rotated, so that the sections were kept in movement and temperature was as homogeneous as possible in every part of the solution. If the well got hot enough to produce a burning sensation in the fingers, the burner had to be removed until that sensation disappeared.

If the impregnation solution was ammoniacal silver, it was kept away from atmospheric oxygen as much as possible. For this reason, the well had to be filled up completely with the reagent and, after immersing the sections, a watch glass was used as a lid to close it. This procedure slowed the decomposition of the reagent by the combined actions of heat and oxygen, but did not impede it, so that the impregnation never exceeded twenty to thirty minutes. As a rule, the solution had to remain colorless or, at the very least, translucent through the process.

(42) The following advice had to be borne in mind in order to succeed in impregnating microglial cells with this method.

    (a) Use pieces obtained from human, rabbit, rat, or mouse brain; microglial cells of some species, such as those of cats, were really difficult to stain with silver carbonate.

    (b) Material needs to be very fresh and the fixation period should not be extended for more than twenty-four hours.

    (c) Although "hyperbromuration" (197, Step 2) was described as optional, it was very difficult to obtain regular results if this step was skipped.

    (d) Sections were collected in 1.3 M ammonia (Step 3) and allowed to stay in this reagent for at least fifteen minutes, changing the bath every five minutes. The action of the last bath could take place overnight.

    (e) Impregnation (Step 5) needed to be carried out in a well surrounded by ice. The length of this step was critical, though it was rather difficult to adjust, because no color changes took place while the sections were immersed in the silver solution. To adjust the impregnation time properly, it was best to impregnate a section for five minutes, and reduce it (Step 6). This section was mounted, coverslipped with glycerin, and examined under the microscope using at least a 25x objective.

    (f) Reduction (Step 5) had to be carried out a section at a time, changing the reducing solution when it turned gray.

(43) This was the method that made possible the identification of oligodendroglia as an independent cell type (Del Río-Hortega, P.: «La glía de escasas radiaciones (oligodendroglía)». Boletín de la Real Sociedad Española de Historia Natural, 21:63–92, 1921). To obtain consistent results with the method, the following cautions had to be taken into account:

    (a) Fixation (Step 1) was carried out at 4°C and for as short a time as possible. Usually, the best results were obtained after twelve to sixteen hours of fixation, while the results yielded after a twenty-four-hour fixation were somewhat inconsistent.

    (b) The sections were collected in 1 M ammonia, rinsed twice in this liquid (five minutes each rinse), and left in it until the next day (in any case, for more than twelve hours).

    (c) The impregnation time was adjusted as in the previous *EN*, but using a 40x objective, because otherwise the delicate oligodendroglial processes were not resolved. For this method, both the impregnation time and the reducing concentration could be modified if complete impregnations of the cells were not obtained. The usual starting point was to impregnate five minutes and then reduce in 10% formalin. Excessive impregnation or reduction resulted in partial astrocytic staining; on the other hand, if the background was covered by an even, grainy precipitate, where the oligodendrocyte somata were barely identified, the impregnation and/or the formalin concentration needed to be raised. When these cell bodies were not stained solid-black, but had a grainy aspect, the concentration of the reducing solution had to be increased without changing the impregnation time. The opposite combination was indicated if the nuclei of these cells were stained.

(d) Reduction was performed a section at a time, leaving the section undisturbed until its color no longer changed. The reductor had to be replaced for each section.

(44) This was done to save silver nitrate, which was one of the most expensive chemicals in the histology lab.

(45) The double embedding in celloidin and paraffin was the only reliable method to obtain 1–2 μm thick sections in Cajal's time. The procedure comprised a regular celloidin embedding (see Chapter 3 of Section One), though the blocks were hardened using chloroform instead of ethanol. The blocks were then immersed for one day in a mixture containing four parts of chloroform, two of origanum oil, four of cedarwood essence, one of absolute ethanol, and four parts of crystallized phenol. Afterward, the blocks were cleared in benzene and immersed in melted paraffin for another twenty-four hours. Finally, the specimen was placed in water in order to solidify the paraffin quickly, and sectioned at the microtome using a type C knife.

(46) Schwann's cells were considered to form a syncytium when they were first described. Although by Cajal's day this assumption had been discarded, the term was still in use.

(47) About the meaning of neurokeratin for Cajal, see 273.

(48) When a nerve is sectioned, especially if the injury is not a clean, straight section, the fibers in the proximal stump degenerate close to their wounded end. The neighboring zone of the nerve, proximal to the degeneration, undergoes functional and morphological changes, which are, however, reversible. This zone, which constitutes the starting point of the regeneration, is called the "metamorphic region."

(49) The peritubular connective sheath is the endoneurium, or, more properly, the fine connective trabeculae that surround the basal membrane of Schwann cells.

(50) Ruffini used the term "ultraterminal branches" to describe a thin expansion in human muscles, which, arising from the arborization of a motor end-plate, runs toward a neighboring muscle fiber, where it ends, forming a rudimentary arborization. Such a finding, although real, must be considered exceptional and pathological." (from Ramón y Cajal, S. and Tello, J. F., *Elementos de histología normal y de técnica micrográfica*. Científico Médica, Madrid, p.403, 1955).

(51) For ammonia, 36° corresponds to 36%.

(52) The "periterminal network" is a structure first described by Boeke, which would connect the neurofibrils in the axonal endings to the neighboring cells' cytoplasm.

(53) "Morphologic" methods are those that demonstrate the morphology of the whole neuron, such as Golgi's or methylene blue staining.

Plates

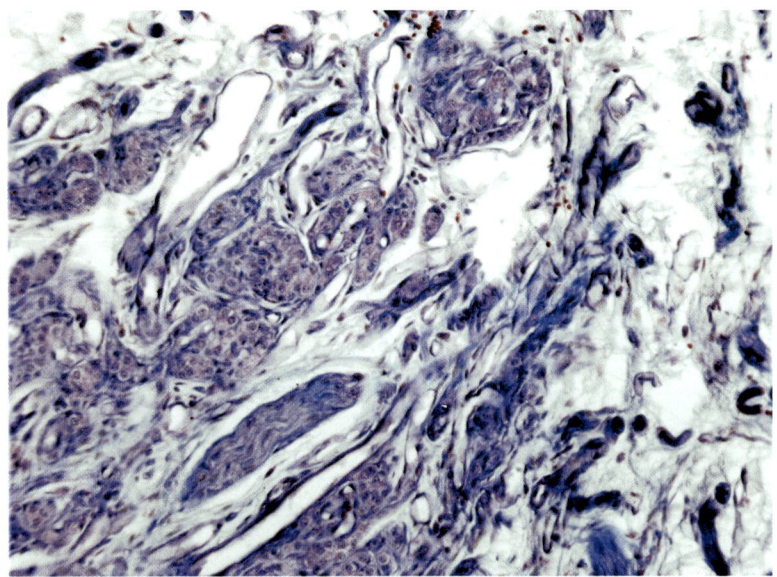

Plate 1. Cajal's trichrome (triple staining with fuchsin or magenta, picric acid and carmine indigo) used by de Castro to stain the glomus caroticum. The ground substance stains light green, collagen bundles and nuclear chromatin dark blue, and the cytoplasm of glomus cells pink. Pericytes and basement membranes stain very dark blue (almost black), highlighting the relationship between cell nests and blood vessels (X20). Photograph obtained from an original slide from Professor Fernando de Castro (Archivo Fernando de Castro).

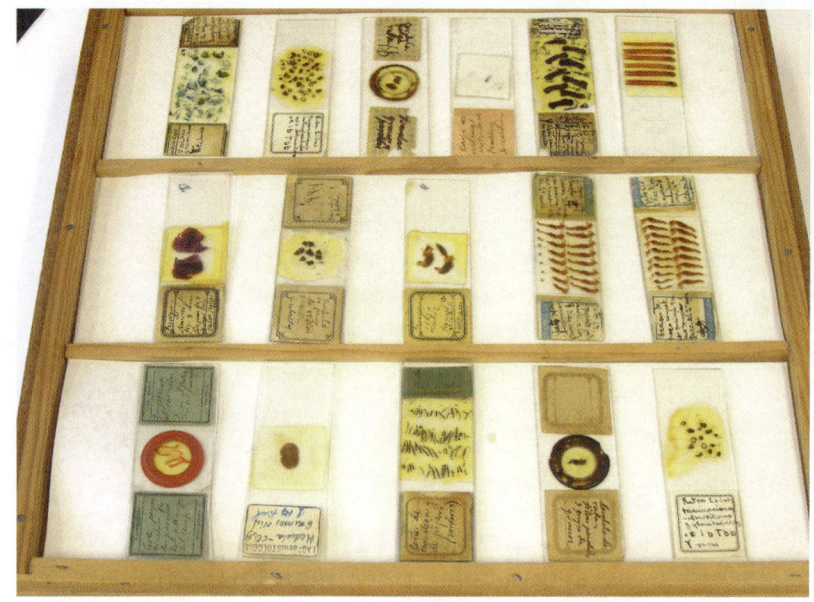

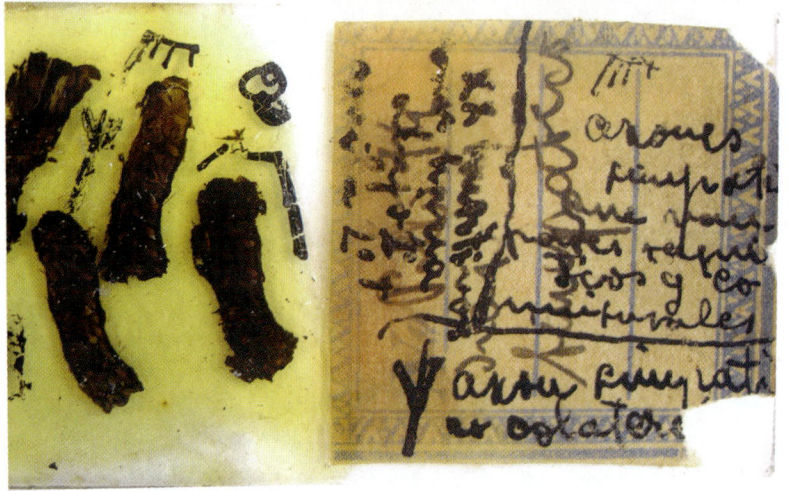

Plate 2. Mounting and conservation of tissue sections. Illustration of original histological slides from the early twentieth century. The sections were covered according to the staining technique. The first slide on the left in the top row has a thin coverslip using Canada balsam as the cover medium, the usual method at the time. The adjacent slide, however, had no coverslip, the tissue being painted over with several layers of Dammar resin dissolved in benzol or xylol. The next slide on the right has a circular coverslip sealed with gum or lacquer.

The lower part of the photograph shows a detail of Section 5 from the top row in order to illustrate the labeling system over sections. The stain is a fast Golgi method of the vertebral axis of an embryo (thick serial sections probably cut with at least a 200 μm setting on the microtome). The label at the slide reads: "Sympathetic axons leading to the rachideal and commissural pairs." In the lower part, next to the trident symbol, the text reads: "Sympathetic axon with collateral branching." Ink lines highlight the most interesting areas, such as the entrance of collaterals in a rachideal ganglion (Figure 2). Photographs obtained from original slides from Professor Fernando de Castro (Archivo Fernando de Castro).

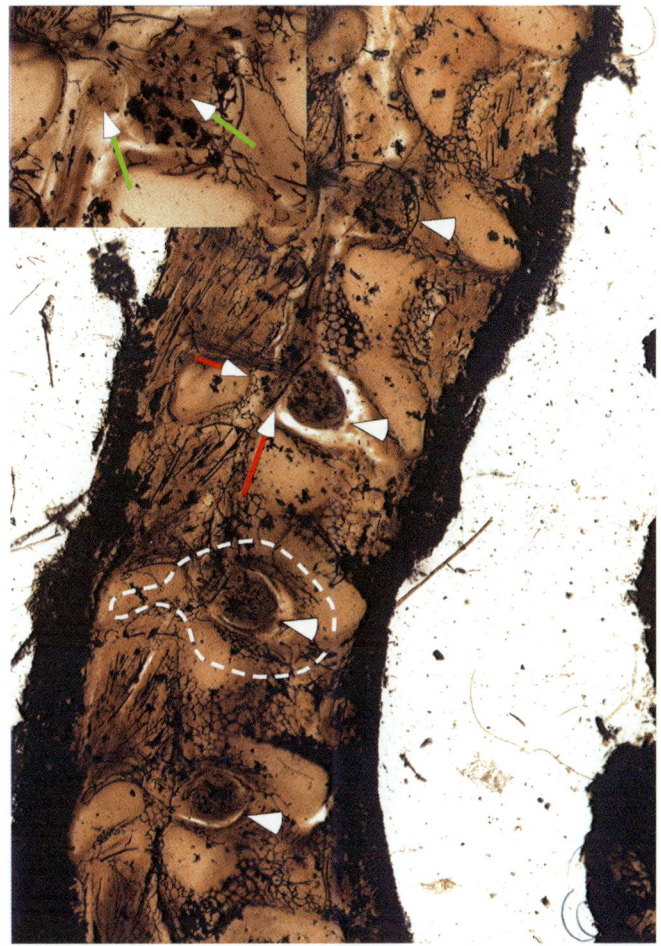

Plate 3. Mosaic of microphotographies (at X10) from the histological slide shown in Figure 1 (bottom part) as a track of the method of study followed by the Cajal school. Arrowheads show the spinal ganglia and the red arrows the chain of sympathetic ganglia. Vertebrae and apophysis clearly define the conjunction holes where ganglia are hosted (white dotted line). The inset shows the sympathetic collateral branches (green arrows, on the left: stellate neurons) and their relationship with the spinal ganglion (rounded neurons: green arrows, on the right). All the images were taken at X10. Photographs obtained from original slides from Professor Fernando de Castro (Archivo Fernando de Castro).

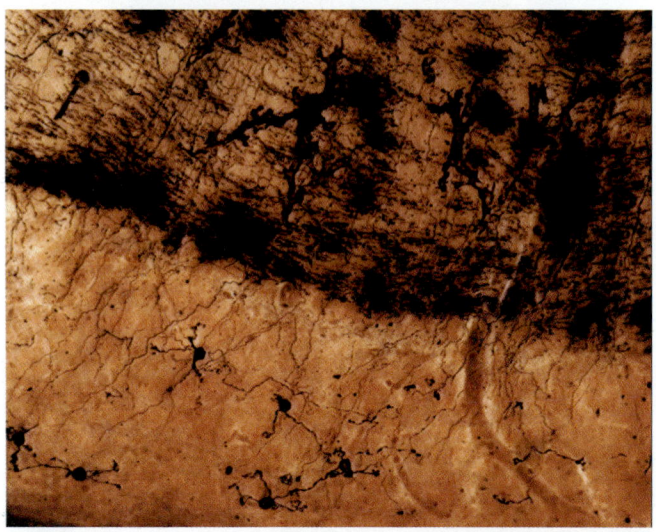

Plate. 4 Methods for the demonstration of neuronal morphology. Golgi method and variants—Fast Golgi. Staining of cerebellar grains and parallel fibers of the molecular layer (X10). Photograph obtained from an original slide from Professor Fernando de Castro (Archivo Fernando de Castro).

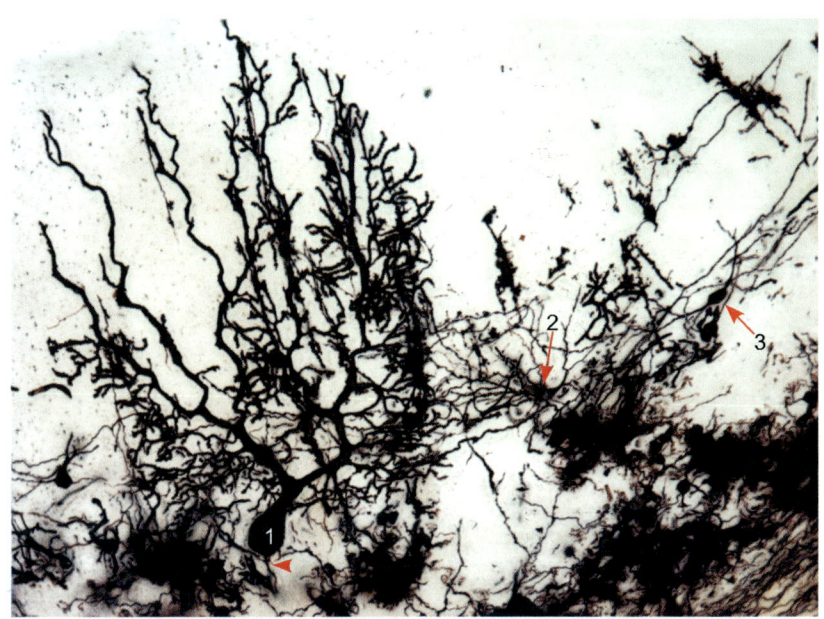

Plate 5. Methods for the demonstration of neuronal morphology. Golgi method and variants—Cox's method. Clear staining allowing the study of various types of neurons in the cerebellum. 1. Purkinje's cell. Arrowhead shows axonal root. 2. Deep stellate cell (basket cell). 3. Lugaro's fusiform cell (X10). Photographs obtained from original slides from Professor Fernando de Castro (Archivo Fernando de Castro).

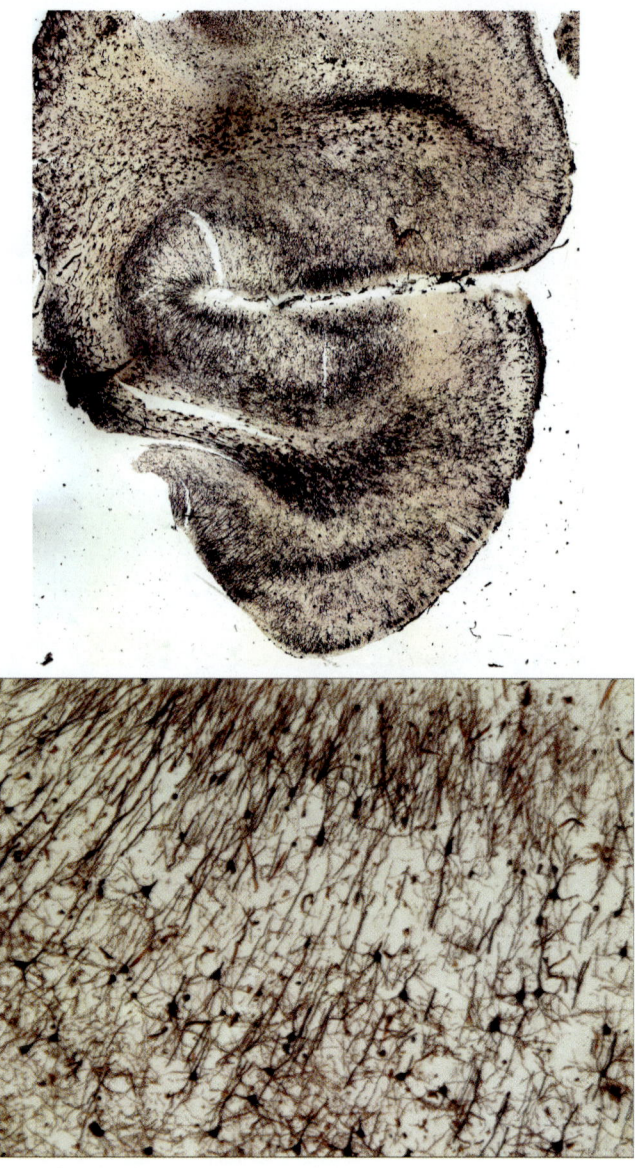

Plate 6. Methods for the demonstration of neuronal morphology. Golgi method and variants—Cox's method applied to the study of cat cerebral cortex (top X5, bottom X10). Photograph obtained from an original slide from Professor Fernando de Castro (Archivo Fernando de Castro).

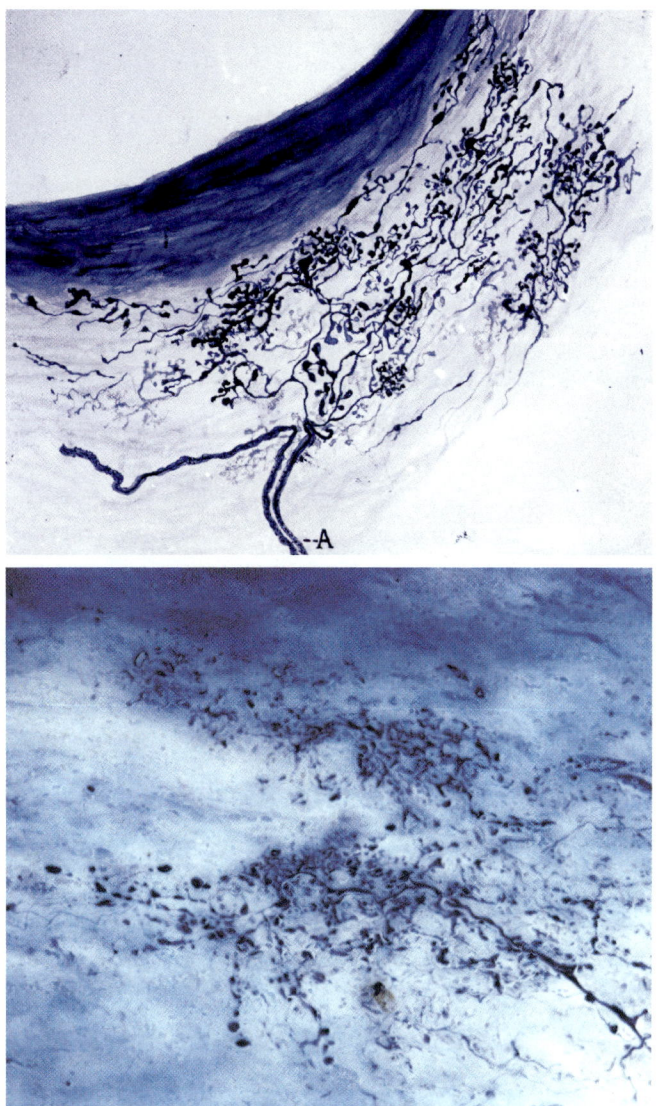

Plate 7. Methods for the demonstration of neuronal morphology. Ehrlich's method and variants using methyl blue. Intravital staining with methyl blue carried out by Professor Fernando de Castro in order to study the fibers of the carotid sinus. (Modification of Cajal's method. Fixed in ammonium molybdate. Adult cat carotid.) In the upper part there is an original pen and ink wash drawing by the author (published in de Castro. F.: "Sur la structure et l'innervation du sinus carotidien de l'homme et des mammifères. Nouveaux faits sur l'innervation et la fonction du glomus caroticum." Trav. Lab. Rech. Biol. 25: 331–380, 1928). Below is a terminal field of fibers in the aortic wall clearly showing characteristic barosensitive meniscus of these fibers. The background blue staining is due to the intravital diffusion of the stain (X20). Photograph obtained from an original slide from Professor Fernando de Castro (Archivo Fernando de Castro), to whom the original drawing also belongs.

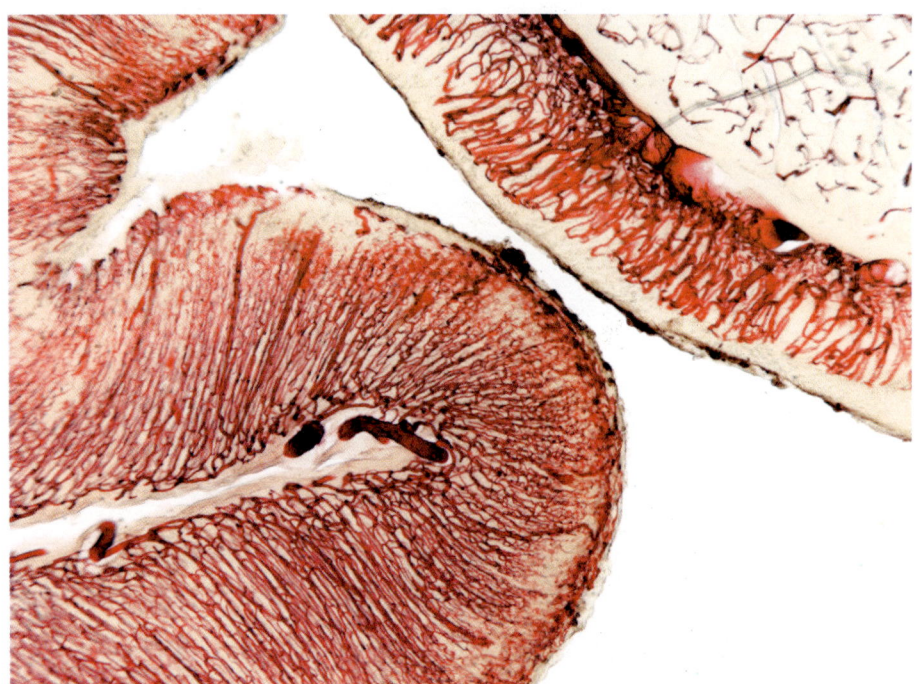

Plate 8. Intravital staining with carmine to analyze blood vessel distribution in the gastric mucosa of the rabbit (X10). Photograph obtained from an original slide from Professor Fernando de Castro (Archivo Fernando de Castro).

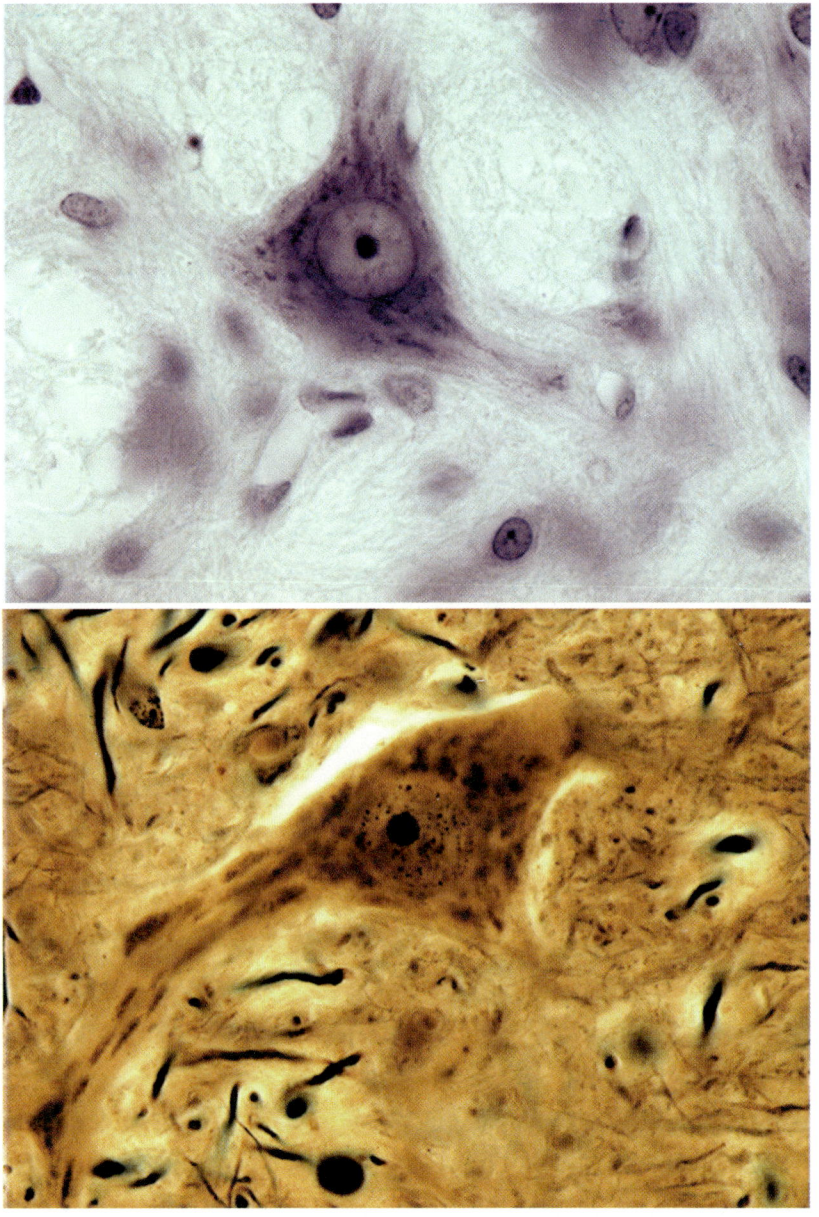

Plate 9. Nervous cell structure. Demonstration of the tigroid substance (Nissl chromatic granules) using anilines (Cresyl violet—top) and silver impregnation (cold silver carbonate –bottom) (X100). Slides from Professor Jaime Merchán Cifuentes.

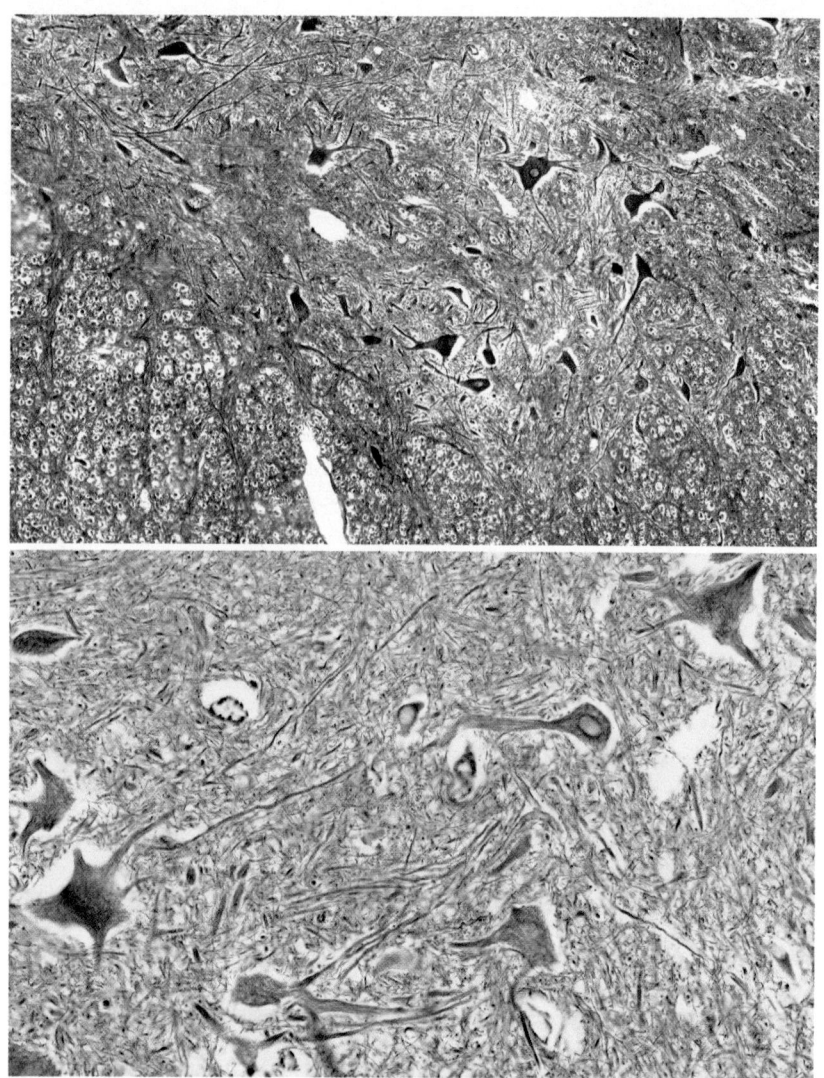

Plate 10. Nervous cell structure. Silver impregnation of neurofibrils. Lamb spinal medulla stained with Bielschowsky's standard procedure (Mosaic X40 –top; X100 –bottom). Slides from Professor Jaime Merchán Cifuentes.

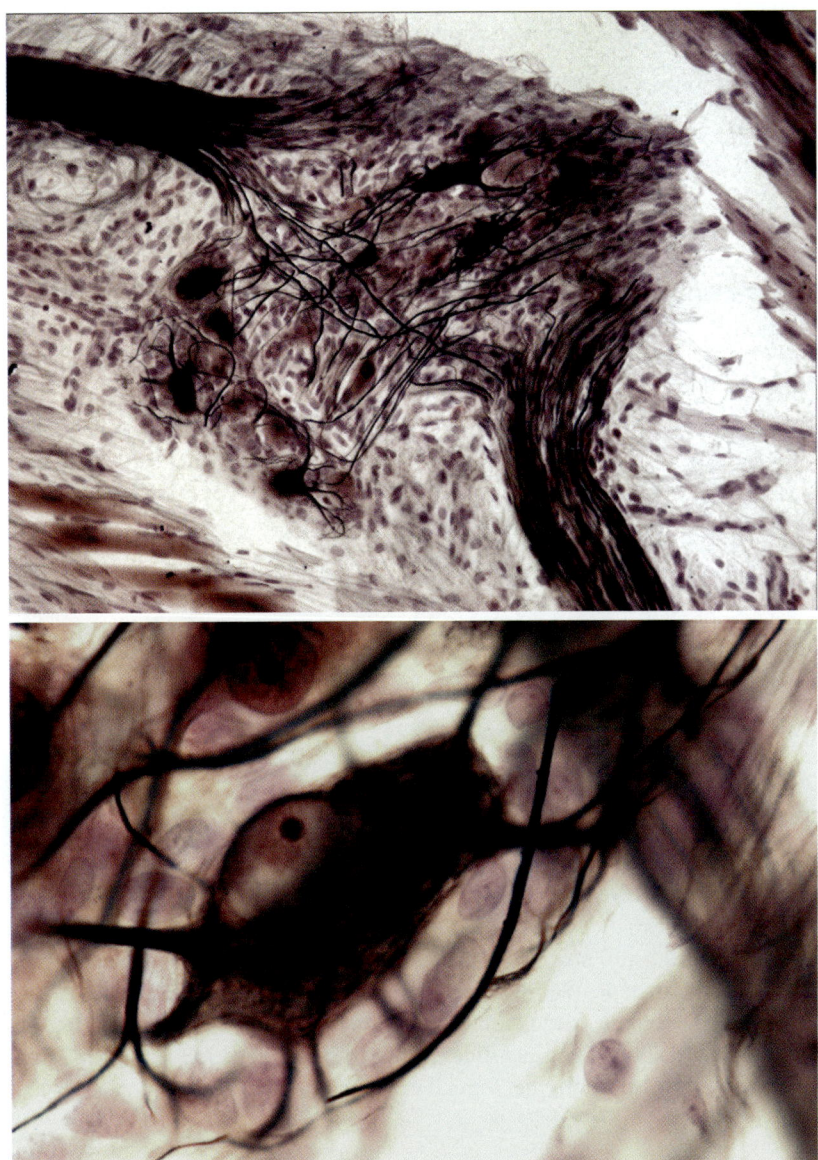

Plate 11. Nervous cell structure. Silver impregnation of neurofibrils. Intramural ganglion (dog esophagus); Gros's method, optimal effect. Top: axonal pathways strongly stained in black; glial capsule, formed by spindle-shaped cells, stained violet (mosaic, X10). Bottom: neuron with somatic cytoplasm and dendrites packed with neurofibrils and surrounded by glial cells (X100). Photographs obtained from original slides from Professor Fernando de Castro (Archivo Fernando de Castro).

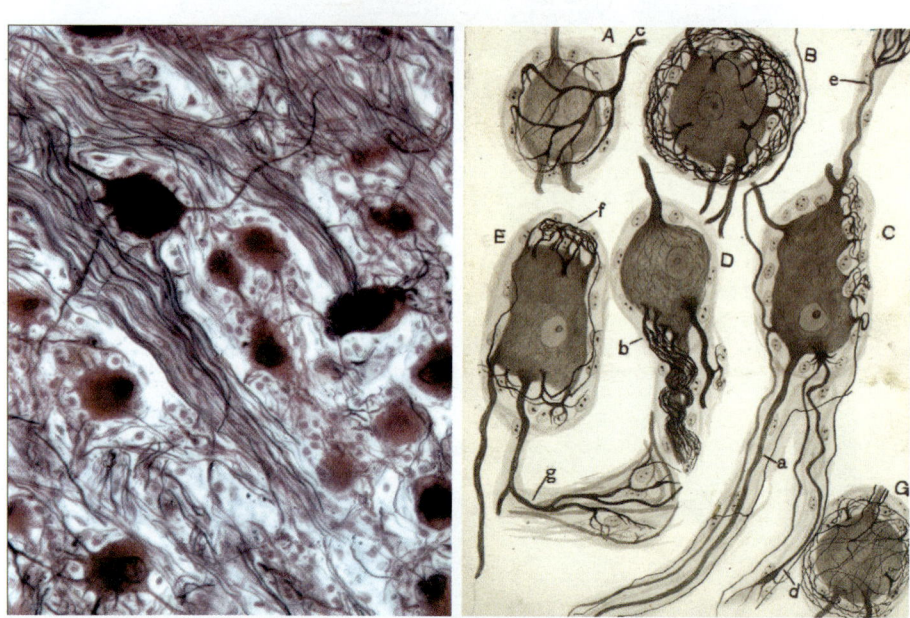

Plate 12. Upper cervical ganglion from a cat (autonomic nervous system) Cajal–Castro's reduced silver impregnation (mosaic X10). On the right, an original sketch by de Castro showing the special features of the dendrites of the cervical sympathetic neurons (published in de Castro. F.: "Sobre la fina anatomía de los ganglios simpáticos, vertebrales y prevertebrales de los simios." Bol. Soc. Esp. Biol. XI: 171–177, 1926). Photograph obtained from original slides from Professor Fernando de Castro (Archivo Fernando de Castro), to whom the original drawing also belongs.

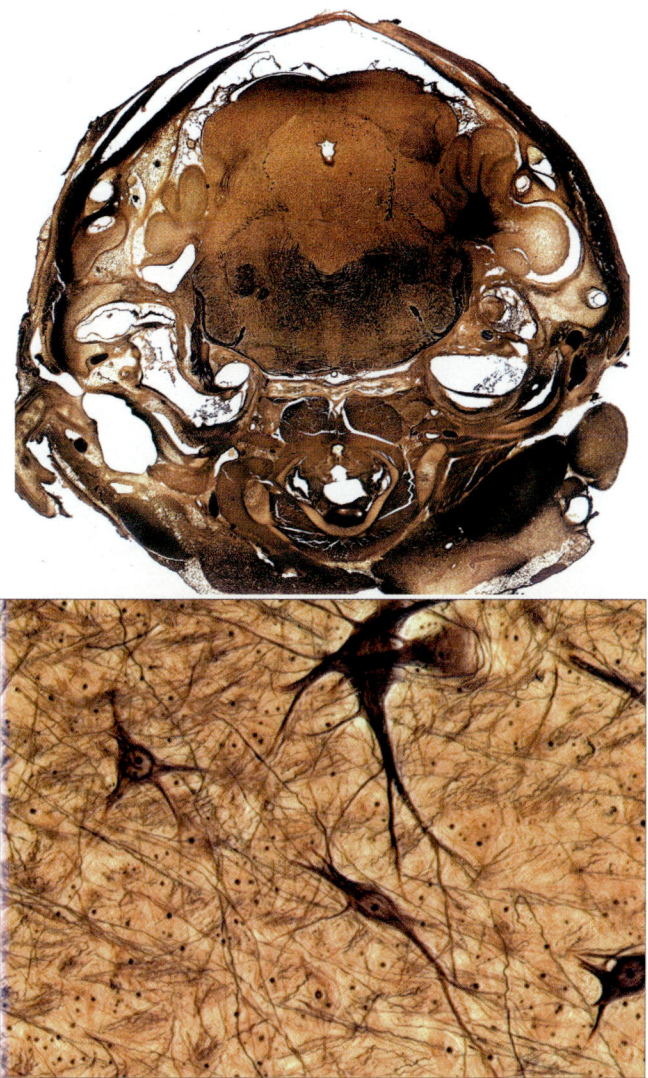

Plate 13. Coronal section from mouse embryo. Cajal–Castro's reduced silver impregnation using somnifene as fixative. These slides were used in the study of morphology and connections of the glomus caroticus. Top: the fibrillary tracts can be clearly seen stained in black against a golden background (X5). Bottom: a high magnification of neurons showing neurofibrils (X40). Photographs obtained from original slides from Professor Fernando de Castro (Archivo Fernando de Castro).

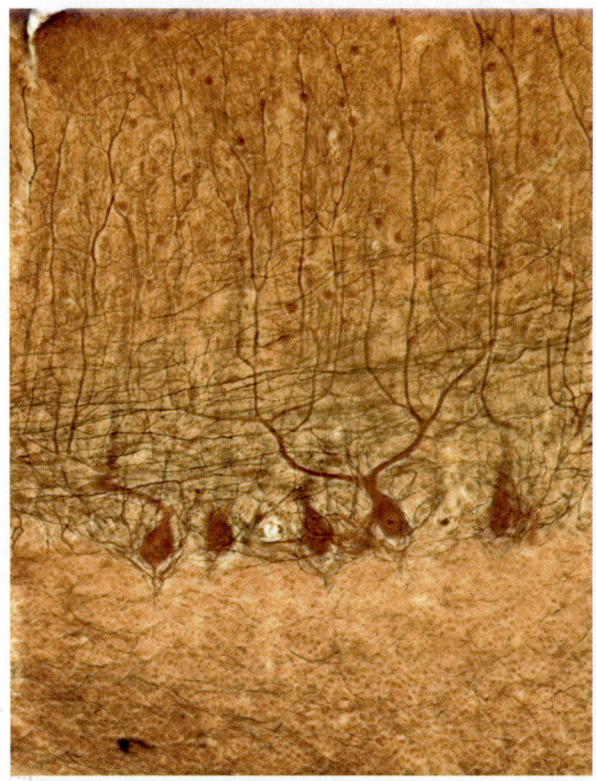

Plate 14. Section of cerebellum impregnated with a hydroquinone-based technique (Ramón y Cajal. S.: "Une formule pour colorer dans les coupes les fibers amedullées et les terminaisons centrales et périphériques." Trab. Lab. Invest. Biol. Univ. Madrid, 23: 237, 1925). The horizontal pathway of the axons of deep stellate cells from the molecular level and the brush axons of Purkinje cells can be clearly seen (X10). Photographs obtained from original slides from Professor Fernando de Castro (Archivo Fernando de Castro).

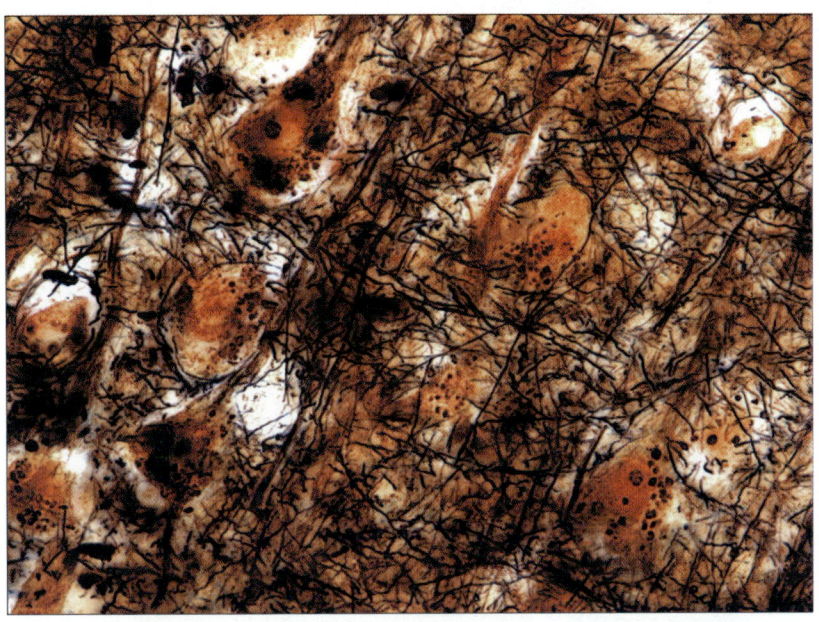

Plate 15. Section of human brain impregnated with an ammonium alcohol (the label reads "brain from an old female"). Lipofuscin granules are seen in the cytoplasm of the neurons from the cortical pyramid (X10). Photographs obtained from original slides from Professor Fernando de Castro (Archivo Fernando de Castro).

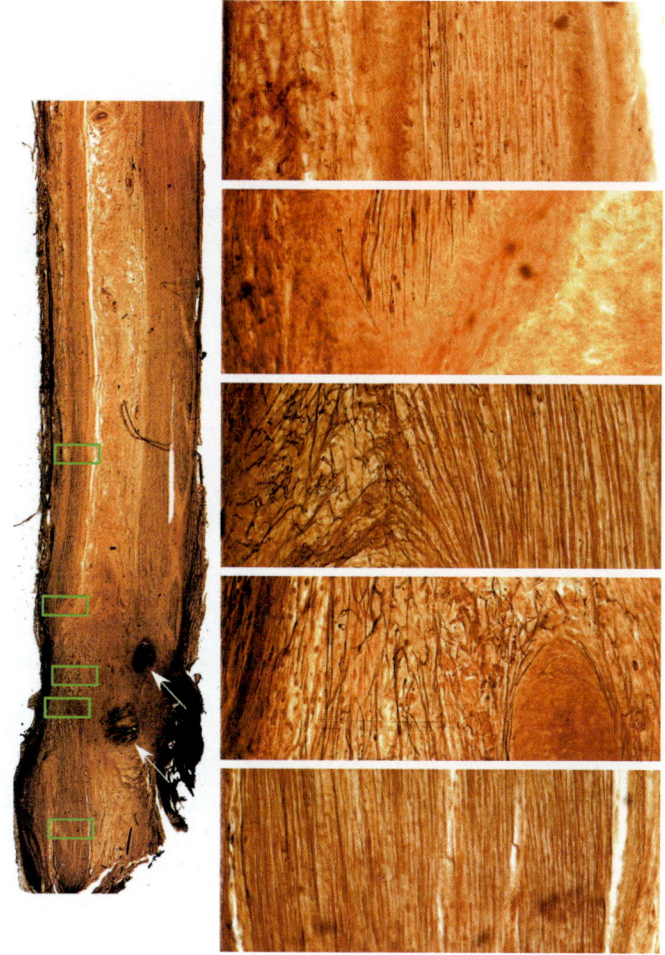

Plate 16. Cajal–Castro's method for the study of peripheral nerve regeneration. Longitudinal section of the sciatic nerve. Arrows show the lesion produced by a suture below the proximal and above the distal end. Green boxes contain details from the right, organized from bottom to top, in a proximal to distal direction (Mosaic X5). Meniscus and dilations possibly represent cones of axonal growth (X20). Photographs obtained from original slides from Professor Fernando de Castro (Archivo Fernando de Castro).

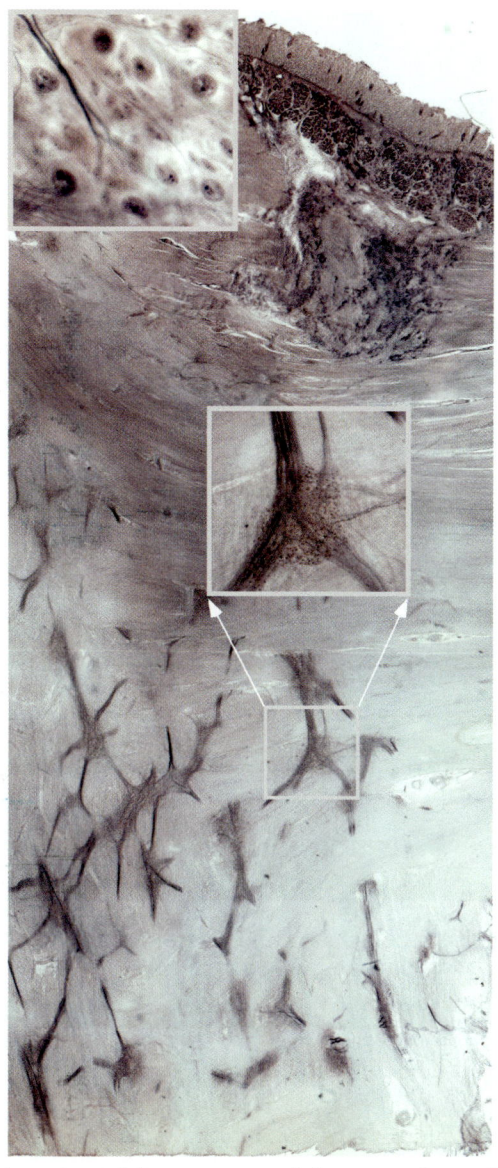

Plate 17. Tangential section of the mucosa and the muscular wall of the stomach of a three-month-old puppy (Mosaic X5). Cajal–Castro's reduced silver impregnation. The intramural plexus make a continuous network of nonmyelinated nerve fibers (Center, X20). Packed cells can be seen in each node of the plexus. Some of these cells may correspond to those named in the current literature as the "interstitial cells of Cajal," which represent motility pacemakers of the intestinal tract (high magnification in the top right corner, X100). Photographs obtained from original slides from Professor Fernando de Castro (Archivo Fernando de Castro).

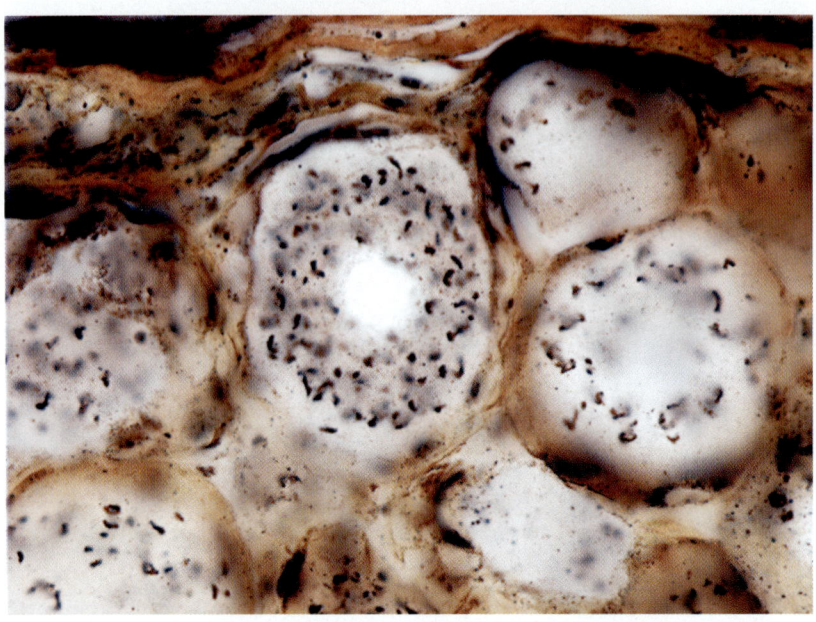

Plate 18. Impregnation of the cellular Golgi complex. Cajal's method using formalin-uranyl nitrate (Ramón y Cajal. S.: "Un sencillo método de coloración selectiva del retículo endoplásmico y sus efectos en los diversos órganos." Trab. Lab. Invest. Biol. Univ. Madrid, 2: 129, 1903). The internal reticular apparatus (terminology in use at the time) is shown. Cajal used this method in exocrine gland cells and proposed, for the first time, its role in cellular secretion (X 100). Original slides from Professor Jaime Merchán Cifuentes.

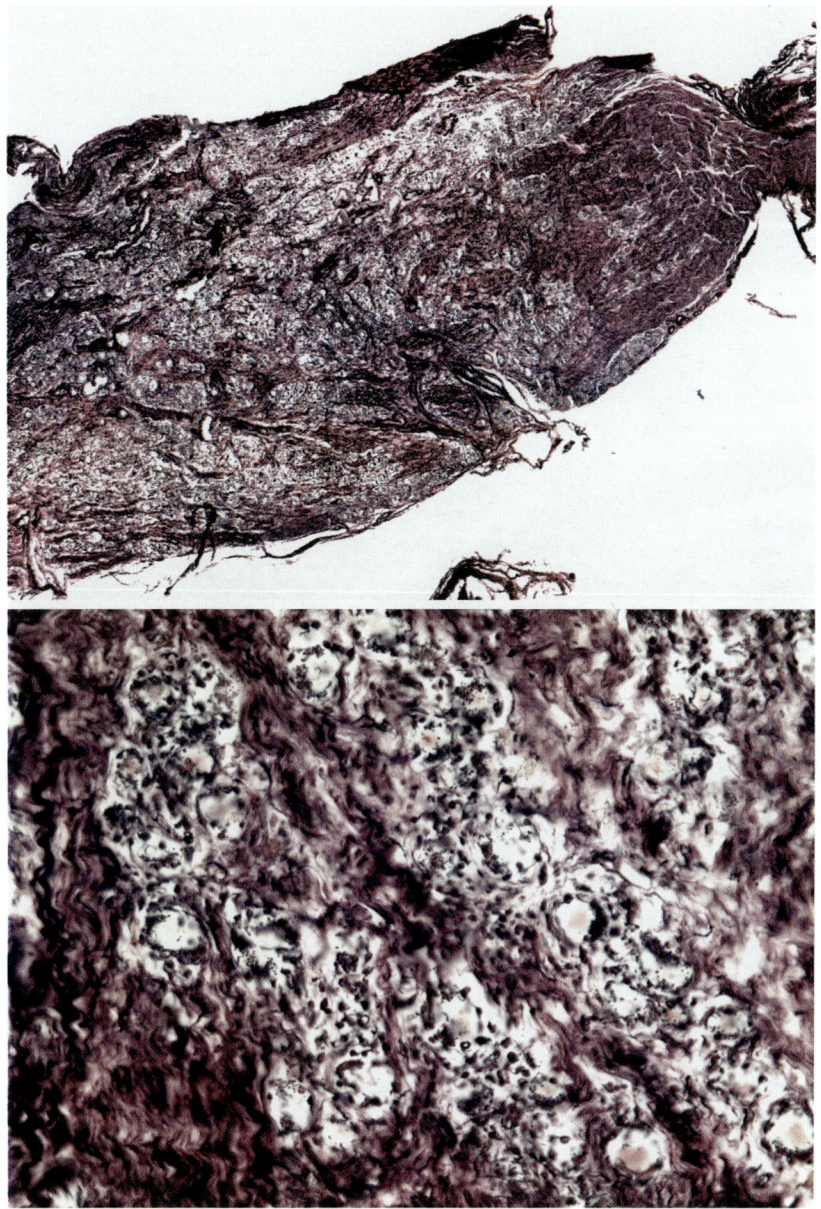

Plate 19. Myelin staining. Del Rio Hortega's method for staining ganglionar glia. Sympathetic ganglion from a cat (X5, X20). Photographs obtained from original slides from Professor Fernando de Castro (Archivo Fernando de Castro).

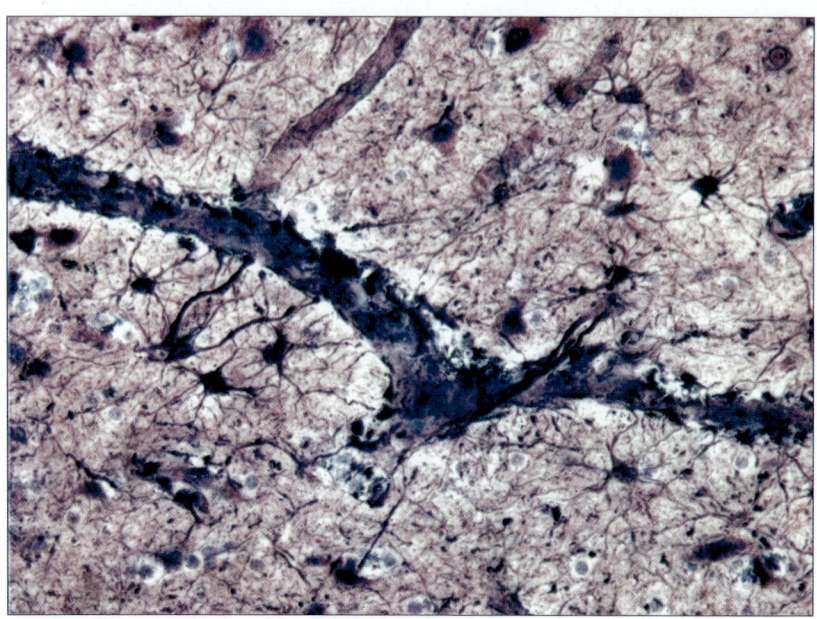

Plate 20. Bolsi's method using Cajal's ammonium silver oxide (Ammonium bromide). Average staining quality. Astrocytes and their "sucking feet" (end feet) attached to a blood vessel wall can be seen (X40). Original slides from Professor Jaime Merchán Cifuentes.

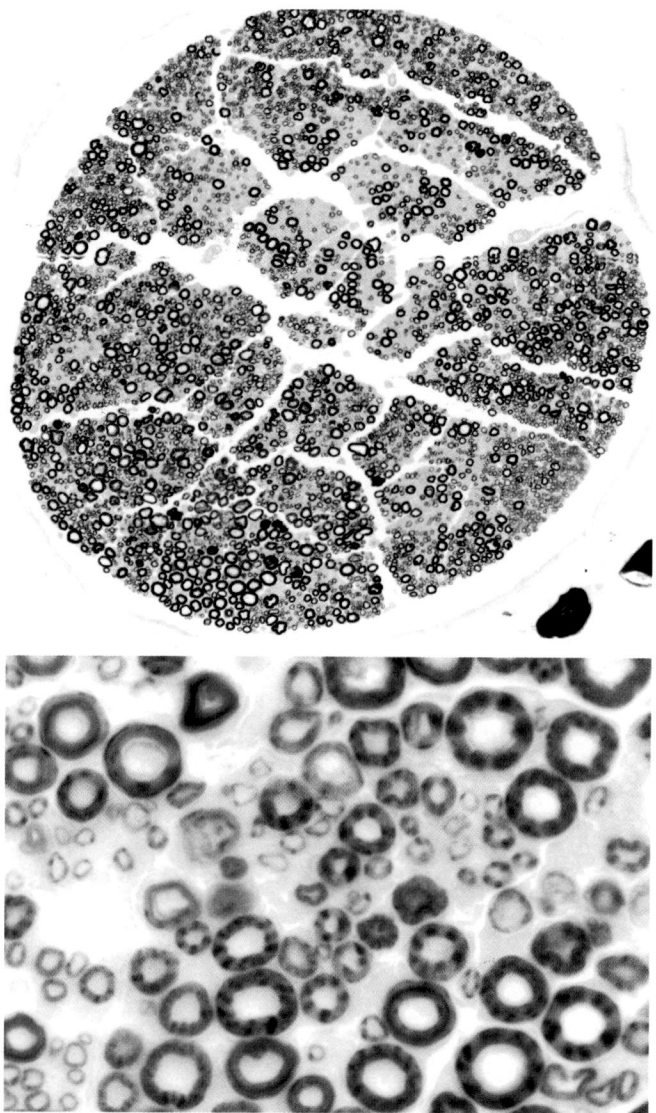

Plate 21. Myelin staining procedures. Osmic acid. Top: low-power image of a peripheral nerve (X10). Bottom: magnification of nodes and paranodes, Schmidt-Lantermann's incisures and spiny bracelet of Nageotte (top left corner X100). Photographs obtained from original slides from Professor Fernando de Castro (Archivo Fernando de Castro).

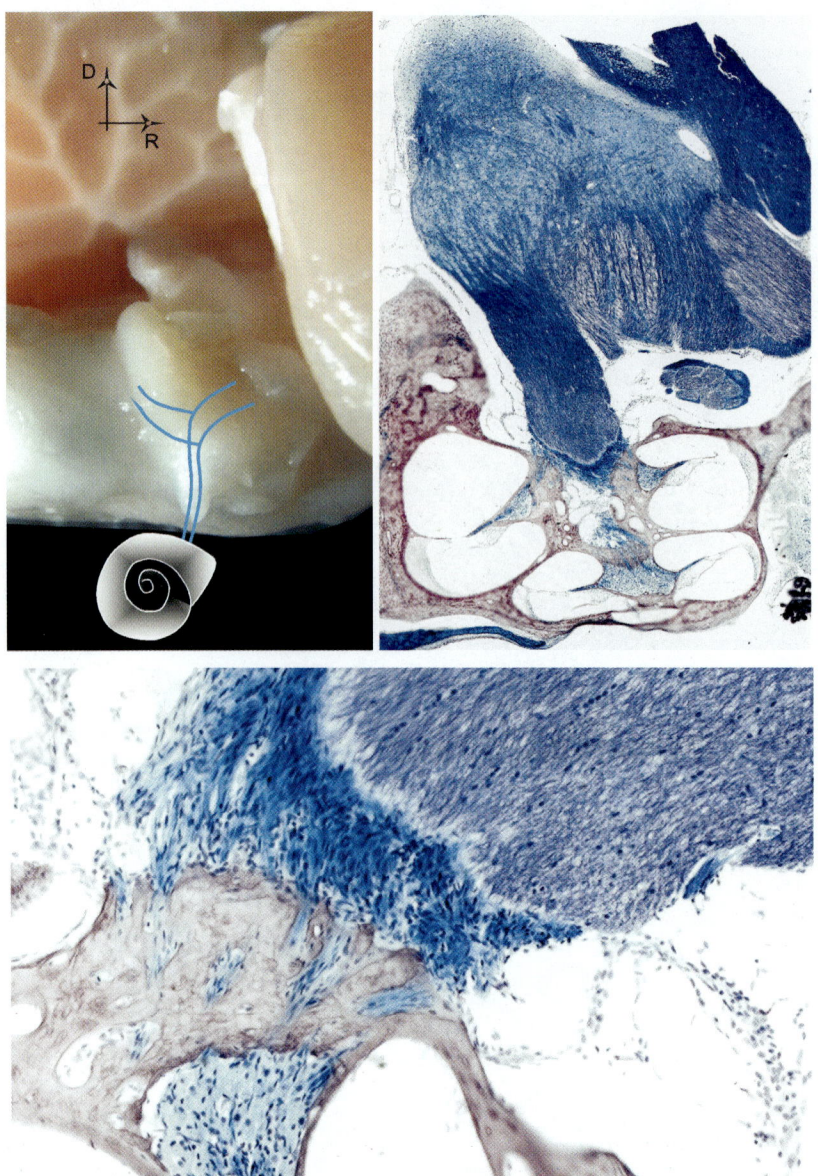

Plate 22. Optimal staining of Kluver Barrera's trichrome method for myelin in a rat auditory nerve. Nitric acid formalin decalcification "used by Cajal for the study of the ear." Top left: cochlear nuclei of rat brain. Right: overview in a sagittal plane of the entire pathway of the cochlea, auditory nerve, and cochlear nuclei. This method highlights the difference in staining between Schwann cells (turquoise) and oligodendrocytes (light blue) (X 10). Bottom: transition zone between central and peripheral glia can be clearly seen (X20). Original slides from Professor Miguel Merchán Cifuentes.

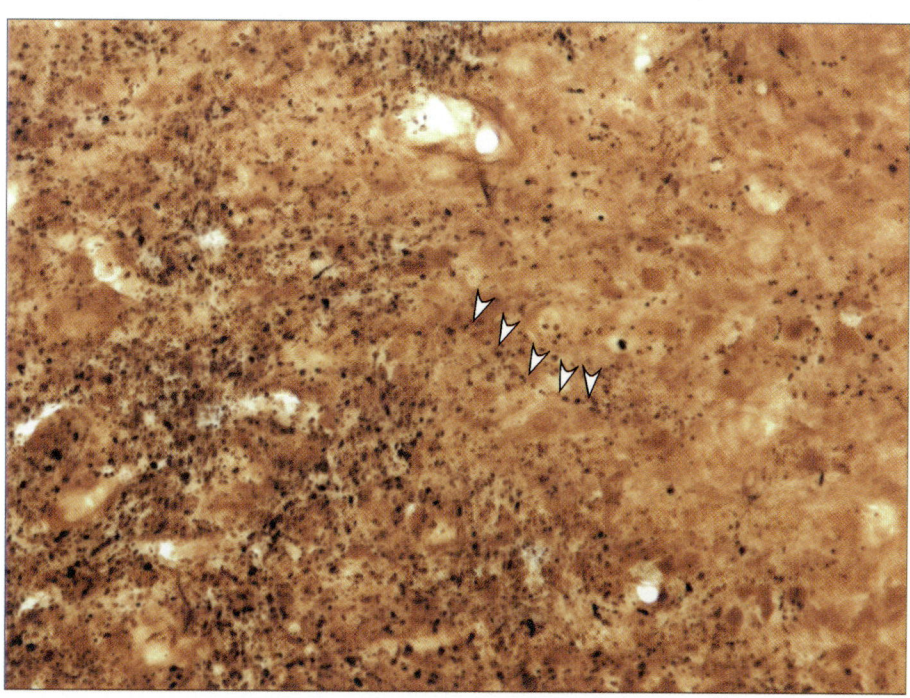

Plate 23. Average quality staining using Fink and Heimer's method for the study of axonal degeneration. Rat's cochlear nuclei subsequent to a small lesion in the cochlea (after seven days). Arrowheads show the fragmented axonal pathway following Wallerian degeneration. Degeneration buds can be selectively seen with this method, which was widely used to analyze nervous system connections before the introduction of tract tracing methods (X 40). Original slides from Professor Miguel Merchán Cifuentes.

VOCABULARY

Balsam. Short for Canada balsam.

Bioblasts. Intracytoplasmic fuchsinophilic granules measuring 0.5–1μm in diameter, first reported by Robert Altmann in 1890 using his own method (**58**). Altmann considered these particles to be the "elementary units of living matter." After the introduction of the first histochemical methods to demonstrate oxidative enzymes, it became clear that the fuchsinophilic granules were mitochondria.

Bügner's bands. Strings of cells that occupy the place of degenerated axons after the transection of a peripheral nerve trunk. They are formed by the proliferation of Schwann cells.

Cajuput. Cajuput (*cajaput, cajuputi*) essence is a hydrated compound of the hydrocarbon $C_{10}H_{16}$, which was formerly obtained from the Malaysian tree kayu-putih (Melaleuca minor).

Candle. In physics, 1 candle is 1/20th of the light emitted by $1cm^2$ of liquid platinum at the temperature of solidification.

Chondrioma. Old term that referred to the entire mitochondrial content of a cell.

Chondriomites. Beaded intracytoplasmic rodlets reported by Benda in 1898 and promptly recognized as a morphological type of mitochondria.

Cyanophilic cells. Plasma cells. In 1896, Cajal reported the existence of a cell type in syphilitic lesions that was characterized by its small size and eccentric nucleus, with chromatin arranged in a cartwheel fashion. The cytoplasm was basophilic, and the cells were thus termed cyanophilic because most of the basic anilines are blue (thionine, toluidine blue, methylene blue, etc.). The same cells were rediscovered three years later by Unna, who was not aware of Cajal's finding. Yet, at the International Medical Congress held in Madrid in 1903, the German pathologist proposed that these cells should be termed, in honor of their discoverer, *cyanophilic cells of Cajal*. The name that finally endured, however, was *plasma cells*.

Diosmotic power. Diffusion capacity.

Eddinger's drawing instrument. This ingenious device (which resembled an upside-down microscope) consisted of a vertical metallic bar that held a microscope stage at 50–60 cm over the table. Above the stage, a powerful light source (an incandescent light bulb, or a voltaic arc lamp) was used to illuminate the preparation. The objectives were located under the stage, and the corresponding intermediate image was enlarged by means of a projecting eyepiece on the drawing table.

Eddinger's macrotome. Instrument used to produce handmade thick brain slices. It consisted of a metal bar that held 4–5 parallel blades, each separated from the next by about one centimeter. A handle was inserted at the opposite side of the bar.

En bloc staining. Bulk staining.

Ezholz granules. Osmiophilic granules appearing in the cytoplasm of the Schwann cells of some animal species. They are identical to Reich's µ granules, and possibly represent myelin metabolic products.

Fibrinoid granules. Cellular inclusions with a fibrin-like stain described by Alzheimer (1910) in the cytoplasm of neuroglial amoeboid cells. These structures appear in the most advanced stages of cell degeneration and probably represent a regressive phenomenon.

Fibrous glial cells. Fibrous astrocytes, white matter astrocytes.

Frohman's striae. These structures, described in 1894, are black, delicate lines, which cross the nerve fiber at right angles to the axon. They are observed when unfixed, mechanically teased peripheral nerve fibers are treated with silver nitrate and then exposed to sunlight. These formations have since been recognized as artifacts.

Fuchsinophilic granules. Another name for bioblasts (*v.s.*).

Glia marginalis. Term coined by Held to name an intricate subpial plexus formed by the processes of astrocytes and ependymal cells. The astrocytic processes form end-feet on the pia and on the leptomeninx, which escort the blood vessels as they penetrate the brain. These end-feet are very close to one another, so it was thought that they formed almost continuous shafts for the pia and the blood vessels; these shafts were known, respectively, as pial limiting membrane and perivascular limiting membrane.

Glial fibers. Astrocytic processes.

Gliocytes. Neuroglial cells. A term also used for sympathetic ganglia satellite cells.

Gliofibrils. See Ranvier-Weigert fibers.

Gliosomes. Intracytoplasmic granules present in the gray matter astrocytes. The existence of cytoplasmic granulations in the astrocytes was reported at the beginning of the twentieth century by Nageotte, Held, Alzheimer, Meves, Mawas, Fieandt, etc., using different methods (**55, 58, 141, 142, 185, 217, 265**). These studies concluded that neuroglial cells contained two types of granules. The first type were highly fuchsinophilic and similar to the mitochondria of other cell types. The second type were formed by larger and less fuchsinophilic structures, which could be stained by the phosphotungstic hematoxylin of Fieandt (**185**) and were thought to be specific to glial cells; the granules were thus called *gliosomes*. In 1910, Nageotte and Mawas suggested that gliosomes were equivalent to secretory granules, thus considering neuroglia "a huge interstitial gland spread throughout the whole central nervous system." The introduction of new procedures by the Madrid Histology School (**173, 175, 177, 186–189**) contributed, paradoxically, to reinforcing this hypothesis. Some of Cajal's students, such as Sacristán (1916) and Del Río-Hortega (1917) even tried to stimulate the glial secretion with tyrosine and pilocarpine, respectively. Although the secretion hypothesis was criticized by some authors (Lugaro, etc.), the current thinking at that time was that protoplasmic astrocytes were actually endocrine cells. In fact, references to this thesis can even be found in some histology textbooks of the 1950s (Levi, Da Costa, Chaves, etc.).

Held's perivascular limitant membrane. See Glia marginalis.

Held's pial limitant membrane. See Glia Marginalis.

Henle's sheath. One of the connective sheaths of the peripheral nerve trunks. The terminology at the time this book was written was rather confusing. The exact meaning of the term Henle's sheath for the authors is as follows: "On their way to the periphery, the nerve trunks divide into their integrating fascicles. The small bundles thus formed ramify even further. The perineurium becomes thinner and transparent and once all the individual nerve fibers are separated from each other, it forms a protecting envelope for each fiber that extends close to the terminal arborization." Henle was the first to describe this thin coat surrounding each fiber and thus Ranvier called it "Henle's sheath" (Ramón y Cajal, S.: *Textura del Sistema Nervioso del Hombre y los Vertebrados*. Vol. I, p. 221. Madrid, 1899).

Hyposulfite. Thiosulfate. Unless otherwise stated, this term is short for sodium hyposulfite (sodium thiosulfate, $Na_2S_2O_3$).

Impregnation. Staining of tissue components by the deposit of metallic salts.

Indurant. Fixative. The term alludes to the hardening action of fixatives on the tissues. Until sectioning techniques were refined, this property of fixatives was as important as the stabilization of the structure itself.

Induration. Fixation.

Interfascicular oligodendroglia. White matter oligodendrocytes.

Internal reticular apparatus. Term coined by Camillo Golgi to designate what is now known as the Golgi complex.

Iris diaphragm. Field diaphragm of a microscope.

Iron and ammonia alum. $(SO_4)_3AlNH_4Fe$.

Jews' pitch. A smooth, asphalt-like black resinous mineral, hard and brittle, which contains several hydrocarbons.

Lecytinoid granules. See Reich's granules.

Leuckart frames. Metal right angles used to shape the melted paraffin into a cube.

Levi's perinucleolar cap. Nucleolus-associated chromatin.

Ligroin. Petroleum ether.

Lime. Lime is, strictly speaking, an alkaline earth, which is the chief constituent of mortar. Chemically, it is a variable mixture of calcium compounds, CaO being the chief one. When this book was written, lime was a colloquial name for calcium oxide, but in some medical texts (especially in the German pathology handbooks) any substance in the body containing calcium that could be detected using histological methods was also known as lime (Kalk, Kalkstein).

Lithium. Colloquialism for lithium. Properly speaking, lithium is a natural product that contains various lithium compounds. In Cajal's day, natural products had been widely replaced at the laboratory by synthetic and/or purified products, but the old (mineralogical) nomenclature sometimes was still used instead of the chemical one.

Lye. Strong alkaline solution used for cleaning. These solutions were named depending on the alkali that was added to the water. Thus, when KOH was used, the solution was called potash lye.

Macroglia. Astrocytes.

Magenta red. Magenta red and red fuchsin were the common names for basic fuchsin in the time of Cajal; this dye is also called aniline red, fuchsin RFN and B-rubin.

Medullated fibers. A term coined by Purkinje (1838) for myelinated nerve fibers. Before it was understood that nerve fibers were connected with what we now call neuronal somata, it was stated that they were formed by an external coat or neurilemma (Schwann cells), a medulla-like sheath (the myelin) and an axial cylinder (axon).

Modus operandi. Latin for protocol.

Modus faciendi. Latin for protocol.

Mordants. Substances, which, although unable to stain when used alone, are capable of forming complexes with tissue components, which can be later stained with specific dyes. Most mordants used in classical histological techniques are salts of aluminum, iron, chromium, or related salts. The metals first form complex ions in the solutions of mordants and then link to the stain by chelation.

Nerve tubes. Nerve fibers.

Neurilemma. This term is somewhat confusing because it can have various meanings. In the Anglo-Saxon neurohistological literature of Cajal's time, the "neurilemma" was made up of all the Schwann cells surrounding an axon, whereas some French authors considered it a connective tissue coat that surrounded each individual axon. Cajal considered the neurilemma to be "[...] a loose connective sheath, rich in blood vessels, which protects the nerves externally, [...] continuous with the pia mater at the point of origin of the nerve. From the inner surface of such sheet, thick connective expansions penetrate inside the nerve, separating the nerve fascicles. In these expansions large arteries and veins, as well as aggregates of adipose tissue, can be identified" (Ramón y Cajal, S.: *Textura del Sistema Nervioso del Hombre y los Vertebrados*. Vol. I, p. 219. Madrid, 1899).

Neurofibrils. In the 1850s, Schultze reported the existence of fine fibrils inside the cytoplasm of nerve cells, which he called neurofibrils. These fibrils were demonstrated more readily by specific methods, such as those of Bethe (**105**), Apáthy (**323**), or Donaggio (**106**), although their existence was only widely accepted after the introduction of the methods of Cajal (**113–130**) and Bielschowsky (**108–112**) in 1903. Electron microscopy studies by Grey and Guillery on tissue stained by Cajal's method showed that the neurofibrils seen with the light microscope were actually microtubules (Journal of Physiology 157: 581–588, 1961).

Neuroglial amoeboid cells. Name coined by Alzheimer (1910) for glial-like cells that appeared in various diseases of the central nervous system (neurosyphilis, rabies, chorea, sleeping sickness, several types of encephalitis, ischemic necrosis, etc.). These cells had a large nucleus and a globular cytoplasm with thick, short protrusions, resembling an amoeba. These cells were initially considered by Alzheimer as astrocytes undergoing regressive changes, although a significant number of pathologists thought that they were a specific cell type capable of phagocytosis, which accumulated around injured regions. Yet, Achúcarro (tannin-silver method, 1911), Cajal (gold-sublimate, 1914) and Del Río Hortega (silver carbonate, 1919) showed that these cells were swollen astrocytes whose expansions were in the process of degeneration ("clasmatodendrosis").

Neurologist. At Cajal's time, anyone studying the nervous system was called a "neurologist."

Neurosomes. Spherical structures (0.5–1 mm in diameter) described by Held in 1895 in the cell body of neurons. This author suggested that they would differ from other cytoplasmic granules (such as mitochondria, plastosomes, or bioblasts), representing the anchorage of the fibrils that run from the soma to the axon terminals.

Nondendritic neuroglial cells. Glial cell category comprising what we now call oligodendroglia and microglia. The analysis of the morphology of the glial cells by the Madrid Histology School began after metallic impregnation procedures were developed for this purpose, such as the tanno-argentic method of Achúcarro (**177**) or Cajal's gold-sublimate (**173**). Both methods rendered superb impregnations of the glial cells, whose basic morphology already had been revealed by Weigert's (**165**) and other aniline stains (**167–172**). None of the available methods, however, stained any processes in a type of cell that was smaller than the glial cells known at that time, and which seemed to be arranged around the neurons and blood vessels and also formed rows in the white matter. The interpretation of these cells became rather troublesome: Some authors (Marinesco, Alzheimer) considered that at least some of them were migratory leukocytes, whereas Robertson stated that the small cells forming rows in the white matter were of mesenchymal origin and named them mesoglia. Cajal (1913) gathered all apolar cells in a single group, which he called the *third element of the nervous centers* (the first and second elements were neurons and glial cells, respectively), a term that did not presuppose the nature of the cells. Nevertheless, some of the components of the *third element* seemed rather similar to neuroglia and were thus considered by Cajal as *non dendritic neuroglial cells*. The controversy ended when Pío Del Río-Hortega, one of Cajal's disciples, developed a new method (**178, 190**) of staining the processes of the third element. In 1919, he classified microglial cells (the "Hortega cells" of the German literature) as an independent cell type, and demonstrated their phagocytic ability and mesenchymal origin (Del Río-Hortega, P.: «El "tercer element" de los centros nerviosos. IV. Poder fagocitario y movilidad de la microglia». Bol. Soc. Esp. Biol. 8: 154–165, 1919). Then, using a modification of the silver carbonate method (**197**), he showed that the cells still remaining in the *non dendritic neuroglial cells* "rag-bag" were what we know at present as oligodendroglia (Del Rio-Hortega, P.: «La glia de escasas radiaciones [oligodendroglia]». *Boletin de la Real Sociedad Española de Historia Natural*, 21: 63–92, 1921). A few years later, he suggested that oligodendroglial cells were homologous to Schwann cells, and responsible for the myelination of the axons (Del Río-Hortega, P.: «¿Son homologables la glía de escasas radiaciones y la célula de Schwann?». *Boletín de la Sociedad Española de Biología*, 10: 1–4, 1922).

Nucleolar spherules. Accessory body of Cajal, usually found in the vicinity of the nucleolus.

Officinal. Solution prepared according to the Pharmacopoeia. The apothecaries at that time stored stock solutions (known as «officinal» or "in the office") with concentrations established by the Pharmacopoeia. Doctors prescribed the proportions in which these «officinal» solutions had to be mixed.

One-third alcohol. Ranvier's one-third alcohol was a 2:1 mixture of water and 40° Cartier alcohol, which was the conventional alcohol grading in use in France at that time. Nowadays, this solution would be prepared mixing 28 cc of absolute ethanol with 72 cc of water.

Perineural endothelial cells. Perineural epithelium.

Pigmentary spherules. Lipofuscin granules.

Plastosomes. Term coined in 1910 by Meves to name a special type of rod-shaped mitochondria. The name alludes to Meves's hypothesis that these rodlets were able to transmit some hereditary characters from the nucleus to the cytoplasm.

Potash. This term is used in the text as a synonym for potassium, although it sometimes refers to potassium hydroxide (**109, 338**). Potash is, strictly speaking, an alkaline substance originally obtained by lixiviating plant ashes and evaporating the solution in large iron pans. The main compound obtained in this way was not potassium hydroxide, but potassium carbonate, which was used mainly in glass production.

Protagonoid granules. See Reich's granules and protagonoid substances.

Protagonoid substances. "Myelin has a very complex chemical composition. According to Kühne and Chittenden, it would contain albumin, collagen, elastin, and nuclein, besides the compounds specific to myelin, such as: cholesterin, protagon, lecithin, cerebrin, and neurokeratin" (Ramón y Cajal, S.: *Textura del Sistema Nervioso del Hombre y los Vertebrados*. Vol. I, p. 199, Madrid, 1899). See also Reich's granules.

Protoplasm. Term coined by Purkinje in 1840 to describe the elemental units of living matter. After the development of the cellular theory, this term became a synonym for cytoplasm, which is how Cajal used it.

Quadrigeminal tubercles. The superior and inferior colliculi. Ranvier-Weigert fibers: See Gliofibrils.

Ranvier crosses. Images that appear at the nodes of Ranvier when unfixed nerve fibers are impregnated with silver nitrate, and later subjected to the reducing action of light. This results in the formation of a cross-shaped precipitate at the nodes, the horizontal arms of which correspond to the axon. The vertical ones are located between adjacent Schwann cells, and are called cementing discs, because it was thought that they would act as a "glue" between consecutive segments of the nerve fiber. Both the "discs" and the "crosses" are nothing more than artifacts, formed by the precipitation of photosensitive silver salts ($AgCl_2$), formed when silver nitrate reacts with chloride ions at the node of Ranvier.

Ranvier-Weigert fibers. Cytoskeleton of the astrocytes. Ranvier-Weigert fibers (also termed *gliofibrils*) were first reported by Louis Ranvier in 1892 after the examination of unstained glial cells when he described highly refringent fibrils, which seemed to form an endless network through the whole nervous system. The cell body of the astrocytes (termed *Deiters' cells* in Cajal's time) were envisioned as the nodes of the network. Ranvier's ideas were supported by Carl Weigert in 1895 with the aid of a special method (**165**). The hypothesis of the gliofibrillar network was criticized by Cajal from 1897, and was abandoned by Ranvier and Weigert after the introduction of the metallic impregnation methods for neuroglia (**173, 175–179**). The existence of intracytoplasmic fibrils in the white matter astrocytes was widely accepted, however, and the name of Ranvier-Weigert fibers was retained in honor of the discoverers of these cellular organelles.

Red fuchsin. See Magenta red.

Reich's granules. In 1903, Reich described two types of granules in the Schwann cells of the human sciatic nerve, based on differences in staining. He thought that these granules would be related to some of the compounds considered then to be specific of myelin (e.g., protagonoid substances). He called the ones that contained lecithin-like lipids ("semilecythins") μ granules, and these were identical to Ezholz's osmiophilic granules (*v.s.*). The other type, named π-granules, would be formed by *protagon* and were metachromatic. The existence of π-granules was confirmed in 1953 by Noback, who demonstrated that they could be stained with the acid-hematein Baker's test, as well as by Blue Nile sulfate, PAS, and Black Sudan (Noback, C.R.: J. Comp. Neurol., 99: 91, 1953). Noback found that these granules are, in fact, metachromatic when stained with toluidine blue.

Remak's fibers. Unmyelinated nerve fibers.

Rezzonico-Golgi apparatus. Spiral filament described by Golgi (1885) and Rezzonico (1879) found inside the Lantermann incisures, when dissociated peripheral nerve fibers are impregnated with silver nitrate. This structure already was considered an artifact by Cajal (*Textura del Sistema Nervioso del Hombre y los Vertebrados*. Vol. I, p. 206. Madrid, 1899).

Rod cells. Term coined by Franz Nissl (*Stäbchenzellen*) for a type of cell that appeared in the cerebral cortex in patients suffering from paretic dementia. They corresponded to hypertrophied microglial cells whose processes became stainable with the Nissl method.

Roux's apparatus. A type of thermostatically controlled oven, in which the air was heated by means of gas lighters and circulated upward.

Segall rings. Artifactual images observed in 1893 by means of silver impregnation. They run circumferentially through the myelin sheath where it is interrupted by Lantermann's incisures.

Semilecythinoid granules. See Reich's granules.

Soda. Colloquial name for sodium, although in some cases (**131**, **145**, **171**, **177**, **310**, **313**) it is used as a synonym for sodium hydroxide. The term originated from the days when the main source of sodium compounds was the mineral known as soda.

Soda hyposulfite. Old name for sodium thiosulfate ($Na_2S_2O_3$).

Sodium hydrate. Obsolete term for sodium hydroxide (NaOH).

Somniféne. Mixture of barbiturates now discontinued but sold until 1960 as a hypnotic by the Swiss firm Hoffman-LaRoche. The composition of *somniféne* is referred in the translator's Note 7, Chapter 3, Section Two.

Spinous double bracelet. This structure was described by Nageotte in 1910 in the region of the nerve fiber now known as the paranode. In this area there would be "some rings which closely surround the axon, and from which parallel crests arise, that seem to act as insertion points for the myelin leaflets" (Ramón y Cajal, S.: *Textura del Sistema Nervioso del Hombre y los Vertebrados*. Vol. I, p. 396. Madrid, 1899; Ramón y Cajal, S., and Tello, J. F.: *Elementos de Histología Normal. Científico-Médica*, Madrid, 1955)

Spiral apparatus of Rezzonico. See Rezzonico-Golgi apparatus.

Sublimate. Mercuric bichloride ($HgCl_2$).

Succinum. Amber.

Succinum tincture. Amber tincture. According to the Spanish Pharmacopoeia (1865), it is made as follows:

Amber	9 drachmas (32 g)
Gentian root	1 drachma (4 g)
Rhubarb	1 drachma (4 g)

Zedoaria	1 drachma (4 g)
Saffron	1 drachma (4 g)
White agaric	1 drachma (4 g)
Theriaca Magna	1 drachma (4 g)
60° Alcohol	7 pounds (1.7 g)

Theriaca Magna (theriac) was a complex drug mixture developed in the fifteenth century by Venetian pharmacists (Theriaca Andromachi Senioris). It was made from seventy-four or more different substances.**Thymol.** A powerful antiseptic obtained from thyme oil and also from the volatile oil of horsemint. It is sold as crystalline, transparent, rhomboidal plates. Chemically it is cymene phenol, $C_{10}H_{130}OH$.

Tonofibrils. Cytoskeleton of epithelial cells (cytokeratin intermediate filaments).

Unmedullated fibers. Unmyelinated nerve fibers (for the origin of the term, see Medullated nerve fibers).

Ventral acoustic ganglion. Ventral cochlear nucleus.

Vermillion. Cinnabar or red crystalline mercuric sulfide, much valued on account of its brilliant scarlet color, used as a pigment or in the manufacture of red sealing wax.

Vesubin. This dye is available nowadays as *Bismarck brown Y*.

NOTES

CHAPTER 1

1. Cajal's original drawings, most of them masterpieces of scientific illustration, are kept in the Museum of the Instituto Cajal, in Madrid (Av. Doctor Arce, 37. 28002 Madrid, España).
2. Cajal continued to make the plates himself until 1900, after which he entrusted the work to Mr. Peláez, the expert engraver of the Tipografía Artística.
3. At that time, postgraduate studies could be carried out at any Spanish university; however, the doctoral thesis had to be read before a Committee of Professors from the Central University in Madrid. Thus, all students were obliged to spend time at their laboratories under supervision.
4. In this paper, on the mucous epithelia and the muscles of insects, he claimed that the tonofibrils connected the cytoplasms of epithelial cells, and that the Z discs of skeletal muscle fibers were continuous between adjacent cells. Curiously enough, these assumptions supported the reticular theory.
5. From a Kölliker letter to Cajal dated November 16, 1889.
6. The optical bases of the microscope image were formulated by Abbe in 1873. In 1889 planapochromatic lenses were not yet available, and the best numerical apertures were about 1.30, as opposed to the 1.60 common today.
7. Mathias-Marie Duval, Professor of Anatomy at La Sorbonne, had large layouts of Cajal's drawings made for his course on the central nervous system. He began the first lecture by saying, "[. . .] a new light on these topics comes from the South, from the noble Spain, the land of the Sun."
8. Because Golgi did not attend the Berlin meeting, Cajal went to Pavia to discuss his results with him, as the inventor of the method. However, Golgi was too busy to receive him and, in fact, they did not meet until the Nobel Prize ceremony.
9. Only a few copies of Cajal's first great treatise, the *Textura,* were published, as Cajal personally paid for the printing. In contrast, *Histologie* was published by the French publisher Maloine, and both the first edition (1909–1911) and the later version (1953) had a wide distribution. At present, all the original editions are out of print, though several English versions are available.
10. Supporting Cajal's research became a matter of honor for the rest of the academic staff. For instance, the Chairman of Gynecology, the Marquis of El Busto, donated his salary for life to Cajal's laboratory and the Chairman of Surgery, Professor Carlos Martín, offered him free accommodation in one of his properties close to the University.

11. His Investiture Lecture was titled, *Reglas y Consejos para la Investigación Biológica* (Rules and Advice for Biological Research) and is one of the most encouraging reference works for young investigators. It was published as a book titled *Los Tónicos de la Voluntad*, and it has recently been translated into English (*Advice for a Young Investigator*).
12. Jorge Ramón developed the formalin-uranyl nitrate method with which he described the cerebellar neuroglial cells named after him.
13. The pathological approach to psychiatry gave excellent results, mainly because the main cause for psychiatric hospitalization at that time was neurosyphilis. Many neuroanatomical and neuropathological findings are still named after the foremost psychiatrists of the time who discovered them, such as Meynert, Gudden, Pierre Marie, Alzheimer, Nissl, and Westphal.
14. The techniques of fixation used at this time gave rise to lineal aggregates of microtubules that were visible with the light microscope. These aggregates were considered to be fibrillar differentiations specific to the cytoplasm and were described in many cells, such as epithelial lining cells (epitheliofibrils), neurons (neurofibrils), and fibroblasts (inofibrils).
15. Enriqueta Levi Rodríguez, "Ketty," was the Instituto's librarian, but also Cajal's secretary, confident, and even his technician. She was deeply admired by the old scientist, who called her "La pequeña" ("little one"). In fact, she was one of the most able and brilliant people at Cajal's side in his later years. Ketty, together with Irene Falcón, were instrumental in the promotion of the feminist movement in Spain. In 1977, she published an admirable essay on Cajal's personality called, "This was Cajal" ("Así era Cajal").
16. The number of scientists who worked at the Institute during Cajal's last years had increased so much that a new, larger building was required. This was completed in 1932. In 1945, however, six years after the end of the civil war, only two people worked there: de Castro (who was also in charge of the library and Cajal's archive of histological preparations) and Tello, who was unpaid but allowed to use one of the many laboratories that had been left unoccupied in the building. Funds were so low that glass slides and coverslips had to be recycled from old preparations.
17. de Castro was very interested in classical music and literature and became an expert in art and antiques.
18. Many students were interested in neurohistology and trained in de Castro's laboratory, but very few remained due to poor working conditions, lack of fellowships, and poor salaries. (de Castro himself had to work as a surgeon's assistant to make a living.). Some of these young scientists emigrated to countries with better opportunities for studying science, while others opted for more profitable jobs.

Chapter 2

1. We shall not deal in this book with either the special types of microscopes (such as those developed for the analysis of submicroscopic particles, or those using ultraviolet light) or with the accessories for microscopy (microtomes, polarizing attachments, etc.), given that these instruments are described in the general treatises on histological technique.
2. A lustrum was a term for a five-year period in ancient Rome.
3. If chloral hydrate shows a slightly acidic reaction, one or two drops of ammonia should be added so that the solution turns neutral or somewhat alkaline (de Castro).

Chapter 7

1. This dye also can be purchased ready for use from some dealers of micrographical products, such as Grübler (Leipzig).
2. See the staining methods for glial cells and connective tissue of the central nervous system.
3. Dr Walker, Professor Schafer's assistant (from Edinburgh), often used this method. Her slides stained with this technique at our laboratory are remarkable.

Chapter 9

1. According to Strong, if lithium bichromate is used instead of potash bichromate, the correct induration degree can be accomplished in three days. However, Luigi Sala, who has tested several bichromates for the slow variation of the Golgi method, suggests that induration in lithium bichromate should last at least ten days. Furthermore, the silver chromate reaction using the bichromate salts of lithium, sodium, calcium, rubidium, magnesium, and copper is not very specific and, in addition, irregular precipitates in the nervous tissue are far more common (Strong: "Lithium bichromate as a new reagent for hardening adult brains in the Golgi method." *New York Academy of Sciences. Biolog. Sec.* 1894; Luigi Sala: "I bicromate di sodio, calcio, magnesio, rubidio, litio, zinco e rame nel metodo de Golgi." *Comunicazione fatta all'Academia di Scienze Mediche e Naturali di Ferrara il 28 Giugno, 1897*).
2. It is advisable to remove the silver precipitate crust of the pieces with a brush before placing them in the second osmium-bichromate mixture.
3. As a rule, bovids and horse retinas render better results than those from rabbits and cats.
4. The amount of osmium in the silver bath must be 1/4 to 1/2 per 100.
5. Strong uses lithium bichromate and formalin for the embryonic nervous system.

Chapter 10

1. Both the induration in formalin and the dehydration must be carried out at a temperature below 12°–15°C.
2. The temperature of the dehydrant must not exceed 15°C.
3. This artifact is rather frequent in all of the methylene-blue-based techniques.

Chapter 11

1. This methylene blue solution is a trademark of the company Buchner & Sohn, from Munich.
2. In the present chapter, only the main variations of the method are discussed; for a more detailed account, see Cajal: Las formulas del nitrato de plata reducido. *Trabajos del Laboratorio de Investigaciones Biologicas*, Vol. VIII, 1910.
3. A simple variation of this procedure was published in *Trabajos del Laboratorio de Investigaciones Biologicas*, Vol. XIX, 1921.
4. This solution is highly alkaline; paraffin sections may detach from the slides if they are not firmly stuck.
5. This may be, however, the normal arrangement in the adult neurons or glial cells.
6. See the use of these dyes in general practice textbooks such as, among others, Cajal and Tello: *Elementos de Histología normal y técnica micrográfica*. Décima edición, 1931.

7. Occassionally, Achúcarro has stained the cell membrane with a modification of his silver-tannin method; unfortunately, the procedure is very inconstant.
8. See our book *Histologie du Systeme Nerveux del Homme et des Vertebres*, French edition, Vol. I, 1909, p. 193.
9. Three or four years ago, Ramón Vinos showed me some Golgi slides where this network appeared not only around the neurons but also enclosing the blood vessels, and even inside them. This finding, together with the well-known fact that this reticulum spans the whole of the gray and white matters, led me to suspect that we are perhaps dealing with a precipitate due to the action of the fixatives. See Ramón y Cajal, S: "Consideraciones críticas sobre la teoría de Bethe." *Trabajos del Laboratorio de Investigaciones Biológicas de la Universidad de Madrid*. Vol. II, Madrid, 1903.

Chapter 13

1. This solution is prepared by dissolving 29 g of Merck's ferric chloride (FeCl3) in 100 cc of distilled water.
2. The usual practice is to prepare a 10 per 100 solution of hematoxylin in 96° ethanol several months in advance; this solution is diluted to a final concentration of 1 per 100 immediately before use.

Chapter 14

1. Methyl blue should not be mistaken for methylene blue.
2. To prepare this solution, place the three components in a porcelain well and then warm gently while stirring with a glass rod; when the sublimate is completely dissolved, let the solution cool and then filter.
3. Microglia will not be shown if the sections are allowed to take a deep yellow or brown color.
4. The well must be gently shaken so that the temperature is homogeneous throughout the solution.
5. First dissolve the hematoxylin in warm water; when this solution has cooled to room temperature, add the other components.
6. Cover the well containing the pyridinated silver carbonate with a watch glass with its convex surface down. Place the flask on a sheet of asbestos paper and heat with a flame just until a burning sensation is felt when holding the glass with bare fingers. The well should be rotated constantly during this step.

Chapter 15

1. Nuclear staining in van Gieson's method should be done with Weigert's iron hematoxylin **(156)**; for this purpose, solution B should be added to 1 per 100 of hydrochloric acid.
2. For this purpose, it is possible to do a rapid staining (ten to fifteen minutes) with basic anilines; afterward, rinse with water and differentiate in 95° alcohol.
3. This fixative is prepared by mixing 30 cc of a saturated solution of picric acid with 10 cc of formalin and 2 cc of acetic acid. Fix for two or three days, rinse with running tap water and store the pieces in 10 per 100 formalin.
4. Commercial formalin is neutralized with chalk for two or three days and then filtered and diluted.
5. Solutions prepared three or four weeks in advance should be discarded, because they may be toxic.

Chapter 16

1. This dye, dissolved in methanol, is sold ready for use by Grübler, from Leipzig.
2. The use of plain formalin should be avoided, because this reagent can dissolve the iron in the tissues.
3. Glassware should be immersed first in hydrochloric acid, then washed with water, and finally immersed in ethanol.
4. This reagent is prepared by mixing 1 g of basic fuchsin, 10 cc of absolute ethanol, and 100 cc of 5 per 100 phenol.

Chapter 17

1. Methyl blue (not methylene blue) should be completely insoluble in absolute alcohol.
2. The staining should be done while heating the slide with a flame until vapor emission appears.
3. A flat wooden toothpick also can be used for this purpose.
4. Generally speaking, the more ammonia added to the ethanol, the paler the medullated axons appear and the better newly formed, regenerating sprouts are shown.

Chapter 18

1. The details of the method were explained to us personally in a letter from Professor Lawrentjew.
2. When large pieces of adult animals are decalcified, the best criterion to assess the end-point of the process is to check for the existence of calcium in the decalcifying liquid.
3. See footnote of section 312.

BIBLIOGRAPHY

Ramón y Cajal, S.: *Recollections of My Life* (E. Horne Craigie with Juan Cano, trans.). Cambridge, MA: The MIT Press, 1996.

Kölliker, A.: Zur feineren Anatomie des Centralen Nervensystems. Ersters Beitrag: Das Kleinhirn. Z. Wissenchaft, Zoologie, tomo 49, n° 4, 1890; Kölliker, A.: Das Rückenmark. Z. Wissenchaft, Zoologie, tomo 51, n° 1, 1890; Kölliker, A.: Der feinere Bau des Verlängerten Marques Anat. Anz. Tomo 4, n° 14 y 15, 1891.

«Estudio sobre la neuroglia de la corteza cerebral del hombre y los animales. I La arquitectura neuróglica y vascular del bulbo olfatorio». Trab. Lab. Inv. Biol. Univ. Madrid 18:1, 1920.

«Estudio sobre la microglía y su transformación en células en bastoncito y cuerpos gránulo-adiposos». Arch. Neurobiol. 1:171, 1920; «Estudios sobre la neuroglía. La glía de escasas radiaciones» Arch. Neurobiol. 2:16, 1921.

Apathy, S.: «Das leitende Element der Nervensystems und seine topographischen Beziehungen zu den Zellen». Mitteil. a. d. Zool. Station zu Neapel., 12: 495–748, 1897.

Bethe, A.: «Ueber die Neurofibrillen und der Ganglienzellen von Wirbelthieren und Beziehungen zu Golginetzen». Arch. f. mikros. Anat., 55: 360–420, 1900.

Ramón y Cajal, S.: «Consideraciones críticas sobre la teoría de Bethe acerca de la estructura y conexiones de las células nerviosas». Trab. Lab. Inv. Biol. Univ. Madrid, 2: 101–128, 1903.

Ramón y Cajal, S.: «Mecanismo de la degeneración y regeneración de los nervios». Trab. Lab. Inv. Biol. Univ. Madrid, 4: 119–210, 1906.

Cajal: See the numerous essays published in Trabajos del Laboratorio de Investigaciones Biológicas de la Universidad de Madrid, and especially the book titled, *Estudios sobre la degeneración y regeneración del sistema nervioso*. Years 1912 and 1914 (with 317 figures).

See, among other treatises: D. Ehrlich, R. Krause, etc., *Enziklopädie der Mikroskopischen Technik*, 1910; A. Pappenheim: *Grundriss der Farbchemie*, etc., 1901; Nietzki, *Chimie des matières colourantes organiques*, Paris, 1901; Damianowich, *Estudio físicoquímico, etc., de las materias colorantes orgánicas artificiales*, Buenos Aires, 1909; Leon Lefevre, *Matières colorantes artificiales*, Paris, 1896, etc.

Ramón y Cajal, S: «Les épines collatérales des cellules du cerveau colourées au bleu de méthylène». *Rev. Trim. Micrográf. Madrid.* Vol. I, , 1896.

Ramón y Cajal, S: «Le bleu de Méthylène dans les centres nerveux». *Rev. Trim. Micrográf. Madrid.* Vol. I, , 1896.

Fajersztajn: «Ein neues Silberimprägnationverfahren als Mittel zür Färbung der Axencylinder». *Neurol. Zentralbl.*, February 1,1901.

Ramón y Cajal, S: «Observaciones microscópicas sobre las terminaciones nerviosas en los músculos voluntarios de la rana». Zaragoza, 1881.

Ramón y Cajal, S: «Sobre un sencillo proceder de impregnación de las fibrillas interiores del protoplasma nervioso». *Archivos latinos de Med. y de Biología*, Number 1, October, 1903. See also an article on the results of this method published in Trab. Lab. Inv. Biol. Univ. Madrid. Volume II, Madrid, 1903.

See Ramón y Cajal, S: «Una fórmula de impregnación argéntica especialmente aplicable a los cortes del cerebelo y consideraciones sobre la teoría de Liesegang, etc.». Trab. Lab. Inv. Biol. Univ. Madrid. Vol. XIX, Madrid, 1921.

de Castro, F: «Quelques formules de fixation pour le méthode de l'argent reduit de Cajal et leurs résultats dans les centres nerveux et les terminaisons nerveuses péripheriques». *Trav. Lab. Rech. Biol. Univ. Madrid.* Vol. XXIII, Madrid, 1925.

See Cajal: Estudios sobre la degeneración del sistema nervioso. Two volumes. Madrid, 1914. *Degeneration and Regeneration of the Nervous System.* Vol. I–II. (R. May, trans.) Oxford: Oxford University Press. The latter text has been considerably extended in certain points.

See Ramón y Cajal, S: «Las fórmulas del nitrato de plata reducido». Trab. Lab. Inv. Biol. Univ. Madrid. Vol. 8, Madrid, 1910.

Liesegang: «Die Kolloidochemie der histologischen Silverfärbung». *Kolloidchem. Beihefte.* Bd. III, Dresden. 1911.

Ramón y Cajal, S: «Une formule pour colourer dans les coupes les fibres amédulleés et les terminaisons centrales et periphériques.» *Trav. Lab. Rech. Biol. Univ. Madrid.*, Volume XXIII, , 1925. A preliminary report on this method was published in Trab. Lab. Inv. Biol. Univ. Madrid, Volume XIX, Madrid, 1921.

For further details about this method, see: G. Marinesco: «Du rôle des ferments oxydants dans les phénomènes de la vie». *Libro en honor de S. Ramón y Cajal*, Vol. I, 1922. See also Seizo Katsunuma: «Intrazelluläre Oxydation und Indophenolblausynthese». *G.Fischer*, Jena, 1924.

See Ramón y Cajal, S: «El núcleo de las células piramidales del cerebro, etc.». Trab. Lab. Inv. Biol. Univ. Madrid. Vol. VIII, Madrid, 1910.

Fajersztajn: «Eir neues Silverimprägnation Verfharen etc». *Neurol. Zentralbl.*, February 1, 1901. This unjustly forgotten scholar was the first to discover the reducing action of formalin on tissues previously soaked either in ammoniacal silver nitrate or in ammoniacal silver oxide.

Ramón y Cajal, S: «Pequeñas comunicaciones técnicas». *Rev. Trim. Micrográf. Madrid* . Vol. V, 1900–1901.

Ramón y Cajal, S: Trab. Lab. Inv. Biol. Univ. Madrid, Vol. XVIII, Madrid, 1920. Idem: «Contribution a la connaissance de la neuroglie, etc». See also Cajal: Trav. Lab. Rech. Biol. Univ. Madrid., Vol. XXIV, 1925.

Ramón y Cajal, S: «Notas técnicas». *Sociedad de Biología.* Session held April30, 1925.

Del Rio-Hortega, P: «La microglía y su transformación en células en bastoncito». Trab. Lab. Inv. Biol. Univ. Madrid, Vol. XVIII Madrid, 1920. Idem: «Histogénesis y evolución normal, éxodo y distribución regional de la microglía». *Archivos de Neurobiología*, 1921.

Del Rio-Hortega, P: «Tercera aportación al conocimiento morfológico e interpretación funcional de la oligodendroglía». *Memorias de la Real Sociedad de Historia Natural*,

Vol. XIV. Madrid, 1928. By the same author, see also: «Estructura y sistematización de los gliomas y paragliomas». *Archivos Españoles de Oncología*, Vol. II. Madrid, 1932.

Ramón y Cajal, S: «Quelques formules de fixation destinées a la méthode au nitrate d'argent». *Trav. Lab. Rech. Biol. Univ. Madrid.*. Vol. V,1907.

Kawamura: *Neue Beiträge Z. Morphol. u. Physhiol. der Cholesterinsteatose*. G. Fischer, Jena, 1927.

See K. Schaffer: Ueber das morphol. Wesen u. die Histopathol. der heriditär-systematischen-Nerven Krankheiten. J. Springer, Berlin, 1926.

See Ramón y Cajal, S: «El azul de metileno en los centros nerviosos». *Rev. Trim. Micrográf. Madrid* Vol. 1,, 1896; see also Histologie du Système Nerveux de l'Homme et des Vertebrés, Vol. 1, p. 273, 1909. Nageotte's bracelet is shown stained in the dorsal roots and white matter of the spinal cord.

Ramón y Cajal, S: «Quelques remarques sur les plaques motrices de la langue des mammiféres». *Trav. Lab. Rech. Biol. Univ. Madrid.*. Vol. XXIII, Madrid, 1925.

Ramón y Cajal, S: «Una fórmula de impregnación argéntica especialmente aplicable a los cortes del cerebelo». Trab. Lab. Inv. Biol. Univ. Madrid Vol. XIX, Madrid, 1921.

INDEX

Achúcarro, N., xii, xiii, 9, 17, 218n36, 226, 227, 234n7
Achúcarro's method
   astrocytes, Del Río-Hortega's variations, 218n36
   centrosomes, Del Río-Hortega's first variation, 119–20, 219n41
   collagen bundles, Del Río-Hortega's third variation, 160
   macroglia, 142–43
   macroglia, fourth variation, 143
   reticulin impregnation, Del Río-Hortega's second variation, 159–60
Alcohol, 25–26, 106, 108–9. *see also* ammoniacal alcohol
Alizarin, 53
Alkaline alcohol, 175
Altmann's liquid, 29
Altmann's staining methods, 60
Alzheimer, A., xi, 226, 227
Alzheimer's method
   basophilic-metachromatic substances, 164–65
   fibrinoid granules, 164
   fuchsinophilic granules, 164
   May-Grünwald stain, cell metabolism alterations, 165
   neuroglial cells, blood vessels, 138
   plastosomes, 118–19, 218n37, 228
Amaurotic idiocy, 165
Amber, amber tincture, 229–30
Ammoniacal alcohol
   cell body bulk staining, 106
   formula, 182–83
   invertebrate nervous tissue, 203

peripheral nerve endings, 190–91, 222n51
peripheral nerve fibers, 182–83
Ammoniacal hematein, 56
Ammoniacal silver carbonate technique, xiii, 9, 160–61, 219n41
Ammoniacal silver oxide method
   macroglia, Bolsi's modification, 145
   microglia, 141–42, 150–51
   principles, 53, 151
Ammonium molybdate fixation, 90–92
Ammonium picrate fixation, 89–90
Ammon's horn, 75, 94, 95
Amyloid substance, 170
Anglade's procedure, macroglia, 135
Aniline violet, 57
Apáthy, S., xii, 10, 89, 226
Apáthy's liquid, 67, 89–90
Apathy's method
   embedding, 42–43
   invertebrate nervous tissue, 202–3
   serial section handling, mounting, 49
Astacus, 36, 211n7
Astrocytes
   ammoniacal silver oxide, 141–42
   Del Río-Hortega's method, 143–44, 218n36
   development of, 9–10, 17
   gliosomes, 224
   gold-sublimate method, 138–40, 219n40
   Ranvier-Weigert fibers, 228
   tanno-argentic method, 227
   techniques, history of, xiii
Autoradiography, xvi
Auxochromes, 53

Axons
  methylene blue, Nemiloff's procedure, 176
  pyridine formula, 183
  reduced silver technique, 113, 125–26
Azan staining, 63–64
Azoulay, L., 6, 7

Barbituric acid, 33
Benda's method
  macroglia, 135–36
  myelin sheaths, 132
Bensley's method, 119
Best's procedure, glycogen demonstration, 169
Bethe, A., xii, 10–11, 90, 226
Bethe's method, neurofibrils, 99–100, 214n28
Bielschowsky, M., xi, 226
Bielschowsky– Agduhr formula, 36, 37
Bielschowsky's method
  connective tissue, 160, 183–84, 222n45
  en bloc staining, Agduhr's modification, 195
  neurofibrils, 10, 101–3, 216n29
  paraffin section toning, 214n28
  peripheral nerve endings, 192
  peripheral nerve endings, Boeke's modification, 192
  peripheral nerve endings, decalcification procedure, 195
  peripheral nerve fibers, Doinikow's modification, 184
  peripheral nerve fibers, Miskolczy's variation, 184
Bioblasts, 60, 211n3, 223, 224, 227
Biondi's liquid, 119, 143, 218n37
Black reaction method, 71
Blood vessels adventitia, 159
Böhmer's hematoxylin, 56
Bolles Lée, 44
Bolsi's method, microglia, 151–52
Brain, spinal cord
  central axons staining, 125
  chloral hydrate fixation, 33, 106–9, 170
  chromatolytic reaction, 123, 218n39
  connective bands demonstration, 159
  gold-sublimate method (Cajal), 138–40, 219n40
  methylene blue (*see* methylene blue)
  Schultze and Stöhr's method, 113–14
  silver chromate procedure (rapid), 72–78
Bügner's bands, 223

Cajal's liquid, iron perchloride, 29–30
Cajal's method. *see* reduced silver nitrate method
Cajal's trichromic staining, 61–62
Cajuput, 223
Calleja, J., 7, 61
Canada balsam, 65–66, 223
Candle, 223
Capillarity, 50
Carmine, 53, 55–56
Castro, F. de, xii–xv, xix–xx, 9, 13–18, 92, 212n19, 232n17
Cedarwood oil, 44, 66–67, 92, 211n13
Cell body
  ammoniacal formalin, 109
  bulk staining, ammoniacal alcohol, 106
  bulk staining, ethanol formula, 105–6
  bulk staining, no fixative, 105
  cell membrane demonstration, 123, 218n39
  centrosomes, 119–20
  chloral hydrate fixation, 33, 106–9
  chondrioma, 119, 223
  formalin, ammoniacal alcohol, 110
  formalin, pyridine, 109
  gold-toning, 110–11, 117, 214n28
  Golgi apparatus (*see* Golgi apparatus)
  hypnotic-based fixatives, 32–33, 106–8
  neurofibrils (*see* neurofibrils)
  neuronal pigment, prepigment, 122
  Nissl chromatic bodies, 97–99, 119, 131
  nuclei, nucleoli, 98
  nucleus coloration, 122–23, 218n39
  oxidative ferments demonstration, 120–21
  pigmentary spherules demonstration, 121–22
  plastosomes, 118–19, 218n37, 228
  pyridine-silver nitrate, 110
  Ranvier-Weigert fibers, 120, 228
  reduced silver technique (*see* reduced silver nitrate method)

reticular membrane (Cajal–Golgi), 123, 218n39, 234n9
silver impregnation methods (*see* silver impregnation methods)
Cell membrane demonstration, 123, 218n39
Cell metabolism alterations
　amyloid substance, 170
　basophilic-metachromatic substances (protagonoid substances), Alzheimer's method, 164–65
　calcareous substances, 171–72
　corpora amylacea, 170–71
　fats, lipoid substances demonstration, 163, 165–67, 222n46
　fatty substances visualization, 163
　ferric pigment demonstration, 167–68
　fibrinoid granules, Alzheimer's method, 164
　fuchsinophilic granules, Alzheimer's method, 164
　glycogen demonstration, 169
　hyaline degeneration, 171
　lecytinoid granules, 167, 225
　May-Grünwald stain, Alzheimer's procedure, 165
　non-ferric pigment demonstration, 168–69
　semilecythinoid granules, 167, 228–29
Centrosomes, 119–20, 219n41
Cerebellum
　bulk staining, ethanol formula, 105–6
　central axons staining, 125
　chloral hydrate fixation, 33, 106–9, 170
　methylene blue, 93, 94
　reduced silver technique, hydroquinone, 112–13
Cerebral cortex
　bulk staining, ethanol formula, 105–6
　methylene blue method, 76–79, 87, 93, 213nn23–24
Chittenden, 228
Chloral hydrate
　Castro's procedure, 36–37
　as fixative, 33, 106–9, 232n3
　invertebrate nervous tissue, 203
　peripheral nerve endings fixation, 191
　peripheral nerve fibers formula, 183
Chondrioma, 119, 223

Chondriomites, 58–64, 223
Chromatophore, 53
Ciaccio's method, fats, lipoid substances demonstration, 166–67
Clove essence, 65–66
CNS impregnation, methylene blue, 93–95
Cochineal, 53, 55–56, 90, 211n8
Collagen bundles, 160
Collidine, 32
Confocal laser-scanning microscopy, xvi
Connective tissue
　acidic dyes, supravital staining with, 161–62
　Bielschowsky's method, 160, 183–84, 222n45
　blood vessels adventitia, 159
　collagen bundles, 160
　cyanophilic cells, 157, 223
　Doinikow's method, 175
　endoneurium, 160
　impregnation methods, 158–61
　neurilemma, 157, 159, 226
　Orcein stain, elastic fibers, 157–58
　principles, 157
　reduced silver nitrate method, 184–85
　resorcin-fuchsin solution preparation, 158
　reticulin impregnation, 159–60
　silver carbonate method (Del Río-Hortega), xiii, 9, 160–61, 219n41
　trypan blue, 161–62
　Van Gieson's picrofuchsin, 58
　Weigert's method, elastic fibers, 158
Corpora amylacea, 170–71
Cowdry, 119, 180
Cox's method, neuronal morphology, 82–84, 212n19
Cresyl violet, 57
Cyanophilic cells, 157, 223
Czokor's cochineal, 55–56

Dahlia violet, 57
D'Ammar resin, 65–66
Decalcifying agents
　Bielschowsky– Agduhr formula, 36, 37
　Castro's procedure, chloral hydrate, 36–37
　Castro's procedure, urethane, 37
　dissociation, 39–40

Decalcifying agents (*Cont.*)
  Ebner's Liquid, 35
  embedding methods (*see* embedding methods)
  Fol's Liquid, 35
  Heidenhain's fixative/decalcifying solution, 36
  Landois's liquid, 40
  nitric acid decalcification, formalin-fixed tissues, 35–36
  nitric acid-formaldehyde formula, 36
  overview, 35
  peripheral nerve endings, 194–97
  Schieffedecker's liquid, 40
  sectioning, 40–41
DeFelipe, J., xii
Deiters' cells, 228
Delafield's hematoxylin, 57
Del Rio Hortega, P., xii, xiii, 9, 10, 16, 119, 122, 140, 143, 145–46, 153, 218n36, 219n40, 224, 226, 227
Del Río-Hortega's method
  gliosomes/mitochondria, 148–49
  microglia, 148–50, 221nn42–43, 222n44
  oligodendroglia, 148–50, 154, 221nn42–43, 222n44
  oligodendroglia, Penfield's modification, 155–56
  oligodendroglia, silver dichromate, 154–55
Dendritic spines, xvi–xvii, 89, 93, 213n25
Diosmotic power, 223
Dissociation
  chemical, 40
  mechanical, 39–40
Dogiel, 85–87, 89, 91, 92, 94, 213n25
Dominici's Liquid, 31
Donnagio, 11, 226
Donnagio's method, neurofibrils, 100–101
During's formula, 81

Ebner's Liquid, 35
Eddinger's drawing instrument, 223
Eddinger's macrotome, 22, 224
Ehrlich's hematoxylin, 57
Ehrlich's method. *see also* methylene blue
  invertebrate nervous tissue, 201–2
  neurofibrils, 181
  spinous double bracelet, 181, 222n48

Embedding methods
  celloidin, collodion, 41–43, 99
  chloroform, 44
  gelatin, 45
  paraffin, 42–44, 99
  paraffin, superficial embedding, 45
  paraffin solvents, 44
En bloc staining methods, 103, 195, 198, 224
Eosin (primrose), 57
Epigraph number 90, 213n22
Epigraph number 100, 213n25
Equivalent neurocytological images, 93, 214nn26–27
Erhlich, P., xi, 85
Ezholz granules, 224

Fajersztajn's procedure, 101–2, 125–26
Fañanás, J. R., 9
Fats, lipoid substances demonstration, 163, 165–67, 222n46
Ferric pigment demonstration, 167–68
Ferrous ferricyanide method, 153, 168
Fibrinoid granules, 164, 224
Fibrous glial cells, 224
Fieandt, 224
Fieandt's method, gliosomes/mitochondria, 147–48
Fixation, 225
Fixatives
  action of, 23–25, 54
  alcohol, 25–26, 106, 108–9
  ammonium molybdate, 90–92
  ammonium picrate, 89–90
  chloral hydrate, 33, 106–9, 232n3
  collidine, 32
  defined, 225
  formaldehyde-based, 25–28, 140
  formalin, 24–25, 80, 109–18, 218nn33–34
  Formalin-Müller (Orth's liquid), 27
  hypnotic-based, 32–33, 106–8
  lineal aggregates, 232n14
  myelin sheaths, 178
  osmic acid, 24, 27–32, 75, 79–80
  picrate/molybdate combined, 92–93
  pyridine (*see* pyridine)
  Regaud's liquid, 27
  specimen collection, preparation, 22–23
  thymol, 27

Flemming's Liquor, 29
FMRI, xvii
Fol's Liquid, 35
Formaldehyde, 24–25, 140
Formaldehyde-ammonium bromide, 25
Formaldehyde-uranyl nitrate, 25
Formalin, 24–25, 80, 109–18, 218nn33–34
Formalin-Müller (Orth's liquid), 27
Formalin/uranyl nitrate
   development of, 232n12
   Golgi apparatus, 116–17
   Golgi apparatus, Da Fano's modification, 118
   macroglia, 140–41
   pathological glial cells, 163
   Schwann cells, 174–75
Formic acid, 73
Frohman's striae, 101, 174, 224
Fuchsin, 53, 57, 225
Fuchsinophilic granules, 164, 224

Gallego, A., xiv, 62
Ganglia
   bulk staining, ethanol formula, 105–6
   hypnotic-based fixatives, 32–33, 106–8
   methylene blue, 76–77
Gans method, microglia, 152–53
Gaskell, N., 45
Gelatin-levulose (Heringa's medium), 103, 216n30
Gene transfer development, xvi
Gentian violet, 57
Glial cells. *see also* macroglia; microglia
   ammoniacal silver carbonate, xiii, 9, 160–61, 219n41
   Heidenhain's iron hematoxylin, 58
Glial fibers, 224
Glia marginalis, 137–38, 224
Glioblasts, 145–46
Gliocytes, 224
Gliofibrillar network hypothesis, 228
Gliofibrils, 134, 136, 138, 162, 173, 224
Gliomata, 140
Gliosomes, 140–41, 146–49, 224
Glycerin, 67
Glycogen demonstration, 169
Gold salts, 53
Gold-sublimate method, macroglia, 138–40, 219n40

Gold-toning
   cell body, 110–11, 117, 214n28
   reduced silver nitrate method, 216n32
   silver impregnation methods, 110–11, 117, 214n28
Golgi, C., xi, 6, 225, 229, 231n8
Golgi apparatus
   arsenious acid method, 115–16
   Cajal, primitive method, 114–15
   defined, 225
   formalin/uranyl nitrate, 116–17
   formalin/uranyl nitrate Da Fano's modification, 118
   Golgi–Veratti's procedure, 114
   impregnation of, 114–18
   Kopsch's method, 117
   Kopsch's method, Kolatschew's modification, 117
Golgi method. *see* rapid Golgi method
Gray reaction method, 71
Grenacher's boracic carmine, 55
Grenacher's carmine, 55
Grey, 226
Gros's procedure, neurofibrils, 103–4, 216n30
Grübler, 63, 64, 86, 88, 95, 98, 134, 176, 208, 211n12
Guillery, 226

Heidenhain, M., 63
Heidenhain's fixative/decalcifying solution, 36
Heidenhain's iron hematoxylin, 58
Heidenhain's procedure, overstained tissues differentiation, 52
Held, 12–13, 224, 226–27
Held's method, glia marginalis, 137–38
Held's perivascular limitant membrane, 224
Held's pial limitant membrane, 224
Hematein staining methods, 60
Hematoxylin, 53, 56–58, 211n10
Hematoxylin and eosin stain, 58
Henle's sheath, 185, 225
Herbst-Grandry corpuscles, 191–92
Heymans, 16
History
   anti- Americanism, 8
   anti-cholera vaccine, 5

History (*Cont.*)
  Cajal epoch, xi–xii
  carotid glomus elucidation, xiv, 14–16
  carotid sinuses elucidation, xiv
  gold sublimate method, 10, 17, 227
  Gründnetz theory, 13
  impulse transmission elucidation, 10–16, 211n3
  nerve regeneration, polygenist theory of, 11
  neuronal polarization, discovery of, 7
  neuron doctrine, xi, xv, 5–7, 10–14
  optic pathways elucidation, 7
  ovens, temperature adjustment, 72, 211n14
  reticular theory, xi, xii, xv, xix–xx, 12, 14, 231n4
  Spanish Civil War, xiv, 16
  Spanish education system, 3–4, 231n3
  Spanish School of Neurohistology, xi–xv, 232n16, 232n18
  synapses, discovery of, 7, 17
  uranyl nitrate method, 9–10
Hollborn, K., 211n12
Holmgrem, N., 74
Holzer's procedure, macroglia, 136
Hyaline degeneration, 171
Hypnotic-based fixatives, 32–33, 106–8
Hyposulfite, 225

Ibáñez, S., 16
Immunocytochemistry, xvi
Impregnation, 225
Indigo, 53
Indurant, 225. *see also* fixatives
Induration, 225
In situ hybridization, xvi
Interfascicular oligodendroglia, 225
Internal reticular apparatus, 225
Intraprotoplasmic granules, 60, 211n3, 223, 224, 227
Invertebrate nervous tissue, 81, 201–3
Iris diaphragm, 225
Iron/ammonia alum, 225

Jahnel, 206–7
Japanese method, 50
Jews' pitch, 225
Jones, T., xii

Köhler illumination, 211n2
Kölliker, 5–6, 213n23
Kopsch's formula, 80–81
Kossa's method, calcareous substances, 171
Kühne, 228
Kulschitzky-Pal's Procedure (Wolters), myelin sheaths, 130
Kultschitzky's method
  embedding, 41–43
  myelin sheaths, 129–30

Lacquers, 52
Lafora, 9, 16, 170
Laguesse's Liquid, 29
Landois's liquid, 40
Lantermann's reticulum, 181
Lawrentjew, 193
Lecytinoid granules, 167, 225
Leuckart frames, 43, 225
Levaditi's method, syphilis, 205–7
Levi's perinucleolar cap, 123, 218n39, 225
Levulose, 216n30
Lhermitte, 98
Liesegang, 111
Liesegang's procedure, reduced silver nitrate method, 111–12
Ligroin, 225
Lime, 225
Lipoid inclusions, 140–41
Lipopigment, 168–69
Lithium, 225
Loyez's method, myelin sheaths, 130–31
Lye, 225

Macroglia. *see also* astrocytes
  Achúcarro's method, 142–43
  Achúcarro's method, fourth variation, 143
  ammoniacal silver oxide, 141–42
  ammoniacal silver oxide method, Bolsi's modification, 145
  Anglade's procedure, 135
  Benda's method, 135–36
  defined, 225
  formalin/uranyl nitrate, 140–41
  glia marginalis, 137–38, 224
  glioblasts, 145–46
  gliomata, 140

gliosomes, 140–41, 146–49, 224
gold-sublimate method (Cajal), 138–40, 219n40
Holzer's procedure, 136
lipoid inclusions, 140–41
Mallory's method, 137
mitochondria (*see* mitochondria)
neuroglial cells, blood vessels, 138
protoplasmic neuroglia, Lugaro's method, 144–45
Weigert's method, 133–34
Weigert's method, Pötter's modification, 134
Magenta red, 225
Mallory's anilines coloration, 63
Mallory's hematoxylin
　phosphomolybdic acid, 59
　phosphotungstic acid, 59–60
Mallory's method, macroglia, 137
Marchi, V., xi
Marchi's method
　embedding, 41–43
　myelin sheaths, 131–32
Marinesco, 227
Mawas, 224
Mayer, P., 127
Medulla oblongata
　bulk staining formulae, 105
　central axons staining, 125
　chloral hydrate fixation, 33, 106–9, 170
　Dogiel's method, 93
　Donnagio's method, 100–101
　gold-sublimate method (Cajal), 138–40, 219n40
　methylene blue, 94–95
　Olt's method, 49
　Schultze and Stöhr's method, 113–14
　Simarro's method, 11–12, 101
Medullated fibers, 226
Melanin pigment, 168–69
Merchán, J., xix–xx
Mercury salts, 53
Mesoglia, 151
Metachromasia, 53
Metallic oxides, 53
Methyl blue, 234n1, 235n1
Methylene blue
　ammonium molybdate fixation, 90–92
　ammonium picrate fixation, 89–90

Apáthy's liquid mounting, 89–90
Bethe's fixation procedure, 90–91
Cajal's dye diffusion method, 93
cedarwood oil, 44, 66–67, 92, 211n13
cerebellum, 93, 94
cerebral cortex, 76–79, 87, 93, 213nn23–24
CNS impregnation, 93–95
D'Ammar resin, 65–66
direct staining by lubrication, 87–88
Dogiel's method, 93
dye diffusion method, 88
Ehrlich original intravascular injection method, 93–94
Ehrlich's method, 85–86, 212n20
flasks, types of, 86, 212n20, 213n22
glycerin mounting, 67
intravascular injection procedure, 86
Kreibich's procedure/rongalite, 95
medulla oblongata, 94–95
Meyer's method, 95
myelin sheath, 92
nuclear staining, 57
oxygenation, 93–94
paraffin, 92
peripheral nerve endings, 189–90
picrate/molybdate combined fixation, 92–93
platinum chloride solution, 91
Pravaz syringe, 88, 213n24
principles of use, 53, 57
room temperature saturated solutions, 94
Schwann cells, Nemiloff's procedure, 176
sensitivity of tissues, 94–95
solutions, types, 86
tissues prone to retraction, 92
in vivo subcutaneous injections procedure, 88–89, 213n25
Methylene blue eosinate, 61
Meves, 224, 228
Meves' procedure, 59
Microglia
　ammoniacal silver oxide, 141–42, 150–51
　Bolsi's method, 151–52
　Del Río-Hortega's method, 148–50, 221nn42–43, 222n44

Microglia (*Cont.*)
  ferrous ferricyanide method, 153
  Gans method, 152–53
  history of, xiii, 9–10
  impregnation, silver oxalate procedure, 152–53
  iron-staining method, pathological specimens, 153–54
  Perls's reaction, 153
  Turnbull's blue method, 153
Microscopy, 21–22, 211nn1–2, 225, 231n6
Mitochondria
  ammoniacal silver carbonate technique, xiii, 9, 160–61, 219n41
  Del Río-Hortega's method, 148–49
  Fieandt's method, 147–48
  Nageotte's procedure, myelin sheaths, 179
  staining methods, 58–64, 146–49, 176, 179, 222n48
Modus operandi/faciendi, 226
Mordants, 52, 54, 226
Motor end-plates/corneal nerves, Ranvier's method, 188
Müller's liquid, 26–27
Myelin sheaths
  ammoniacal alcohol formula, 182–83
  artificial distortions, 181
  Benda's method, 132
  bulk impregnation formulae, reduced silver nitrate method, 182
  chloral hydrate formula, 183
  degeneration, 178–79
  fixatives, 178
  Kulschitzky-Pal's Procedure (Wolters), 130
  Kulschitzky's method, 129–30
  Lantermann's reticulum, 181
  Loyez's method, 130–31
  Marchi's method, 131–32
  methylene blue, 92
  mitochondria, Nageotte's procedure, 179
  neurofibrils, Bethe and Mönckeberg's method, 181–82
  neurokeratin framework, 181
  Pal's method, 128–29
  regeneration phenomena, 182
  Schultze osmic acid procedure, 178
  Schultze's method, 131
  Spielmeyer's method, 130
  Weigert's method, 127–28

Nageotte, J., xi, 173, 224, 229
Nageotte's method
  Schwann cells, 174
  spinous double bracelet, 180–81, 222n48
  spiral apparatus, 180, 229
  syncytium/unmyelinated fibers, 177–78
Negri bodies, 208–9
Nerve endings. *see* peripheral nerve endings
Nerve tubes, 173, 226
Neurilemma, 157, 159, 226
Neurofibrils
  Bensley's method, 119
  Bethe and Mönckeberg's method, 181–82
  Bethe's method, 99–100, 214n28
  Bielschowsky's method, 10, 101–3, 216n29
  definitions, 226
  Donnagio's method, 100–101
  Ehrlich's method, 181
  gold-sublimate method, 10, 17, 227
  Golgi-impregnated sections, 74
  Gros's procedure, 103–4, 216n30
  history of, xii–xiii, 10–13
  invertebrate nervous tissue, 202–3
  periterminal network, 14–15, 192, 222n52
  pyridine formula, 183
  reduced silver nitrate method, 11–15 (*see also* reduced silver nitrate method)
  Schultze and Stöhr's method, 113–14
  Simarro's method, 11–12, 101
Neuroglial amoeboid cells, 119, 226
Neuroglial elements staining, 76–77
Neurokeratin framework, 181
Neurologist, 226
Neuronal morphology
  artifacts, consistency, 212n19
  bichromate induration, 72, 233n1
  black reaction method, 71
  cerebral cortex (*see* cerebral cortex)
  combined method, 78–79
  Cox's method, 82–84, 212n19

During's formula, 81
Golgi's method (see rapid Golgi method)
   gray reaction method, 71
   invertebrate nervous tissue, 201–2
   Kopsch's formula, 80–81
   rolling method, 76–77
   Sánchez's formula for invertebrates, 81
   silver chromate procedure (see silver chromate procedure)
   silver nitrate immersion, 72
   Strong's formula, 81
Neuronal nucleolus staining, 54
Neuron doctrine, xi, xv, 5–7, 10–14
Neurosomes, 226–27
New Concept of the Histology of the Nervous System The (Cajal), 5–7
Nile blue sulfate method, fats, lipoid substances demonstration, 166
Nissl, F., xi, 229
Nissl chromatic bodies, 97–99, 119, 131
Nissl method
   alcohol fixatives, 25–26, 106, 108–9
   cedarwood oil, 44, 66–67, 92, 211n13
   D'Ammar resin, 65–66
   embedding, 41–43, 45, 99
   equivalent images, 98
   equivalent neurocytological images, 93, 214nn26–27
   protocols, 97–99
   serial section handling, mounting, 48
Nitric acid decalcification, formalin-fixed tissues, 35–36
Nitric acid-formaldehyde formula, 36
Nó, R. L. de, xii, 9, 16, 197
Noguchi's method, syphilis, 206
Nondendritic neuroglial cells, 227
Non-ferric pigment demonstration, 168–69
Nuclear chromatin staining, 54
Nucleolar spherules, 122–23, 218n39, 227
Nucleus coloration, 122–23, 218n39

Obrégia's procedure, 48–49
Officinal solution, 128, 158, 211n5, 227
Olfactory bulb staining, 76–78
Olfactory mucous staining, 76–78
Oligodendroglia

ammoniacal silver carbonate technique, xiii, 9, 160–61, 219n41
   definitions, 225
   Del Río-Hortega's method, 148–50, 154, 221nn42–43, 222n44
   Del Río-Hortega's method, Penfield's modification, 155–56
   Del Río-Hortega's method, silver dichromate, 154–55
   Golgi method, bichromate-formalin variations, 155
   history of, xiii, 10
   silver oxalate impregnation, 156
Olt's method, 49
One-third alcohol, 227
Optic nerve fibers staining, 76–77
Origins of Inflammation (Cajal), 4–5
Orth's liquid (Formalin-Müller), 27
Orth's lithium carmine, 56
Osmic acid
   fats, lipoid substances demonstration, 165
   as fixative, 24, 27–32, 75, 79–80
   principles of use, 53
Osmium-bichromic mixture, 28–29
Outer plexiform layer staining, 76–77
Oxidative ferments demonstration, 120–21

Pal's method, myelin sheaths, 128–29
Pappenheim's staining methods, 62
Paranode, 229
Pathological conditions. *see* cell metabolism alterations; *specific conditions*
Perineural endothelial cells, 184–85, 227. *see also* connective tissue
Peripheral nerve endings
   alcohol/formic acid, Dogiel's formula, 191–92
   ammoniacal alcohol formula, 190–91, 222n51
   Bielschowsky-Gros method, 193–94
   Bielschowsky's decalcification procedure, 195
   Bielschowsky's procedure, 192
   Bielschowsky's procedure, Boeke's modification, 192
   chloral hydrate fixation, 191
   decalcification, 194–97

Peripheral nerve endings (*Cont.*)
  Ehrlich-Dogiel's supravital staining
    method, 189–90
  en bloc staining, 103, 195, 198, 224
  fixative mixtures, 191
  floating sections Cajal's method, 198–99
  formalin-fix specimens, section
    staining, 198–99
  gold chloride methods, 187–89
  Golgi's methods, 189
  Herbst-Grandry corpuscles, 191–92
  hypnotics/nitric acid fixation, 191
  interstitial sympathetic neurons, 189
  Loewit-Fischer's procedure, 187–88
  motor end-plates/corneal nerves,
    Ranvier's method, 188
  principles, 187, 190
  pyridine fixation, 191
  reduced silver nitrate method,
    190–92, 196–97
  reduced silver nitrate method, frozen
    sections, 194
  reduced silver nitrate method, Golgi's
    modification, 192
  Ruffini's procedure, 188–89, 222n51
  Schultze and Stöhr's method, 113–14
  Schultze's method, 194
  sympathetic, dorsal root ganglia,
    76–79, 198–99
Peripheral nerve fibers
  ammoniacal alcohol formula, 182–83
  Bielschowsky's method, 160, 183–84
  Bielschowsky's method, Doinikow's
    modification, 184
  Bielschowsky's method, Miskolczy's
    variation, 184
  bulk impregnation formulae, reduced
    silver nitrate method, 182
  chloral hydrate formula, 183
  fresh examination, 173
  Lantermann's reticulum, 181
  myelin (*see* myelin sheaths)
  nerve tubes, 173, 226
  neurokeratin framework, 181
  peritubular connective sheath,
    185, 222n50
  protagonoid (π) granules, 176–77, 228
  pyridine formula, 183
  Ranvier crosses, 174, 228

Reich's granules, 177, 228–29
Remak's fibers, 176–77, 229
Rezzonico-Golgi apparatus, 176,
  180, 229
Schmidt-Lantermann incisures,
  179–80, 222n48
Schwann cells, 174–78
Segall rings, 180, 229
silvering method, 174
spinous double bracelet, 176, 180–81,
  222n48, 229
spiral apparatus, 180, 229
Periterminal network, 14–15, 192, 222n52
Peritubular connective sheath,
  185, 222n50
PET-scan, xvii
Picrate/molybdate combined
  fixation, 92–93
Pigmentary spherules, 227
Pigmentary spherules
  demonstration, 121–22
Plastosomes, 118–19, 218n37, 228
Platinum salts, 53
Poljak, 74
Potash, 228
Pravaz, C. G., 88, 213n24
Primrose (eosin), 57
Protagonoid (π) granules, 176–77, 228
Protagonoid substances, 164–65, 228
Protoplasm, 228
Protoplasmic neuroglia, Lugaro's
  method, 144–45
Prussian blue reaction, ferric pigment
  demonstration, 168
Purkinje, 228
Purkinje cells
  bulk staining, ethanol formula, 105–6
  methylene blue staining, 94–95
Pyramidal cells
  bulk staining, ethanol formula, 105–6
  methylene blue staining, 94–95
Pyridine
  as fixative, 24, 32, 103, 108–9,
    218n34, 219n40
  invertebrate nervous tissue, 203
  peripheral nerve endings fixation, 191
  peripheral nerve fibers formula, 183
  uranyl-nitrate/pyridine method,
    syphilis, 207

Quadrigeminal tubercles, 77, 228

Rabies, 208–9
Rabl's Mixture, 31
Ramón y Cajal, P., 9, 90–91, 95, 104, 223, 226, 227
Ramón y Cajal, S., xi–xii, xiv–xv, xix–xx, 3–14, 17, 181, 231n7, 231nn1–3, 231nn9–10, 232n11
Ranvier, L., xi, 228
Ranvier crosses, 174, 228
Ranvier's method, motor end-plates/corneal nerves, 188
Ranvier-Weigert fibers, 120, 228
Rapid Golgi method
  applications of, xvii, 72, 212n15, 212n19
  D'Ammar resin, 65–66
  development of, xi–xii, 5, 7–10, 212n19
  double impregnation procedure (Cajal), 74
  formalin fixation, 24–25, 80, 109–18
  invertebrate nervous tissue, 201
  mercuric bichloride, 81–82
  methylene blue in, 7–8
  peripheral nerve endings, 189
  Timofejew's modification, 80
Reduced silver nitrate method
  applications of, xvii, 216n32
  axons, 113, 125–26
  calcareous substances, 171–72
  connective tissue, 184–85 (*see also* connective tissue)
  D'Ammar resin, 65–66
  decalcification procedures, 196–97
  development of, xii
  embedding methods, 41–43
  fixation, 216n32
  fixatives, nerve endings, 190–91
  floating sections, peripheral nerve endings, 198–99
  gold-toning, 216n32
  hydroquinone formula, 112–13
  impregnation, 216n32
  invertebrate nervous tissue, 203
  Liesegang's procedure, 111–12
  neurofibrils, 11–15
  paraffin section toning, 214n28
  peripheral nerve endings, 190–92, 196–97
  peripheral nerve endings, frozen sections, 194
  peritubular connective sheath, 185, 222n50
  post-fixation treatment, 216n32
  protocol, 104–5
  reduction, embedding, 216n32
  regeneration phenomena, 182
  ripening of the reaction, 104
  Schmidt-Lantermann incisures, formalin-pyridine-manganese, 180
  Schultze and Stöhr's method, 113–14
  section staining, 111–14
Regaud's liquid, 27
Reich's μ granules, 177, 224, 228–29
Remak's fibers, 176–77, 229
Resorcin-fuchsin solution preparation, 158
Reticular membrane (Cajal–Golgi), 123, 218n39, 234n9
Reticular theory, xi, xii, xv, xix–xx, 12, 14, 231n4
Reticulin impregnation, 159–60
Retina staining, 76–78
Rezzonico, 229
Rezzonico-Golgi apparatus, 176, 180, 229
Robertson, 227
Rod cells, 229
Rodríguez, E. L., 232n15
Roehl's method, calcareous substances, 171
Rolling method, 76–77
Romanowski's method, 61
Roncoroni's intranuclear rodlet, 123, 218n39
Roussy, 98
Roux's apparatus, 93, 229
Ruffini's procedure, peripheral nerve endings, 188–89, 222n51
Russel's method, hyaline degeneration, 171

Sacristán, 224
Safranin, 53, 57
Sánchez, D., xii, 9
Sánchez's formula for invertebrates, 81
Sandarac, 83, 212nn18–19
Scarlet red stain
  fats, lipoid substances demonstration, 165–66
  glycerin mounting, 67

Schaffer's method, fats, lipoid substances
    demonstration, 167, 222n46
Schallibaum's liquid, 50
Schieffedecker's liquid, 40
Schmidt-Lantermann incisures,
    179–80, 222n48
Schmorl's technique, tuberculosis, 210
Schultze, 226
Schultze and Stöhr's method,
    neurofibrils, 113–14
Schultze's method, myelin sheaths, 131
Schwann cells
    Doinikow's method, 175
    formalin/uranyl/ammoniacal
        silver, 174–75
    methylene blue, Nemiloff's
        procedure, 176
    Nageotte's method, 174
    protagonoid (π) granules, Reich's
        method, 176–77, 228
    Reich's granules, 177, 228–29
    Remak's fibers, 176–77, 229
    supporting network, 176, 222n49
    syncytium/unmyelinated fibers,
        Nageotte's procedure, 177–78
    Unna-Pappenheim method, 176
    Unna's method, 176
Sealing wax method, 50
Section mounting, preservation
    aniline-stained, 66
    Apáthy's liquid, 67
    Canada balsam, 65–66, 223
    cedarwood oil, 44, 66–67, 92, 211n13
    celloidin-embedded specimens, 65–66
    clove essence, 65–66
    D'Ammar resin, 65–66
    double impregnation procedure,
        74, 212n16
    encrustation procedure, 66
    frozen section procedure, 40–41
    glycerin, 67
    Golgi-impregnated sections, 74
Segall rings, 180, 229
Semilecythinoid granules, 167, 228–29
Serial section handling, mounting
    albumin procedure, 50
    Apathy's procedure, 49
    capillarity, 50
    celloidin-based materials, 47–49

Japanese method, 50
Obrégia's procedure, 48–49
Olt's method, 49
paraffin-embedded materials, 50
Schallibaum's liquid, 50
sealing wax method, 50
Weigert's methods, 48
Silver carbonate method, connective tissue, xiii, 9, 160–61, 219n41
Silver chromate procedure
    Juschtschenko's modification, 79–80
    rapid, 72–78
    rapid indirect, 79
    slow, 72
Silver impregnation methods
    ammoniacal, 101–5
    cell body structures, 101–5
    general procedure, 214n28
    gold-toning, 110–11, 117, 214n28
    microglia, silver oxalate
        procedure, 152–53
    oligodendroglia, silver oxalate
        procedure, 156
    reduced silver nitrate (*see* reduced silver
        nitrate method)
    warm, 119–20, 220n41
Silver salts, 53
Simarro, L., 5
Simarro's method, neurofibrils, 11–12, 101
Sleeping sickness, 208
Soda, 229
Soda hyposulfite, 83, 225
Sodium hydrate, 229
Sodium thiosulfate, 225
Somniféne, 229
Spielmeyer's method, myelin sheaths, 130
Spinous double bracelet, 176, 180–81,
    222n48, 229
Spiral apparatus of Rezzonico, 180, 229
Spongioblasts staining, 76–77, 212n17
Staining methods. *see also specific methods
    by name*
    adjective, 52
    aniline dyes, 57
    bichromatic, trichromatic, 55–57
    bioblasts, 60, 211n3, 223, 224, 227
    Cajal's trichromic, 61–62
    chondriomites, 58–64
    defined, 53

double, triple, 57–58
dye source, composition, 53–54
en bloc, 103, 195, 198, 224
hematein, 60
impregnation, 53
iron-hematoxylin modifications, 58–64
Mallory's anilines coloration, 63
Meves' procedure, 59
mitochondria (*see* mitochondria)
mordants, 52, 54, 226
Negri bodies, 208–9
overstained tissues differentiation, 52
Pappenheim's, 62
principles, 51–52
progressive, 52
regressive, 53
tuberculosis, 209–10
Strong's formula, 81
Stümer, 171
Sublimate, 30, 229
Sublimate-acetic acid, 31
Succinum, succinum tincture, 229–30
Sudan III stain, glycerin mounting, 67
Sympathetic/auditory endings staining, 76–79, 198–99
Sympathetic ganglia staining, 76–79
Syncytium/unmyelinated fibers, Nageotte's procedure, 177–78
Syphilis, 205–8

Tanin ammoniacal silver method, xiii
Tanno-argentic method, astrocytes, 227
Tello, F., xii, 16, 197
Texture of the Nervous System in Man and the Vertebrates, The (Cajal), 7
Theriaca Magna (theriac), 230
Thionine, 44, 53, 66–67, 92, 211n13
3D techniques, xvi
Thymol, 27
Toluidine blue, 53, 57
Tonofibrils, 230

Treponema, 205–8
Trypanosomes, 208
Tuberculosis, 209–10
Turnbull's blue method, 168
Two-photon laser-scanning microscopy, xvi–xvii

Unmedullated fibers, 230
Unna's polychrome blue, 44, 66–67, 92, 211n13
Uranyl/formalin. *see* formalin/uranyl nitrate
Uranyl-nitrate/pyridine method, syphilis, 207
Urethane, 33, 37

Van Gieson's method
    hyaline degeneration, 171
    triple stain, 60–61
Ventral acoustic ganglion, 110, 230
Vermillion, 50, 230
Veronal, 33
Vesubin, 230
Vesuvine, 57

Wässle, H., xvii
Weigert, C., xi, 228
Weigert's method
    corpora amylacea, 170–71
    elastic fibers, 158
    embedding, 41–43
    glial cells, 227
    macroglia, 133–34
    myelin sheaths, 127–28
    overstained tissues differentiation, 52
    serial section handling, mounting, 48
Windle, W., xi

Zenker's Fixative, 30–31
Ziehl-Neelsen's method, tuberculosis, 209